HIKE LIST

D0872933

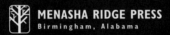
MENASHA RIDGE PRESS
Birmingham, Alabama

60 HIKES WITHIN 60 MILES

CLEVELAND

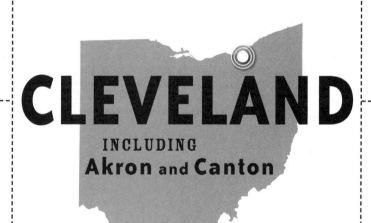

INCLUDING
Akron and Canton

SECOND EDITION

DIANE STRESING

60 Hikes Within 60 Miles: Cleveland

Copyright © 2011 by Diane Stresing
All rights reserved
Printed in the United States of America
Published by Menasha Ridge Press
Distributed by Publishers Group West
Second edition, first printing

Library of Congress Cataloging-in-Publication Data

Stresing, Diane, 1966–
  60 hikes within 60 miles, Cleveland : including Akron and Canton /
  Diane Stresing.— 2nd ed.
     p. cm.
  Includes bibliographical references and index.
  ISBN-13: 978-0-89732-611-7
  ISBN-10: 0-89732-611-3
  1. Hiking—Ohio—Cleveland Region—Guidebooks. 2. Cleveland Region
  (Ohio)—Guidebooks. I. Title. II. Title: Sixty hikes within sixty miles,
  Cleveland.
  GV199.42.O32C547 2011
  917.71—dc22

                                                2011007750

Cover and text design by Steveco International
Cover photo of downtown Cleveland © David Liu
Maps by Scott McGrew and Diane Stresing
All photographs by Diane Stresing unless otherwise noted

Menasha Ridge Press
P.O. Box 43673
Birmingham, AL 35243
www.menasharidge.com

DISCLAIMER

This book is meant only as a guide to select trails in the Cleveland area and does not guarantee hiker safety in any way—you hike at your own risk. Neither Menasha Ridge Press nor Diane Stresing is liable for property loss or damage, personal injury, or death that result in any way from accessing or hiking the trails described in the following pages. Please be aware that hikers have been injured in the Cleveland area. Be especially cautious when walking on or near boulders, steep inclines, and drop-offs, and do not attempt to explore terrain that may be beyond your abilities. To help ensure an uneventful hike, please read carefully the introduction to this book, and perhaps get further safety information and guidance from other sources. Familiarize yourself thoroughly with the areas you intend to visit before venturing out. Ask questions, and prepare for the unforeseen. Familiarize yourself with current weather reports, maps of the area you intend to visit, and any relevant park regulations.

FOR ALL THOSE WHO DEDICATE THEIR TIME TO PRESERVING OHIO'S NATURAL BEAUTY SO THAT WE ALL MAY ENJOY IT

TABLE OF
CONTENTS

ACKNOWLEDGMENTS

Every book is the result of collaboration, and I feel very fortunate to have teamed up with some great people on this one.

Amber Kaye Henderson wrangled the 60-odd files (and several hundred pictures) I sent into a manageable text. (Thanks, Amber.) Molly Merkle handled the big-picture stuff and the minor details with equal care. In fact, everyone at Menasha Ridge Press made working on this book a pleasant experience. It's only right to acknowledge Bud Zehmer too, who was trusting enough when he was with Menasha Ridge Press to offer this great project to an unknown little writer with a new pair of hiking boots.

Here at home, my family and friends were supportive and encouraging. My husband hiked many trails with me (when he'd rather have been on his bike!) and contributed several photos. My daughter didn't complain when I insisted on "just a quick hike" on our way here, or home from there, even when it interfered with a shopping trip. My son enthusiastically pointed out a few thousand beetles, butterflies, fish, and rocks and identified some very interesting faces in trees that I'd have missed had I been alone on the trail. He was also the only person who was absolutely certain I'd make my deadline. (Thanks, Dude!)

I thank my father for giving me the hiking gene, the inclination to hit the trail for no other reason than to see whatever may be waiting there to be seen. (Thanks, Dad!) I am also grateful for decades of my mother's advice. Because of it, I was careful, wore sunscreen and good shoes, always carried a snack, and drank plenty of water along the way. (Thanks, Mom. See, I was listening.) Michelle Schultz has been not only encouraging to a fault but also a very astute market analyst. (Shelly, I didn't follow all of your advice, but between you and me, you're probably right.)

I am also indebted to dozens of people in the field, so to speak, who shared with me their time, enthusiasm, and incredible knowledge as I worked on this book. Jean Backs, Chris Craycroft, and Chris Smith deserve special mention. Finally, though it may seem out of context, I feel I should acknowledge the Portage County Animal Protective League. The weak and frightened puppy rescued at West Branch Reservoir so many years ago remains my favorite hiking buddy. Spike was always eager to hit the trail and never complained about revisiting a section or an entire hike, and if he ever suspected I lost my sense of direction, he didn't say a word.

—DIANE STRESING

FOREWORD

Welcome to Menasha Ridge Press's *60 Hikes within 60 Miles,* a series designed to provide hikers with information needed to find and hike the very best trails surrounding cities usually underserved by good guidebooks.

Our strategy was simple: First, find a hiker who knows the area and loves to hike. Second, ask that person to spend a year researching the most popular and very best trails around. And third, have that person describe each trail in terms of difficulty, scenery, condition, elevation change, and all other categories of information that are important to hikers. "Pretend you've just completed a hike and met up with other hikers at the trailhead," we told each author. "Imagine their questions; be clear in your answers."

An experienced hiker and writer, author Diane Stresing has selected 60 of the best hikes in and around the Cleveland metropolitan area. This second edition includes new hikes. Stresing provides hikers (and walkers) with a great variety of hikes—and all within roughly 60 miles of Cleveland—from urban strolls on city sidewalks to aerobic outings in the Cuyahoga Valley.

You'll get more out of this book if you take a moment to read the Introduction explaining how to read the trail listings. The "Maps" section will help you understand how useful topos will be on a hike and will also tell you where to get them. And though this is a "where-to," not a "how-to" guide, those of you who have not hiked extensively will find the Introduction of particular value.

As much for the opportunity to free the spirit as well as to free the body, let Diane Stresing's hikes elevate you above the urban hurry.

**All the best,
The Editors at Menasha Ridge Press**

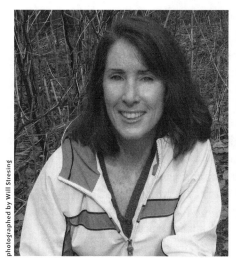

photographed by Will Stresing

Diane Stresing grew up in Columbus, moved to the Cleveland area in 1989, and currently lives in Kent. A genuine Buckeye, Stresing received a B.A. in journalism from Ohio State University. When she's not hiking, biking, or spending time with her family, Stresing works as a commercial freelance writer, providing newsletter copy, Web content, and news and magazine features to a variety of clients.

PREFACE

What's the difference between a hike and a walk? I fielded this question often while I was writing this book. Refer to your dictionary and you'll find that *hike* comes right after *hijack,* begging a word-association game. Is a hike just a walk, hijacked by wanderlust? Perhaps.

The folks at Merriam-Webster define *hike* as "a long walk especially for pleasure or exercise," and also "to travel by any means." But walking is a mode of transportation too. Clearly, the difference between a hike and a walk is subject to individual interpretation.

My interpretation, then, is that walking is *primarily* a means of transportation, a point-A-to-point-B kind of thing. Hiking is more a means of *exploration*—even when the ground you're exploring lies between point A and point B. When you define hiking as a means of exploration, you can turn a walk into a hike by altering your perspective. Your perspective will be different than mine, even on the same trail. That's part of the fun of hiking—finding out where the trail takes you.

LAND OF PLENTY (OF VARIETY)

Every hiker has a favorite topography. When I began this book, I was a hill lover—the steeper and rockier, the better. A view from on high was a bonus, but I was really in it for the climb. I recognize that lake loops have a serene quality, and forests offer a comfort of their own. But to my surprise, as I gathered a variety of hikes for this book, I developed a genuine appreciation—a love, really—for wetlands. The sticky goo of a bog and the temporary squishiness of a vernal pool create something like a giant petri dish, growing the strangest stuff!

Whatever land type is your favorite, you can probably find it here in northeastern Ohio. Between the gluey bogs and slippery marshes and the edge of Lake Erie, you'll find pretty waterfalls,

steep outcrops of shale and Sharon conglomerate, boreal forests, and glacial formations including kames and kettle lakes.

Most of these hikes travel over Ohio's glaciated Western Allegheny Plateau, and
a few tread along the Great Lakes eco-region. When you consider an eco-region, you
must take into account both land and water systems. The land in the Western Allegheny
Plateau is dotted with short, gravelly, dome-shaped hills called kames. These bumps
in the landscape were formed by converging glacial lobes. Some of the cool cavelike
spots, such as those found at Nelson-Kennedy Ledges and Gorge Metropark, even
support species native to Canada. The Western Allegheny Plateau also boasts some
remaining wetlands, most of which are protected as state nature preserves, such as the
Kent (Cooperrider) Bog and Herrick Fen.

In considering our water systems, the crooked Cuyahoga River gets a great deal of
attention, but Grand River and Tinker's Creek watersheds are of equal importance, as
each hosts a significant number of rare and endangered plants and animals.

To learn more about Ohio's eco-regions and the unique species they shelter, spend
some time at The Nature Conservancy's website, nature.org, or call the Ohio chapter
office at (614) 717-2770.

HISTORY UNDERFOOT: FROM TERRIBLE FISH TO TRAINS

About 360 million years before the glaciers made their mark on Ohio's landscape,
there was no landscape. All of Ohio was under water. When you visit the Rocky River
Reservation, you'll see *Dunkleosteus,* the "terrible fish" that was considerably larger
than a shark—it probably ate sharks for breakfast! The nature center at Rocky River is
a great place to learn about Ohio's ancient history and more recent events as well.

The first white settlers in northeastern Ohio came here to create the Connecticut
Land Company's Western Reserve. Those hardy easterners built homes, churches,
colleges, roads, and railroads when they arrived, and many of these original structures
can be seen along the trails described in this book. These settlers also built stations on
the "invisible" Underground Railroad—you can take a glimpse into the lives of the
abolitionists when you visit Austinburg in Ashtabula County (see page 66).

The folks who settled here made their mark in other ways too. Lifesaver candies
were invented in Garrettsville, for example, and artist Henry Church of Chagrin Falls
left his "signature" on Squaw Rock (see page 54). Many famous Ohioans are buried
at Lake View Cemetery and in dozens of smaller, but equally historical, burial sites in
the area. In traipsing and researching these trails, I learned more about Ohio's history
than I did in all of my school days. What's more, I found these lessons fascinating. I
hope you do too.

SEASONS ON THE TRAIL

"Winter hiking? Are you crazy?"

All four seasons offer scenic sights on northeastern Ohio trails. Don't let a little number (such as -4°) keep you inside. Properly outfitted, you can be comfortable, have fun, and enjoy something that's hard to find on the trail in the summer months: solitude.

Hike the same trail in each season and you'll discover that it has multiple personalities. What was a serene lake in June is the scene of a raucous party of migrating waterfowl in November. If you think that the woods look dead and drab in the winter, look again. As soon as the leaves fall off the trees, they already have their spring buds. Look closely and you'll see how much tree bud structures differ from each other. And you don't have to look closely in the winter months to spot other features: bird, squirrel, and insect nests (galls) are easy to notice on bare limbs. So are the unusual shapes and growth patterns of many branches.

Before spring officially arrives, many wildflowers poke through the snow to reach for the sun. Get out and see if you can identify them by their leaves, before they bloom.

In the summer, poison ivy, black flies, and mosquitoes may make you think twice before you leave home. Don't let them ruin your fun; the proper repellent will deter them. And here's more good news: Poison ivy is just about the only plant you have to fear. Learn to identify its distinctive leaves and habits (it climbs trees as much as it creeps along the ground) and you'll be able to avoid it. Poison oak usually isn't a problem in Ohio, and if you stay away from the mushiest parts of a bog, you're almost certainly safe from poison sumac as well.

People, unfortunately, are far more dangerous to plants than plants are to us. As tempting as it may be, never pick anything along the trail. Even the seemingly innocent action of picking a wildflower on one part of a trail and leaving it on another can hasten the progression of a hostile species. Many nonnative species are aggressive (purple loosestrife, for example) even though they are also pretty. Leave them where they are. In some places, wildlife management experts have decided to control or eradicate the aggressive plants; in others, they remain under observation. In any case, the hiker is bound to follow the trail mantra: "Take only pictures; leave only footprints."

WHAT DO TIMBERDOODLES DO, AND ARE NUTHATCHES REALLY NUTTY?

You don't have to be a bird guru to find bird-watching fascinating. The common robin has one of the most beautiful songs of all North American birds. The often-heard catbird can imitate the songs of more than 200 other birds. It can also do impressions of other noises, such as a rusty gate hinge or a crying baby. At Tinker's Creek, I had a rather eerie feeling as I listened to a repeated, panicked call: "Wah! Wah!" If I hadn't been watching the catbird as he called, I would have been certain that I was hearing a human infant! Another time, walking along a city sidewalk, I spotted a backyard-variety blue jay flying very low. He was weighted down by his catch: a fat mole. (Imagine the feast in that nest!)

Birds, both common and rare, offer great entertainment. If you want to learn about them but are overwhelmed by the volumes of bird-watching books, I recommend picking up a chart that identifies a few local varieties for starters. Or visit the children's section of your local bookstore, where you'll find the thinner books an easy starting point. (Several examples are listed in Appendix D. It was from one of these children's books that I learned nuthatches, unlike other birds, can walk both up *and down* tree trunks and branches. Now, I'm always on the lookout for a bird walking the "wrong" way down a tree.) It doesn't take much effort—or much information—to get hooked on birds.

Another great way to learn about our feathered friends is to attend a naturalist-led outing. The rangers and naturalists I've met over the years have all been great sources of information, as well as patient and not the least bit stuffy. Watch your local park listings for events and go, ask questions, and delight in the answers.

I had the good luck to meet Christine Craycroft of the Portage Park system this way. Several years ago, Craycroft led an educational program on the American woodcock, also called the timberdoodle, at Towner's Woods. During the short, enjoyable presentation and walk, I learned more about birds (and frogs, and a few other things) than I had in the previous year. So if you are able to attend any similar programs, by all means, go! And don't worry that you'll be surrounded by experienced ornithologists—chances are, you won't be the only new bird-watcher in the group.

"BEARLY" MENTIONED MAMMALS

Are bears coming back to Ohio? Well, maybe if we're lucky. Are coyotes really common in the Cleveland Metroparks? Probably more so than you think.

Even if you hike each of these trails several times, it's unlikely that you will see a bear or a coyote. On the other hand, you are quite likely to spot deer, raccoons, and even foxes along these trails. You can also see beavers at work and watch bats zigzagging about in the early evenings.

For more information about bears that occasionally explore our neck of the woods or the coyote population around us, visit the Ohio Department of Natural Resources website (**dnr.state.oh.us**) or that of Cleveland Metroparks (**clevelandmetroparks.com**). And try to avoid making snap judgments about either of these "dangerous" animals. After all, if Floridians reside with alligators and crocodiles, we can probably live in harmony with our native species too.

HERE A PARK SYSTEM, THERE A PARK SYSTEM, EVERYWHERE . . .

In northeastern Ohio, we enjoy the benefits of many strong park systems and conservation-minded organizations. Most of the hike descriptions in this book include contact information so you can learn more about the area and the park system that manages it. But if you're really interested in learning about a particular area, the *best* way is to volunteer in it.

Volunteers in parks have increasingly important positions. There's a role for every person and personality too. Whether you're inclined to lead a hike, ring up sales in a nature shop, create posters, build a trail, or file paperwork, you'll be greatly appreciated. I have volunteered in city and county park systems and also in the Cuyahoga Valley National Park. Each experience has proven extremely rewarding. Volunteers have the opportunity to learn from a talented pool of workers and other volunteers, and then share their knowledge with others. No matter how much or how little time you may offer, a creative volunteer coordinator can help you find your niche. Start by calling your local parks and recreation office or any of these organizations:

ASHTABULA COUNTY PARKS
ashtabulacountyparks.org
(440) 576-0717

BUCKEYE TRAIL ASSOCIATION
buckeyetrail.org

CLEVELAND METROPARKS
clevelandmetroparks.com
(216) 635-3200

CUYAHOGA VALLEY NATIONAL PARK
dayinthevalley.com or
nps.gov/cuva
(330) 657-2350

GEAUGA PARK DISTRICT
geaugaparkdistrict.org
(440) 285-2222

LAKE METROPARKS
lakemetroparks.com
(440) 358-7275

LORAIN COUNTY METRO PARKS
loraincountymetroparks.com
(800) 526-7275

METRO PARKS SERVING SUMMIT COUNTY
summitmetroparks.org
(330) 867-5511

THE NATURE CONSERVANCY
nature.org
(614) 717-2770

PORTAGE PARK DISTRICT
portageparkdistrict.org
(330) 297-7728

STARK PARKS
starkparks.com
(330) 477-3552

Finally, no matter where you hike or visit, take the time to learn where you are and to understand the rules that govern that particular trail. Rules vary. State nature preserves, for example, prohibit pets and anything with wheels, while most state parks welcome pets (on a leash) and even bikes (on some trails). Some city parks do not allow pets; others welcome canine visitors. The rules of the trail are created for a reason; following them makes outings more pleasant for everyone.

TAKE A HIKE

In assembling a variety of hikes for this book, I walked through parks and creek beds, on city sidewalks and around the zoo. Everywhere I went, I discovered something. In the hike profiles, I've tried to convey some of the wonder I felt in those discoveries. Now it's your turn. I hope that this book serves as a list of good suggestions, a set of starting points from which you'll discover many pleasures of your own.

Happy trails.

HIKING RECOMMENDATIONS

BUSY HIKES

HIKES FEATURING WATERFALLS

HIKES FEATURING WILDFLOWERS

HIKES FEATURING WILDFLOWERS (CONTINUED)

HIKES GOOD FOR CHILDREN

HIKES GOOD FOR SOLITUDE

HIKES GOOD FOR WILDLIFE VIEWING

HIKES FEATURING NATURE CENTERS

HIKES WITH STEEP SECTIONS

HISTORICAL TRAILS

LAKE HIKES

LAKE HIKES (CONTINUED)

SCENIC HIKES

TRAILS GOOD FOR MOUNTAIN BIKES

TRAILS GOOD FOR RUNNERS

URBAN HIKES

HIKES WITH LESS THAN 1 MILE OPTIONS

HIKES 1–3 MILES

HIKES 1–3 MILES (CONTINUED)

HIKES 3–6 MILES

HIKES LONGER THAN 6 MILES

6 0 HIKES
WITHIN 6 0 MILES

C L E V E L A N D
INCLUDING
AKRON AND CANTON

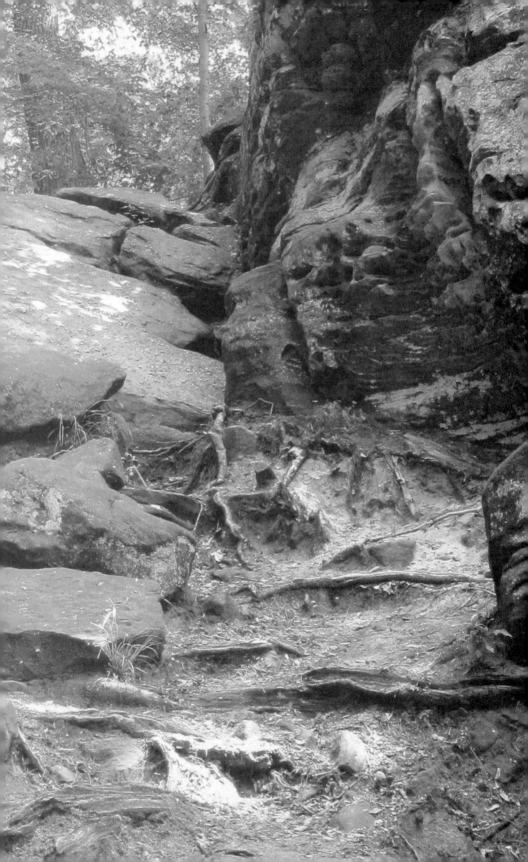

INTRODUCTION

Welcome to *60 Hikes within 60 Miles: Cleveland!* If you're new to hiking or even if you're a seasoned trailsmith, take a few minutes to read the following introduction. We'll explain how this book is organized and how to get the best use of it.

HIKE DESCRIPTIONS

Each hike contains six key items: a brief description of the trail, a key at-a-glance information box, directions to the trail, a trail map, an elevation profile, and a more detailed trail description. Many hikes also include information about nearby activities. Combined, the maps and information provide a clear method to assess each trail from the comfort of your favorite reading chair.

IN BRIEF

A taste of the trail. Think of this section as a snapshot focused on the historical landmarks, beautiful vistas, and other interesting sights you may encounter on the trail.

AT-A-GLANCE INFORMATION

The At-a-Glance information boxes give you a quick idea of the specifics of each hike. Fourteen basic elements are covered.

LENGTH The length of the trail from start to finish. In almost all cases there are options to shorten or extend the hikes, but the mileage corresponds to the described hike. Consult the hike description to help decide how to customize the hike for your ability or time constraints.

CONFIGURATION A description of what the trail might look like from overhead. Trails can be loops, out-and-backs (that is, along the same route), figure eights, or balloons. Sometimes the descriptions might surprise you.

DIFFICULTY The degree of effort an "average" hiker should expect on a given hike. For simplicity, difficulty is described as *easy, moderate,* or *difficult.*

SCENERY Rates the overall environs of the hike and what to expect in terms of plant life, wildlife, streams, and historical buildings.

EXPOSURE A quick check of how much sun you can expect on your shoulders during the hike. Descriptors used are self-explanatory and include terms such as *shady, exposed,* and *sunny.*

TRAFFIC Indicates how busy the trail might be on an average day, and if you might be able to find solitude out there. Trail traffic, of course, varies from day to day and season to season.

TRAIL SURFACE Indicates whether the trail is paved, rocky, smooth dirt, or a mixture of elements.

HIKING TIME How long it took the author to hike the trail. She is a fast hiker who stops frequently to take in unusual sights, to take pictures, and to take a sip of water. Her average hiking speed is 2.5 miles per hour.

DRIVING DISTANCE This is how far to drive from a given point—in this case, from the I-77/I-480 exchange.

ACCESS A notation of fees or permits needed to access the trail (if any) and whether the trail has specific hours.

WHEELCHAIR TRAVERSABLE Notes whether the trail is wheelchair compatible.

MAPS Which map is the best for this hike and where to get it.

FACILITIES What to expect in terms of restrooms, water, and other amenities available at the trailhead or nearby.

CONTACT INFORMATION Gives you contact information, including phone number and website, in case you want to do additional research.

DESCRIPTIONS

The trail description is the heart of each hike. Here, the author provides a summary of the trail's essence and highlights any special traits the hike offers. Ultimately, the hike description will help you choose which hikes are best for you.

NEARBY ACTIVITIES

Not every hike will have this listing. For those that do, look here for information on nearby sights of interest.

MAPS

The maps in this book have been produced with great care and, used with the hiking directions, will help you stay on course. But as any experienced hiker knows, things can get tricky off the beaten path.

The maps in this book, when used with the route directions present in each chapter, are sufficient to direct you to the trail and guide you on it. However, you will find superior detail and valuable information in the United States Geological Survey's 7.5-minute series topographic maps. Topo maps are available online in many locations. The easiest single Web resource is located at **msrmaps.com.** You can view and print topos of the entire Unites States there and view aerial photographs of the same areas. The downside to topos is that most are outdated, having been created 20–30 years ago. But they still provide excellent topographic detail.

If you're new to hiking, you might be wondering, "What's a topographic map?" In short, a topo indicates not only linear distance but elevation as well, using contour lines. Wavy contour lines spread across topo maps, each line representing a particular elevation. At the base of each topo, a contour's interval designation is given. If the contour interval is 200 feet, then the distance between each contour line is 200 feet. Follow five contour lines up on a map and the elevation has increased by 1,000 feet.

Let's assume that the 7.5-minute series topo reads "contour interval 40 feet," that the short trail we'll be hiking is two inches in length on the map, and that it crosses five contour lines from beginning to end. What do we know? Well, because the linear scale of this series is 2,000 feet to the inch (roughly 2¾ inches representing 1 mile), we know that our trail is approximately four-fifths of a mile long (2 inches are 4,000 feet). But we also know that we'll be climbing or descending 200 vertical feet (five contour lines are 40 feet each) over that distance. And the elevation designations written on occasional contour lines will tell us if we're heading up or down.

In addition to outdoor shops and bike shops, you'll find topos at major universities and some public libraries, where you might try photocopying the ones you need instead of buying them. But if you want your own and can't find them locally, visit the United States Geological Survey website at **topomaps.usgs.gov** or other vendors mentioned in the appendix as resources for topographic maps and software.

THE OVERVIEW MAP AND KEY

Use the overview map on the inside front cover to find the exact location of each hike's primary trailhead. Each hike's number appears on the overview map, on the hike list facing the overview map, and in the table of contents. As you flip through the book, you'll see that a hike's full profile is easy to locate by watching for the hike number at the top of each page. The book is organized by region, as indicated in the table of contents. A map legend that details the symbols found on trail maps appears on the inside back cover.

REGIONAL MAPS

The book is divided into regions, and prefacing each regional section is an overview map of that region. The regional map provides more detail than the overview map does, bringing you closer to the hike.

TRAIL MAPS

Each hike contains a detailed map that shows the trailhead, route, significant features, facilities, and topographic landmarks such as creeks, overlooks, and peaks. The author gathered map data, which was then downloaded into the digital mapping program Topo USA and processed by expert cartographers to produce the highly accurate maps found in this book. Each trailhead's GPS coordinates are included with each profile (see below).

ELEVATION PROFILES

Each hike contains a detailed elevation profile that corresponds directly to the trail map. The elevation profile provides a quick look at the trail from the side, enabling you to visualize how it rises and falls. Note the number of feet between each tick mark on the vertical axis (the height scale). To avoid making flat hikes look steep and steep hikes appear flat, height scales are used throughout the book to provide an accurate assessment of each hike's climbing difficulty.

GPS TRAILHEAD COORDINATES

In addition to highly specific trail outlines, this book also includes the latitude and longitude coordinates for each trailhead. The latitude and longitude grid system is likely quite familiar to you, but here is a refresher.

Imaginary lines of latitude—called parallels and approximately 69 miles apart from each other—run horizontally around the globe. Each parallel is indicated by degrees from the equator (established to be 0°): up to 90°N at the North Pole and down to 90°S at the South Pole.

Imaginary lines of longitude—called meridians—run perpendicular to latitude lines. Longitude lines are likewise indicated by degrees: Starting from 0° at the Prime Meridian, in Greenwich, England, they continue to the east and west until they meet 180° later at the International Date Line in the Pacific Ocean. At the equator, longitude lines also are approximately 69 miles apart, but that distance narrows as the meridians converge toward the North and South poles.

Each degree can be divided into 60 minutes and each minute into 60 seconds. This system provides a precise location by the coordinates of the latitude and longitude lines.

For more on GPS technology, the USGS offers a good deal of information regarding UTM coordinates at its website, **usgs.gov.**

WEATHER

Spring, summer, and fall have obvious allure for hikers in northeastern Ohio. On average, August has the clearest days, followed closely by July, September, and October. If there is a best month to hike around here, it might be October. Most of the summer bugs are gone, but some of the late summer and fall wildflowers remain. Temperatures tend to be quite nice in the afternoons, and the trees are at their colorful best. But there is no reason to stay inside during any month. Consider your destination in terms of the day's weather. A wetland trail may be impassable on a wet spring day, yet stunningly beautiful in December. Black flies bite hard (really hard!) in August; you may want to hit an urban trail then. Wear mosquito repellent when you're on the trail afternoons and evenings, from April through October.

AVERAGE DAILY TEMPERATURES BY MONTH FOR CLEVELAND, OHIO			
JAN	FEB	MAR	APR
24.8°F	27.2°F	37.3°F	47.6°F
MAY	JUN	JUL	AUG
58.0°F	67.6°F	71.9°F	70.4°F
SEP	OCT	NOV	DEC
63.9°F	52.8°F	42.6°F	30.9°F

TRAIL ETIQUETTE

Whether you're on a city, county, state, or national park trail, always remember that great care and resources (from nature as well as from your tax dollars) have gone into creating these trails. Treat the trail, wildlife, and fellow hikers with respect.

Here are a few general ideas to keep in mind while on the trail.

1. **Hike on open trails only. Respect trail and road closures (ask if not sure); avoid possible trespass on private land; obtain all permits and authorization as required. Also, leave gates as you found them or as marked.**

2. **Leave no trace of your visit other than footprints. Be sensitive to the dirt beneath you. This means staying on the trail and not creating any new ones. Be sure to pack out what you pack in. (Note: Some people believe that there's a special place in heaven for hikers who gather rubbish while on the trail and pack that out too.)**

3. **Never spook animals. An unannounced approach, a sudden movement, or a loud noise startles most animals. A surprised snake or skunk can be dangerous for you, for others, and to themselves. Give animals ample time and space to adjust to your presence.**

4. **Plan ahead. Know your equipment, your ability, and the area in which you are hiking—and prepare accordingly. Be self-sufficient at all times; carry necessary supplies for changes in weather or other conditions. A well-executed trip is a satisfaction to you and to others.**

5. **Be courteous to other hikers, or bikers, you meet on the trails.**

WATER

"How much is enough? One bottle? Two? Three?! Who wants to carry the extra weight!" One simple physiological fact should convince you to err on the side of excess when it comes to deciding how much water to pack: A human working hard in 90° heat needs approximately ten quarts of fluid every day. That's two and a half *gallons*—12 large water bottles or 16 small ones. In other words, pack along one or two bottles even for short hikes.

Serious backpackers hit the trail prepared to purify water found along the route. This method, while less dangerous than drinking it untreated, comes with risks. Many hikers pack along the slightly distasteful tetraglycine hydroperiodide tablets (sold under the names Potable Aqua, Coughlan's, and others). Some invest in portable, lightweight purifiers that filter out the crud. Unfortunately, both iodine and filtering are now required to be absolutely sure you've killed all the nasties you can't see. *Giardia,* for example, may hit one to four weeks after ingestion. It will have you bloated, vomiting, shivering with chills, and living in the bathroom. But there are other parasites to worry about, including *E. coli* and *cryptosporidium.* (Affectionately known as "crypto," it's even harder to kill than *giardia.*)

For most people, the pleasures of hiking make carrying water a relatively minor price to pay to remain healthy. If you're tempted to drink found water, do so only once you thoroughly understand the purification method and the risks involved.

FIRST-AID KIT

A typical kit may contain more items than you might think necessary. But these are just the basics:

Ace bandages or Spenco joint wraps

Antibiotic ointment (Neosporin or the generic equivalent)

Aspirin or acetaminophen

Butterfly-closure bandages

Band-Aids

Benadryl or the generic equivalent —diphenhydramine (an antihistamine, in case of allergic reactions)

Gauze (one roll and a half-dozen 4-inch-by-4-inch compress pads)

Hydrogen peroxide or iodine

Matches or pocket lighter

Moleskin/Spenco Second Skin

A prefilled syringe of epinephrine (for those known to have severe allergic reactions to things such as bee stings)

Snakebite kit

Sunscreen

Water purification tablets or water filter (see note above)

Whistle (more effective in signaling rescuers than your voice)

Pack the items in a waterproof bag such as a zip-top bag or a similar product. You will also want to include a snack for hikes longer than a couple of miles. A bag full of GORP (good ol' raisins and peanuts) will kick up your energy level fast.

HIKING WITH CHILDREN

No one is too young for a hike in the woods or through a city park. Be careful, though. Flat, short trails are probably best with an infant. Toddlers who have not quite mastered walking can still tag along, riding on an adult's back in a child carrier. Use common sense to judge a child's capacity to hike a particular trail, and always keep in mind the possibility that the child will tire quickly and need to be carried.

When packing for the hike, remember the needs of the child as well as your own. Make sure children are adequately clothed for the weather, have proper shoes, and are protected from the sun with sunscreen. Kids dehydrate quickly, so make sure you have plenty of fluid for everyone.

To assist an adult with determining which trails are suitable for children, a list of hike recommendations for children is provided on pages xvi–xvii.

Finally, when hiking with children, remember the trip is bound to be a compromise. A child's energy and enthusiasm alternates between bursts of speed and long stops to examine snails, sticks, dirt, and other attractions.

THE BUSINESS HIKER

Whether in the Cleveland area on business as a resident or visitor, these 60 hikes offer perfect, quick getaways from the busy demands of commerce. Many of the hikes are classified as urban and are easily accessible from downtown areas. Instead of eating inside, pack a lunch and head out to one of the many links in the Emerald Necklace (Cleveland Metroparks) for a relaxing break from the office or convention. Or plan ahead and take a small group of your business comrades on a nearby hike in Cleveland Lakefront State Park or along the canal. A well-planned, half-day getaway is the perfect complement to a business stay in northeastern Ohio.

ANIMAL AND PLANT HAZARDS

TICKS

Ticks like to hang out in the brush that grows along trails. Hot summer months seem to explode their numbers, but you should be tick-aware during all months of the year. Ticks, which are arthropods and not insects, need a host to feast on in order to reproduce. The ticks that light on you while hiking will be very small, sometimes so tiny that you won't be able to spot them. Primarily of two varieties, deer ticks and dog ticks, both need a few hours of actual attachment before they can transmit any disease they may harbor. Ticks may settle in shoes, socks, or hats, and they may take several hours to actually latch on. The best strategy is to visually check every half hour or so while hiking, do a thorough check before you get in the car, and then, when you take a post-hike shower, do an even more thorough check of your entire body. Ticks that haven't attached are easily removed but not easily killed. If you pick off a tick in the woods, just toss it aside. If you find one on your body at home, dispatch it and then send it down the toilet. For ticks that have embedded, removal with tweezers is best.

MOSQUITOES

Although it's not a common occurrence, individuals can become infected with the West Nile virus by being bitten by an infected mosquito. Culex mosquitoes, the primary varieties that can transmit West Nile virus to humans, thrive in urban rather than in natural areas. They lay their eggs in stagnant water and can breed in any standing water that remains for more than five days. Most people infected with West Nile virus have no symptoms of illness, but some may become ill, usually 3–15 days after being bitten.

In the Cleveland area, late spring and summer are the times thought to be the highest risk periods for West Nile virus. At this time of year—and anytime you expect mosquitoes to be buzzing around—you may want to wear protective clothing, such as long sleeves, long pants, and socks. Loose-fitting, light-colored clothing is best. Spray clothing with insect repellent. Remember to follow the instructions on the repellent and to take extra care with children when using a repellent with DEET.

SNAKES

Some of the venomous snakes found in the United States, including the rattlesnake, cottonmouth, copperhead, and coral snake, all live in the Cleveland area and can be found on virtually every hike in this book. However, most of your snake encounters will be with the 100-plus nonvenomous species and subspecies. Although you could spend some time studying the snakes in the area, the best rule is to leave all snakes alone and give them a wide berth as you hike past.

BLACK BEARS

It's unlikely that you will meet a bear on any of these trails; there are still very few in Ohio, and in most cases, the bear will detect you first and leave. That said, there are no definite rules about what to do if you meet a bear. Should you encounter a bear, here is some advice, based on suggestions from the National Park Service:

- **Stay calm.**
- **Move away, talking loudly to let the bear discover your presence.**
- **Back away while facing the bear.**
- **Avoid eye contact.**
- **Give the bear plenty of room to escape; bears will rarely attack unless they are threatened or provoked.**
- **Don't run or make sudden movements; running will provoke the bear, and you cannot outrun a bear.**
- **Do not attempt to climb trees to escape bears, especially black bears. The bear will pull you down by the foot.**

- **Fight back if you are attacked. Black bears have been driven away when people have fought back with rocks, sticks, binoculars, and even their bare hands.**
- **Be grateful that it is not a grizzly bear.**

POISON IVY, POISON OAK, AND POISON SUMAC

Recognizing poison ivy, oak, and sumac and avoiding contact with them is the most effective way to prevent the painful, itchy rashes associated with these plants. Poison ivy ranges from a thick, tree-hugging vine to a shaded groundcover, three leaflets to a leaf; poison oak occurs as either a vine or shrub, with three leaflets as well; and poison sumac flourishes in swampland, each leaf containing 7–13 leaflets. Urushiol, the oil in the sap of these plants, is responsible for the rash. Usually within 12–14 hours of exposure (but sometimes much later), raised lines and/ or blisters will appear, accompanied by a terrible itch. Refrain from scratching because bacteria under fingernails can cause infection and you will spread the rash to other parts of your body. Wash and dry the rash thoroughly, applying a calamine lotion or other product to help dry the rash. If itching or blistering is severe, seek medical attention. Remember that oil-contaminated garments, pets, or hiking equipment can easily cause an irritating rash on you or someone else, so wash not only any exposed parts of your body but also clothes, gear, and pets.

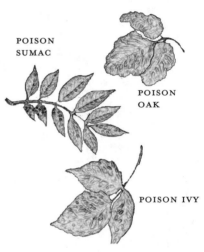

POISON SUMAC

POISON OAK

POISON IVY

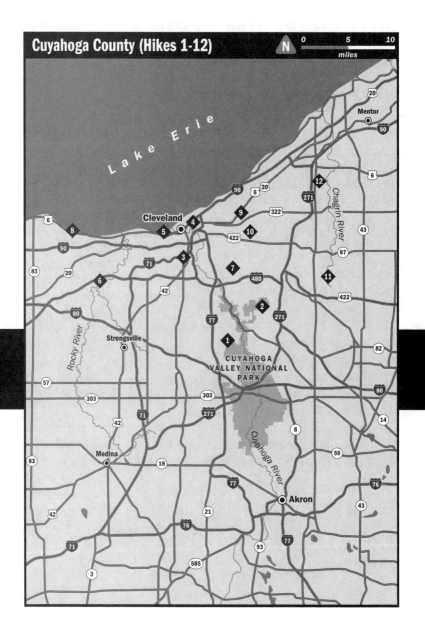

Cuyahoga County (Hikes 1-12)

N

0   5   10
              miles

Lake Erie

Mentor

Cleveland

Strongsville

Rocky River

Medina

Chagrin River

CUYAHOGA
VALLEY NATIONAL
PARK

Cuyahoga River

Akron

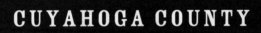

CUYAHOGA COUNTY

01 BRECKSVILLE RESERVATION

KEY AT-A-GLANCE INFORMATION

LENGTH: 3.5–4.9 miles

CONFIGURATION: Three loops with optional connector trail

DIFFICULTY: Salamander Loop Trail, moderate–difficult; other trails, easy

SCENERY: Prairie with wildflowers, vernal pool, great views of Chippewa Creek and Gorge

EXPOSURE: Prairie is exposed; other trails are shaded.

TRAFFIC: Short trails are well traveled; Salamander Loop Trail and My Mountain Overlook offer solitude.

TRAIL SURFACE: Prairie Loop Trail is asphalt and grass; other two are loose dirt and gravel.

HIKING TIME: 1 hour

DRIVING DISTANCE: 8 miles from I-77/I-480 exchange

ACCESS: Daily, 6 a.m.–11 p.m. except where otherwise posted

WHEELCHAIR TRAVERSABLE: Harriet Keeler Memorial, yes; other trails, no

MAPS: USGS Northfield; also at nature center and clevelandmetroparks.com

FACILITIES: Restrooms and water

CONTACT INFORMATION: Call the Brecksville Nature Center at (440) 526-1012 or visit cleveland metroparks.com.

IN BRIEF

Three short complementary loops in Cleveland Metroparks's Brecksville Reservation give visitors a good leg stretching and several picture-perfect views. Prairie fields, a vernal pond, and a forest trail to a lovely "mountain" give the budding naturalist (and casual sightseer) plenty to think about.

DESCRIPTION

Start the first of two short loop trails from the Harriet L. Keeler Memorial parking area on the south side of Chippewa Creek Drive. Follow the paved Prairie Loop Trail west to the Keeler Memorial. Keeler graduated from Oberlin College in 1870 and then moved to Cleveland. She was a suffragette and a Cleveland public school teacher, and she eventually became the system's superintendent. Keeler was also a prolific nature writer. For all of these accomplishments, she is honored here. Likewise, several of northeastern Ohio's different plant communities are also honored in this reservation.

From the memorial, you'll head south on a path of short grass, through a peaceful tall-grass prairie. The path gradually turns eastward, passing an intersection with the Wildflower Loop Trail. Continue forward,

GPS Trailhead
Coordinates

Latitude   41° 19.099259'

Longitude 81° 37.152121'

Directions

Follow I-77 South and take Exit 149A/OH 82, merging onto OH 82/East Royalton Road. Follow OH 82 east past OH 21 through Brecksville, turning right onto Chippewa Creek Drive. The Harriet L. Keeler Memorial/Overlook parking area is about 0.2 miles south of the park entrance.

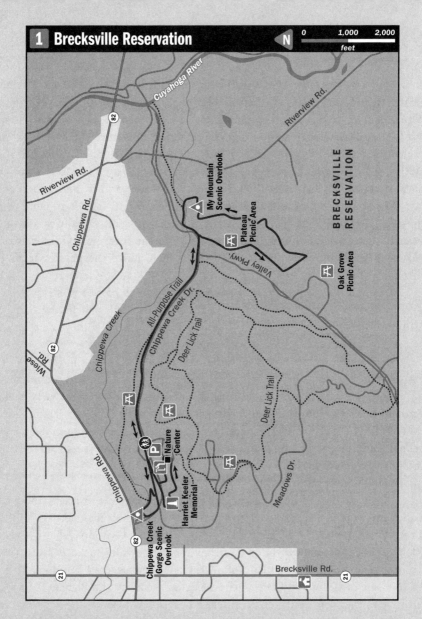

0   1,000   2,000

N

feet

Cuyahoga River

Riverview Rd.

82

Riverview Rd.

Chippewa Rd.

BRECKSVILLE RESERVATION

My Mountain Scenic Overlook

Plateau Picnic Area

Valley Pkwy.

Oak Grove Picnic Area

All-Purpose Trail

Chippewa Creek Dr.

Chippewa Creek

Deer Lick Trail

Deer Lick Trail

82

Wiese Rd.

Chippewa Rd.

P

Nature Center

Harriet Keeler Memorial

Meadows Dr.

82

Chippewa Creek Gorge Scenic Overlook

21

Brecksville Rd.

21

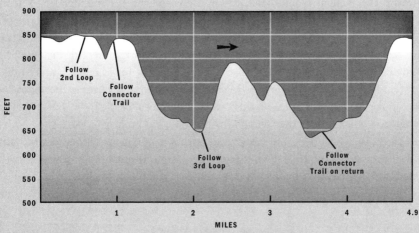

900

850

800

750

700

650

600

550

500

FEET

Follow 2nd Loop

Follow Connector Trail

Follow 3rd Loop

Follow Connector Trail on return

1   2   3   4   4.9

MILES

and soon after the mown grass trail meets asphalt, you'll find the nature center. (*Note:* Deer Lick Cave Loop Trail is a popular, longer trail that leaves from the nature center; if you wish to extend your hike at this time, go inside for a map.) Walk around the nature center clockwise, and as you leave the building, you'll notice some of the trees along this paved trail are labeled for easy identification. With a bit of studying, you can learn to tell your dawn redwoods from your black cherries. Farther west, the trail leads to a raised prairie observation deck.

This prairie is managed so it won't become a forest. It is dominated by tall grasses and brightened by wildflowers most of the year. Foxgloves and other beardtongue varieties bloom May through mid-summer; pretty Shreve's irises bloom in June and July. Tall sunflowers stretch above the grasses from July through early fall, and goldenrods gild the prairie August–October.

Continue west on the paved trail (this is the north half of Wildflower Loop Trail) and you'll see that a few of the trees are not only labeled by name but also noted for their utility. (*Note:* Pioneers made chewing gum from the sap of sweet gum trees.)

You'll have walked about 0.7 miles when you return to the Keeler Memorial. Start a new loop here, Hemlock Loop Trail, by crossing to the north side of Chippewa Creek Drive and walking down to the creek overlook (where you'll want to pull out your camera!). The path turns right then left again, sloping downhill. The path here is generally shady; during the fall, your feet noisily crunch over the oak leaves. You'll hear the creek before you see it; once it comes into view, you will follow its path. Eventually, you'll part ways—the creek ducks under OH 82 and out of sight.

Take a sharp left, heading back up the hill on a carpet of leaves and gravel. Follow the trail southwest, back to the All Purpose Trail, then across Chippewa Creek Drive to visit "your" mountain—My Mountain Overlook, that is—via the Metroparks's Salamander Loop Trail and the statewide Buckeye Trail. (*Note:* To reach the mountain, you can follow the All Purpose Trail running along the eastern side of Chippewa Creek Drive to Valley Parkway and Plateau Picnic Area or drive to the picnic parking area; let your legs decide.)

From the Plateau Picnic Area, follow signs for the Salamander Loop Trail and the blue blazes of the Buckeye Trail. From the picnic area parking lot, begin walking toward the shelter. About 100 yards in front of the shelter, you'll enter the rugged path. Once known as My Mountain Trail, it is now named for the amphibians that this area supports, and is also a simple delight for hikers who like hills. This area, like the prairie below, is managed by thinning the forest periodically to encourage the growth of rare wildflowers. Chippewa Creek Drive falls away to your right as you head up the steep path. You'll be glad that you wore your boots here—the going is slippery and uneven due to roots and gravel. The narrow path follows the ridge of the hill (it's not really a mountain) until the roadway lies 40 feet below. Then the trail bends left, looking over the picnic shelter below.

Things are pretty quiet up here, and you can imagine that it truly is your

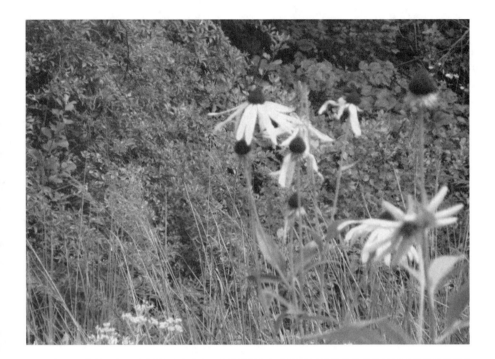

A tallgrass prairie buzzes with life.

mountain if you wish. The only sound you'll hear may be the squish of your boots as you near the vernal pool. This oak-hickory forest was thinned in the 1990s to encourage wildflower growth. Here, evidence of thinning is obvious, an aid to hikers to get a good look at the usually wet area.

Formed like puddles in contained basin depressions, vernal pools have no permanent aboveground outlets. They typically follow the water table—rising with winter and spring runoff, drying in summer, and filling and freezing in fall and winter. Because they dry out, they cannot support fish. But vernal pools support other species, such as frogs, salamanders, and fairy shrimp, which lay eggs in the pools. Depending on the species, the eggs either hatch before the pool dries out or they incubate throughout the wet-dry-freeze cycle, hatching the next year. While these temporary pools look like puddles, they are important ones.

On the western side of the pool, about 0.3 miles into the trail, you'll make a sharp left and see the blue blazes of the Buckeye Trail again. Soon, the trails split, and Salamander Loop Trail veers left, heading west. Almost a mile into your jaunt, the trail offers you a short spur to the overlook—take it, if you're not afraid of heights. From the top end of this steep and narrow path, you'll have a bird's-eye view of Riverview Road and the OH 82 bridge.

Retrace your steps down, taking a sharp right to rejoin the loop and continue counterclockwise. This last leg of the trail offers great wildflower displays in the spring. Your legs, perhaps tired of climbing, will welcome the downhill

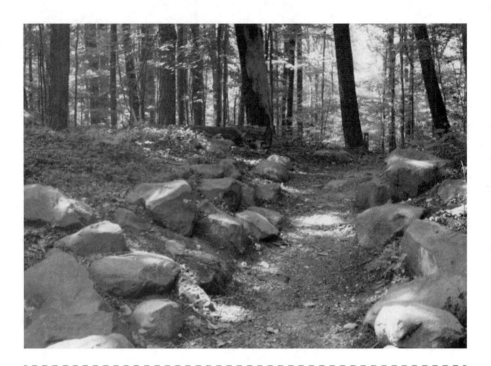

Brecksville Reservation offers hikers great trail variety.

portion of the loop at about 1.4 miles. A short set of wooden steps leads to the bottom of the picnic area driveway. Turn left to return to the parking area if you drove; if you walked, turn right and cross the parkway to follow the All Purpose Trail over a pretty bridge and Chippewa Creek.

NEARBY ACTIVITIES

Brecksville Reservation offers several other trails with nice hills—Deer Lick Cave Loop Trail, for example, is about 4 miles long. Stop at the nature center, visit **clevelandmetroparks.com,** or call (440) 526-1012 for more information.

History buffs might want to visit the Squire Rich Home & Museum, built in 1835 using local walnut trees. Located inside Brecksville Reservation and managed by the Brecksville Historical Society, the museum hosts annual festivals and is open for tours. Call (440) 526-7165 for a schedule.

BRIDAL VEIL FALLS AND TINKER'S CREEK GORGE

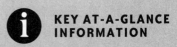

IN BRIEF

An easy hike with a big-view payoff: enjoy cascades and waterfalls on the way to Ohio's grandest canyon, nearly 200 feet deep.

DESCRIPTION

Cross the parkway and enter the trail, following 65 wooden steps down to the overlook. Along the way there are several places to stop and admire the water gently bathing the shale as it trips along to the falls.

At the bottom of the steps, the walking and bridle paths cross. Horses cross the shallow water on hoof; the rest of us use the bridge. As you look north from the bridge, notice the layers of Bedford shale that line the side of the hill.

At the bottom of the 85-foot drop, you'll find a small observation deck with benches. Stop here to enjoy the view.

Once you've had a good look, get off the deck and step onto the Bridle Trail, continuing west. You'll roll up and down several gentle hills, under the shade of thick maple, oak, and hemlock trees. The eastern hemlock is common in this area, often simply lumped in with the evergreen family. Hemlocks can be distinguished by their tiny opposing leaves, deep green in color, that lie flat along their

KEY AT-A-GLANCE INFORMATION

LENGTH: 2 miles

CONFIGURATION: Loop

DIFFICULTY: Easy

SCENERY: Waterfall, gorge, lush forest, fall color, wildflowers in spring

EXPOSURE: Completely shaded except for overlook

TRAFFIC: Moderate–heavy

TRAIL SURFACE: Dirt and gravel trail on north side, paved on south

HIKING TIME: 45 minutes

DRIVING DISTANCE: 12 miles from I-77/I-480 exchange

ACCESS: Daily, 6 a.m.–11 p.m.; parking lots that close at sunset are clearly posted.

WHEELCHAIR TRAVERSABLE: No, but the overlook is accessible from Cleveland Metro Parkway

MAPS: USGS Shaker; also available at clevelandmetroparks.com

FACILITIES: Pay phone, water, and restroom at Egbert Road ranger station; portable restrooms at the gorge overlook; water and restrooms at Hermit's Hollow Picnic Area

CONTACT INFORMATION: Call the Garfield Park Nature Center at (216) 341-3152 or see cleveland metroparks.com. Emergency phones are along the parkway.

Directions

From I-480 East, take I-271 south to Exit 23/Broadway Avenue/Forbes Road and head west on OH 14/Broadway. Turn right onto Forbes Road and then right onto Broadway. Turn left on Bedford Chagrin Parkway/Egbert Road and make a quick right onto Cleveland Metro Parkway. Head west about 2 miles to the parking area for Bridal Veil Falls Overlook, on the left.

GPS Trailhead Coordinates

Latitude 41° 22.312982'

Longitude 81° 32.936103'

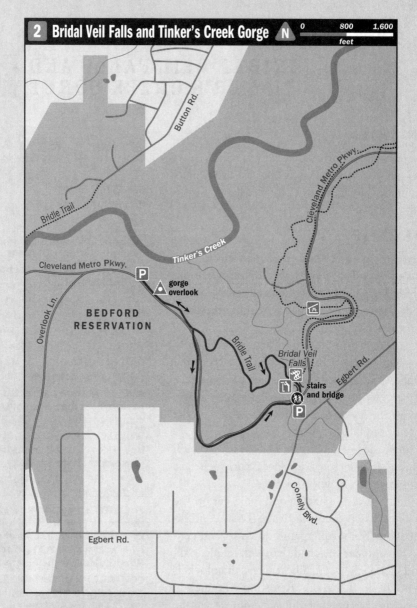

2 Bridal Veil Falls and Tinker's Creek Gorge

N

0   800   1,600
feet

Button Rd.

Cleveland Metro Pkwy.

Bridle Trail

Tinker's Creek

Cleveland Metro Pkwy.

P

gorge
overlook

Overlook Ln.

BEDFORD
RESERVATION

Bridle Trail

Bridal Veil
Falls

stairs
and bridge

Egbert Rd.

P

Conelly Blvd.

Egbert Rd.

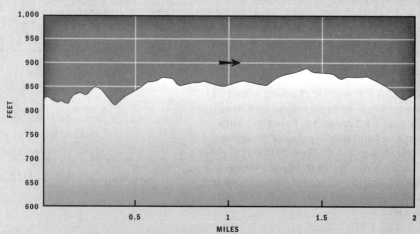

1,000
950
900
850
800
750
700
650
600

FEET

0.5   1   1.5   2

MILES

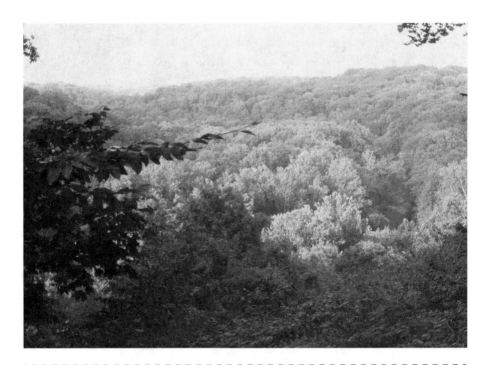

No dam to see at this National Natural Landmark

branches. Look for narrow white stripes on the leaves' undersides.

The wide dirt-and-gravel trail you're on performs double duty here. It is both the park district's Bridle Trail and a portion of the Buckeye Trail, and it is well marked. A mile west of the falls, you'll rise up to meet the parkway again, soon reaching the gorge overlook.

The overlook itself is wheelchair- and stroller-accessible (parking is available directly off Cleveland Metro Parkway). The view is the main attraction, of course, but the history is also interesting.

Tinker's Creek, the largest tributary to the Cuyahoga River, begins in Kent, Ohio—about 15 miles southeast. Once it reaches this area, it winds its way nearly 5 miles through Bedford Reservation. In 1965 public officials planned to dam the gorge, intending to flood it to create a large inland lake they would call Lake Shawnee. A five-year study by naturalist William F. Nimberger, however, highlighted the valley's unique blend of plant and animal species. Public opinion, swayed in large part by Nimberger's study, convinced politicians to abandon their plans to dam the gorge. Today the gorge is a National Natural Landmark.

To return to your car, retrace your steps on the Bridle Trail or cross the parkway to the south and take the All Purpose Trail back to the parking area at Bridal Veil Falls. The difference in the two paths is negligible—about 0.1 mile.

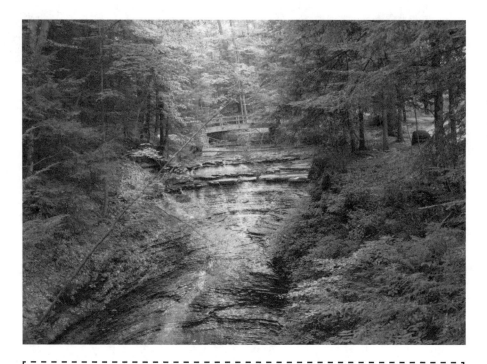

Bridal Veil Falls

NEARBY ACTIVITIES

Shawnee Hills Golf Course is just south of here; enter from Egbert Road. To arrange a tee time, call (440) 232-7184. Or follow the parkway east a few miles to South Chagrin Metropark (see page 54), where another chapter of the area's history has been preserved.

CLEVELAND METROPARKS ZOO 03

IN BRIEF

Is this a hike or an amusement park? Both. And where else in Cleveland can you see polar bears *and* kangaroos?

DESCRIPTION

The zoo dates back to 1882, when Jeptha Wade donated 73 acres in the University Circle area where the Western Union Telegraph Company kept a small herd of deer. Over the years, other local animals such as Canada geese and raccoons were added to the collection. Eventually, plans to establish the Cleveland Museum of Art in Wade Oval meant that the menagerie must move. From 1907 to 1914, the animals were relocated to the zoo's current site, then called Brookside Park. The Works Progress Administration (WPA) completed many projects at the zoo during the Depression era. Since then the zoo has had several caretakers: The Cleveland Museum of Natural History from 1940 to 1957, the Cleveland Zoological Society from 1957 to 1975, and the Cleveland Metroparks since 1975. Each has added to the zoo's history and attractions; each addition seems more fascinating than the last.

Inside the RainForest's two-acre habitat you'll find some of the world's strangest animals. Wolf Wilderness exposes us to a pack of gray wolves, a beaver dam, and a variety of other species both indoors and out. Australian Adventure, closed in winter (though you can

KEY AT-A-GLANCE INFORMATION

LENGTH: 3.5 miles (add The RainForest for a total of 4 miles)

CONFIGURATION: Connecting loops

DIFFICULTY: Easy, except a long hill

SCENERY: African savanna, desert, beaver dam, greenhouse, outdoor sculptures, rain forest building

EXPOSURE: Path is mostly exposed; exhibits provide shade and shelter.

TRAFFIC: Moderate, with crowds for special events

TRAIL SURFACE: Asphalt

HIKING TIME: 4 hours to see it all

DRIVING DISTANCE: 7 miles from I-77/I-480 exchange

ACCESS: Daily, 10 a.m.–5 p.m.; closed January 1 and December 25. Admission, April–October: Adults, $10; children ages 2–11, $7; children age 1 and younger, free. Admission, November–March: Adults, $7; children ages 2–11, $5; children age 1 and younger, free.

WHEELCHAIR TRAVERSABLE: Yes

MAPS: USGS Lakewood; also available at entrance gate

FACILITIES: Restrooms, water, and pay phone at Welcome Plaza

CONTACT INFORMATION: Visit clemetzoo.com or call (216) 661-6500.

Directions

Take I-480 West to Exit 16/OH 94/State Road. Follow State Road north until it dead-ends at Pearl. Turn right and follow Pearl approximately 0.5 miles; then turn left onto Wildlife Way, which leads to the zoo's main entrance.

GPS Trailhead Coordinates

Latitude 41° 26.821260'

Longitude 81° 42.695639'

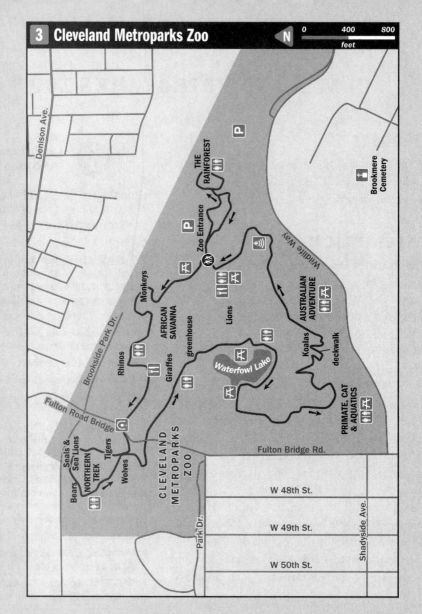

0   400   800

feet

N

Denison Ave.

P

THE RAINFOREST

Zoo Entrance

P

Brookmere Cemetery

Wildlife Way

Monkeys

AUSTRALIAN ADVENTURE

AFRICAN SAVANNA

Lions

greenhouse

Koalas

deckwalk

Rhinos

Giraffes

Waterfowl Lake

PRIMATE, CAT & AQUATICS

Brookside Park Dr.

Fulton Road Bridge

Fulton Bridge Rd.

Seals & Sea Lions

Bears

NORTHERN TREK

Tigers

Wolves

CLEVELAND METROPARKS ZOO

Park Dr.

W 48th St.

W 49th St.

W 50th St.

Shadyside Ave.

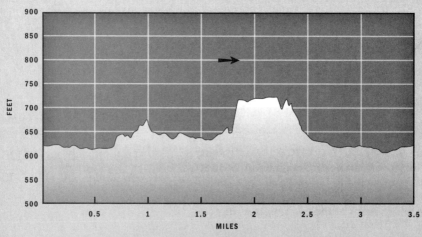

FEET

900
850
800
750
700
650
600
550
500

0.5   1   1.5   2   2.5   3   3.5

MILES

still visit the kangaroos), invites visitors to take a walk—or a train ride—through the outback. So lace up your boots, mate, and walk this way.

From the Welcome Plaza, head north (right) to the African Savanna. As the path curves to the west, you'll encounter gazelles, great African cranes (some of the largest birds in the world), and finally, the Masai giraffes. The Masais are hard to miss: they are the tallest animals on earth, reaching 16–18 feet. A female born here in August 2008 was 6 feet tall and weighed 140 pounds at birth! If they aren't near the fence as you round the park's northern edge, don't worry; observation decks on both sides of the exhibit give you plenty of chances to catch them, if only on camera. Once you've visited with the black rhinos and strolled under the impressive Fulton Road Bridge, you'll have logged more than 0.5 miles.

Following the signs to the Northern Trek section, a right turn leads you to some of the zoo's older exhibits. The sea lion and polar bear pools were both built of native stone quarried from Euclid Creek Reservation. Climb the steps between the two exhibits to watch both from above.

Continuing through the Northern Trek, you'll walk by the placid Bactrian camels (two humps) before reaching Wolf Wilderness. Step inside the cabin-style building to see a variety of exhibits, including turtles, fish, and beavers. Watch for the Mexican gray wolves from behind the cabin's glass wall. They are hard to spot until they move; be patient and you can get a good look. Leave the cabin for the center of the Northern Trek to visit with several bear species, tigers, and reindeer. Heading east, back under the Fulton Bridge, you'll pass the African Savanna again. The greenhouse, at about 1.5 miles, is a must-stop spot for gardeners. For several months each year, it's also home to hundreds of butterflies. Opposite the greenhouse is the original zoo building—Wade Hall. Relocated from Wade Park in the mid-1970s and completely refurbished in 1992, today it is a Victorian-style ice cream parlor.

On your right you'll find a towering birdcage. It has to be towering because it houses Andean condors, some of the world's highest flyers, along with vultures and other large birds.

Once you reach the southern edge of Waterfowl Lake, turn left and then right to visit the koalas in GumLeaf Hideout. On your right, just past the koalas, looms the only serious hill in the park: a 1,250-foot-long boardwalk climbing 800 feet up from Australian Adventure to the land of primates, big cats, and big fish above. Before you tackle that, head for the land down under.

Australian Adventure is serious fun. The Boomerang Railway railroad track encircles a walk-through lorikeet aviary, kangaroos and wallabies, and a 55-foot tree house. You'll "climb" inside the man-made baobab tree on a swingy suspension bridge. Bats, snakes, and a creepy animatronic crocodile await your entrance. The exit is a slide, disguised as a long snake. (*Note:* Much of the Australian Adventure area is wheelchair accessible; the tree house isn't.)

Next, you'll take the 1,250-foot boardwalk up 800 feet to the southwest corner of the park. (You can take the tram instead, but then you'll miss the only serious aerobic workout of the hike.) Steps in the middle of each zigzag along

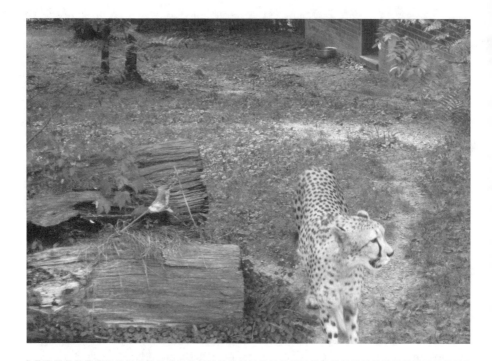

Prowl around the zoo for exercise, and leave with an education.

the ramp allow walkers a bit of a shortcut, while strollers and wheelchairs roll up. At the top of the climb, you've logged about 2.5 miles and several dozen species. Pause to enjoy a shady view of the Big Creek ravine before proceeding to the Primate, Cat & Aquatics Building. Heading north from the top of the park, follow the path as it winds by Waterfowl Lake. Flamingos will signal your return to the entrance. Now you have about 3.5 miles on your sneakers and, probably, a head full of freshly gained knowledge.

If you leave the zoo and head east to The RainForest building, you'll add at least 0.7 miles to your hike, as well as a new perspective on rain forest habitats. Consider this: in Ohio, the average ten-acre plot of land is home to about 34 different species; on ten acres in Ecuador's rain forest you'll find about 200.

Inside the dome-shaped exhibit, you can watch as dozens of bats feed, fly, and crawl about a red-lit room. If you're more interested in birds than bats, you'll enjoy the exhibit highlighting the Southern Hemisphere species, such as the yellow-billed cuckoos, which make their summer homes in Ohio. Beyond bats and birds, the rain forest is home to hundreds of other animals; many are exhibited here.

Between African Savanna, the Northern Trek, Australian Adventure, and the RainForest, it's quite possible that a zoo hike will provide you with more information than you can process in one day. Don't worry–there's no quiz later, and you can always return to refresh your memory.

DOWNTOWN CLEVELAND HIGHLIGHTS 04

IN BRIEF

How many hikes start at a historical landmark and shopping mall? This one does. Whether you have out-of-town guests who want to see the north coast, or you haven't been downtown for a while, this mini-tour will put you in a Cleveland state of mind, with stops at stately Public Square, the anything-but-square Rock and Roll Hall of Fame and Museum, and other highlights. The Terminal Tower observation deck, offering panoramic views of the city, reopened to the public in the summer of 2010. In addition to Cleveland's man-made skyline, you may also spot some of the peregrine falcons that nest on ledges of the building's exterior.

DESCRIPTION

From Tower City's lower lot, go inside Tower City Center and up the escalator and wander north through the fabulous shopping center. When the Van Sweringen brothers planned the 52-story tower in the 1920s, they worked to sway both public opinion and political decisions to have it constructed to their desired specifications. Built to be the main tower in the Cleveland Union (railroad) Terminal, it was the tallest building outside of New York City from its opening in 1930 until 1967. Today, the tower cum mall-and-office space

KEY AT-A-GLANCE INFORMATION

LENGTH: 3 miles
CONFIGURATION: Loop
DIFFICULTY: Easy
SCENERY: Landmark buildings (both old and new), our Great Lake, public art, pigeons, peregrine falcons
EXPOSURE: Mostly exposed
TRAFFIC: Moderately heavy
TRAIL SURFACE: City sidewalks
HIKING TIME: 1.5 hours
DRIVING DISTANCE: 9 miles from I-77/I-480 exchange
ACCESS: Most shops, museums, and attractions are open daily.
WHEELCHAIR TRAVERSABLE: Yes, except cemetery and historical ships
MAPS: USGS Cleveland North and Cleveland South; Downtown street maps posted at each RTA stop
FACILITIES: Public restrooms at Tower City and Galleria (East Ninth Street and Lakeside Avenue)
CONTACT INFORMATION: Purchase tickets for the observation deck at the information desk at Terminal Tower. To learn more about the peregrine falcons at the tower, see falconcam-cmnh.org/news.php or inquire at the information desk. See "Nearby Activities" on page 29 for additional contact information.

Directions

From I-77 North take Exit 163/East Ninth Street. From East Ninth Street, merge onto East 14th Street, turning right at Orange Avenue and following signs to Public Square/Stadium. Then go north on Broadway. Turn left onto West Huron Road to park at the Tower City Center parking garage.

GPS Trailhead Coordinates
Latitude   41° 29.810700'
Longitude   81° 41.634958'

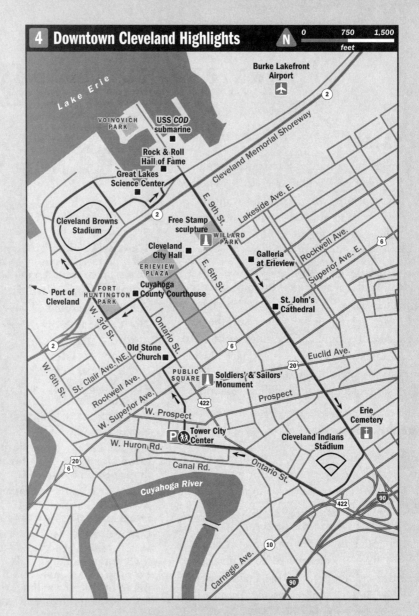

N

0   750   1,500
feet

Burke Lakefront
Airport

Lake Erie

Cleveland Memorial Shoreway

2

VOINOVICH
PARK

USS *COD*
submarine

Rock & Roll
Hall of Fame

Lakeside Ave. E.

Great Lakes
Science Center

E. 9th St.

Rockwell Ave.

6

Cleveland Browns
Stadium

2

Free Stamp
sculpture

WILLARD
PARK

Superior Ave. E.

Cleveland
City Hall

E. 6th St.

Galleria
at Erieview

ERIEVIEW
PLAZA

Port of
Cleveland

FORT
HUNTINGTON
PARK

Cuyahoga
County Courthouse

St. John's
Cathedral

W. 3rd St.

Ontario St.

6

Euclid Ave.

2

Old Stone
Church

20

St. Clair Ave. NE.

PUBLIC
SQUARE

Soldiers' & Sailors'
Monument

W. 6th St.

Rockwell Ave.

Prospect

W. Superior Ave.

422

Erie
Cemetery

W. Prospect

20

W. Huron Rd.

Tower City
Center

P

Cleveland Indians
Stadium

6

Canal Rd.

Ontario St.

Cuyahoga River

422

90

Carnegie Ave.

10

90

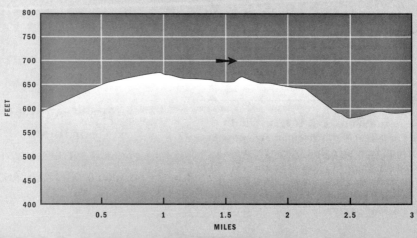

800

750

700

650

FEET

600

550

500

450

400

0.5   1   1.5   2   2.5   3

MILES

has far outlived the railroad line for which it was planned, yet it remains a signature flourish on Cleveland's skyline.

Exit Tower City Center onto Euclid Avenue and find yourself on Public Square. The Soldiers' and Sailors' Monument, built in 1894, sits to your right, on the eastern side of Ontario. The monument to the 10,000 Cleveland-area soldiers who served in the Civil War is open inside; you can walk right into it if you like.

Continue north across Public Square to the Old Stone Church. The church was established here on the corner of Ontario and Rockwell in 1834; it has been rebuilt a couple of times since. The building you see today dates back to 1855. If your timing is good (don't interrupt a wedding!), you can go in to appreciate its ornate interior. Follow Ontario north, across St. Clair, to the Cuyahoga County Courthouse. As you approach, crane your neck to take in six stately sculptures atop the building's facade. The marble figures were created by Herbert Adams in 1911; each honors an individual for his contributions to English law. Simon de Montfort (1200–1265) for example, helped establish the House of Commons. Below, Alexander Hamilton and Thomas Jefferson sit on opposite sides of the main entrance steps.

With a nod to Misters Hamilton and Jefferson, turn left in front of the courthouse and follow Lakeside Avenue west about half a block; turn right onto West Third. From the top of the hill, you'll catch a glimpse of Lake Erie. Follow West Third downhill, passing the Port of Cleveland on your left, and wind around the 31-acre site of Cleveland Browns Stadium. This may be a good place to get some landscaping ideas: an estimated 24,700 trees, plants, and flowers grow on the stadium grounds, and the field, sporting Kentucky bluegrass, is heated to extend its growing season.

Follow West Third east as it bends right, heading south into Erieside—the 171-foot-tall stadium now stands to your right. Turn left onto North Marginal, walking east past the Great Lakes Science Center and the Rock and Roll Hall of Fame and Museum. Be sure to peer behind the Science Center to marvel at the 618-foot-long *William G. Mather* steamship, a piece of history in striking visual contrast to the futuristic Rock and Roll Hall of Fame and Museum, designed by architect I. M. Pei. Here you'll also notice signs advertising tours on the *Goodtime III*. When visiting Cleveland, the *Mather, Goodtime,* and nearby USS *COD* submarine offer a comprehensive education in the city's unbreakable connection to the Great Lakes. Tours on any of the three are enjoyable, but the hands-down best choice for hikers is a walk-and-crawl-through tour of the USS *COD*. (See "Nearby Activities" on page 29.) Continue your walk from here by turning right, going south on East Ninth Street. Cross over busy OH 2, also known as the Shoreway, and begin to head uphill.

Just south of Lakeside Avenue, you'll find the Galleria. The beautiful mall, modeled to honor Cleveland's history of interior arcades, lost many retail occupants after the prestigious Tower City Center opened, but the food court inside the Galleria remains popular with downtown workers and visitors.

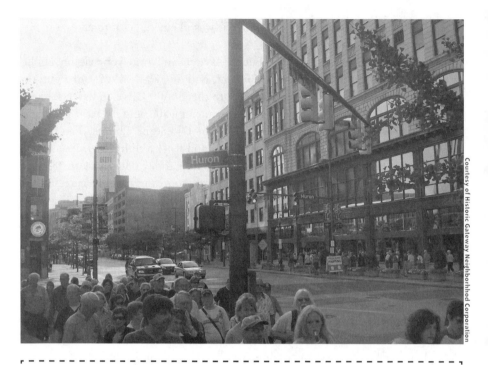

Courtesy of Historic Gateway Neighborhood Corporation

Urban hikers can go inside many Cleveland landmarks.

Farther down East Ninth, you'll see the always-good-for-a-conversation-starter *Free Stamp* sculpture at Willard Park, on the north side of St. Clair. Ahead and on your left, at the corner of East Ninth and Superior, is St. John's Cathedral. Originally constructed from 1848 to 1852, the current church is part of a complete rebuilding that took place from 1946 to 1948.

Continue south (crossing Vincent, Chester, Euclid, and Prospect) to reach Bolivar. Progressive Field (known for years as Jacobs Field), home of the Cleveland Indians, is on your right. To see some of the interesting sculptures designed for the new ballpark in 1994, take a brief detour and follow Eagle Street west. Several of the sculptures function as fashionable benches: *Who's on First, Meet Me Here,* and the abstract *Sports Stacks.* (Between you and me, I see a baseball bat in there, but you decide for yourself.) Once you've peered inside the gates of Progressive Field, return to East Ninth and turn right, heading south again.

On the eastern side of East Ninth (on your left) is old Erie Street Cemetery. How old is it? Created in 1826, when Erie Street was constructed, it was the city's first official cemetery. Many bodies buried at church cemeteries were relocated here when Erie Street opened. And there lies Chief Thunderwater, the most likely inspiration for the city's baseball tribe. Thunderwater appeared in *Buffalo Bill's Wild West Show* and was known as the "official" Cleveland Indian. Today, Thunderwater shares the grounds with Cleveland's earliest permanent settlers, Lorenzo and Rebekah Carter, and other folks notable in the city's history.

From the cemetery, take East Ninth to Carnegie and head west past the front of Progressive Field, where you'll face the oft-photographed entrance to Hope Memorial Bridge, which opened in 1932 as the Lorain-Carnegie Bridge. Impressive stone carvings on each entrance represent the progression of transportation. The figures hold various icons—a covered wagon, stagecoach, car, and several trucks. Water transportation isn't represented by the figures, but the bridge itself reminds us—it was built 93 feet above water level to allow for shipping clearance.

With your feet now on Broadway, turn right (north) to Huron, and return to the parking garage at Tower City Center.

NEARBY ACTIVITIES

It's OK to act like a tourist here, even if Cleveland is your hometown. Grab your camera and go see the USS *COD*, for starters. Open May–September, the World War II submarine tour is only for the agile. Visitors enter and exit through original hatches and climb ladders over equipment inside. For information call (216) 566-8770 or visit **usscod.org**. Less constraining is the *William G. Mather*, the 1925 flagship of the Cleveland-Cliffs Iron Company, which is now operated by the Great Lakes Science Center as a floating maritime museum; call (216) 694-2000 for information. You can cruise the Cuyahoga River aboard the *Goodtime III*, enjoying fabulous views of Cleveland's industrial flats and the area's many different bridges. So (ahem) for a *Goodtime*, call (216) 861-5110 or visit **goodtimeiii.com**. For a hike offering a different view of the skyline, visit Edgewater Park (see page 30).

Thanks to Thomas Yablonsky for reviewing this hike. Yablonsky is the executive director for the Historic Gateway Neighborhood Corporation (HGNC). HGNC offers a series of award-winning walking tours called Take a Hike! More information can be found at historicgateway.org or by calling (216) 771-1994.

05 EDGEWATER—CLEVELAND LAKEFRONT STATE PARK

KEY AT-A-GLANCE INFORMATION

LENGTH: 2.5 miles

CONFIGURATION: Figure eight

DIFFICULTY: Easy

SCENERY: Lake Erie views, Cleveland skyline, bird-watching opportunities from the western end of the trail

EXPOSURE: Mostly exposed

TRAFFIC: Moderately heavy

TRAIL SURFACE: Paved parcourse trail and dirt path

HIKING TIME: 1 hour

DRIVING DISTANCE: 14 miles from I-77/I-480 exchange

ACCESS: Daily, 6 a.m.–11 p.m.

WHEELCHAIR TRAVERSABLE: Partially—the paved fitness/bike path is accessible.

MAPS: USGS Lakewood; also available at dnr.state.oh.us

FACILITIES: Restrooms at nature center, beach area, and fishing pier

CONTACT INFORMATION: To find out more about the beach, fishing pier, and marina, visit dnr.state.oh.us or clevelandlakefront.org, or call (216) 881-8141.

IN BRIEF

Edgewater offers pleasant hiking along the Lake Erie shore, good fishing, and a 900-foot-long public swimming beach. It also provides the best seat in the house for Cleveland's annual Independence Day fireworks display.

DESCRIPTION

Edgewater Park sits between downtown Cleveland and the city of Lakewood, perhaps not a location many would consider scenic. But it is! To see it is to believe it.

Starting from the scenic overlook parking lot, follow the paved trail east. At the west end of the parking lot, you'll meet German composer Richard Wagner. Actually, it's just his statue, a gift to the city from many of Cleveland's German immigrants. From the base to the top of his hat, Wagner stands 18 feet tall, and he's been looking out over the lake and the skyline since 1911. If only he could talk. . . .

Continue east on the bike path. Several unmarked paths on your left lead down to a sandy dirt trail about 25 feet closer to the lake, and as many feet below you. Stay on the paved path; the path below you is your return route.

The paved fitness/bike path offers striking lake views to the north as it continues east

GPS Trailhead Coordinates

Latitude   41° 29.314020'

Longitude   81° 45.050819'

Directions

Take I-77 North to Exit 163/I-90 East. Follow signs to Erie, PA, and merge onto I-90 East. Take Exit 174B to merge onto OH 2 west, toward Lakewood. Continue onto US 20 West/US 6 West, exiting and turning right, then left into the Edgewater/Cleveland Lakefront State Park lot.

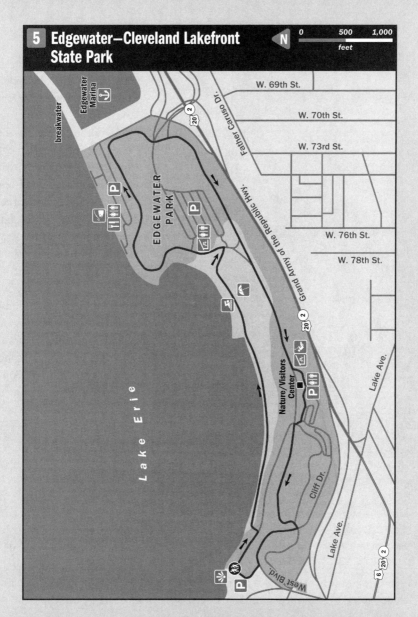

N

0   500   1,000
feet

breakwater

Edgewater Marina

W. 69th St.

W. 70th St.

W. 73rd St.

Father Caruso Dr.

EDGEWATER PARK

P

P

W. 76th St.

W. 78th St.

Grand Army of the Republic Hwy.

20 2

20 2

Lake Ave.

Lake Erie

Nature/Visitors Center

P

Cliff Dr.

Lake Ave.

6 20 2

West Blvd.

P

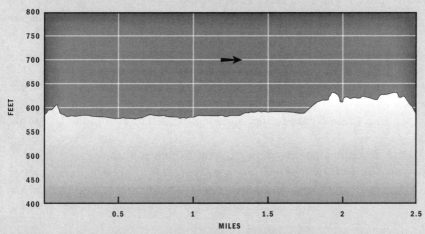

800

750

700

650

600

550

500

450

400

FEET

0.5   1   1.5   2   2.5

MILES

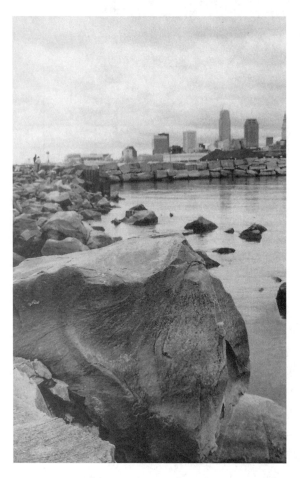

Look for clamshells in the water along the breakwater.

past a small playground. The path grows shadier by the step as you make your way to the picnic pavilion. The melon-colored pavilion, built in 1951, is listed on the National Register of Historic Places. A statue of Conrad Mizer also lends a note on history. Mizer, who moved to Cleveland in the late 1800s, hosted free public concerts here at Edgewater. He also founded the Cleveland Grand Orchestra, which eventually became the Cleveland Symphony Orchestra. With a nod to Mizer, continue on the path that begins to slope downhill as it ventures east, toward the beach.

The swimming beach at Edgewater is 900 feet long, and on warm summer afternoons, you'll hear it long before you see it. It's a popular spot for swimming and just hanging out. In the off-season, you'll hear the coos and cries of hundreds of other visitors: seagulls. They are some of the only wildlife you'll spot here most days, but they make up for lack of variety with their sheer numbers.

Continue on the path downhill, veering to the left at the triangle intersection. This is the middle of the figure eight of the hike formation; you'll cross this way again on your return. Walk past the beach house and head toward the lakeshore. The path curves to the right, and from here you'll have a great view of the city skyline and the Cleveland West Pierhead Light. The 30-foot-tall lighthouse was built in 1911, adjacent to the fog signal building built in 1910. It remains a U.S. Coast Guard facility, marking the entrance from the lake to the Cuyahoga River.

Follow the path along the shore, past the fishing pier, and as far east on the breakwater as you dare. The old, uneven sidewalk is popular with anglers; on good days, they catch perch and walleye here. The footing can be challenging, but if you are willing to take a few giant steps over breaks in the path, you can continue to the end. As always, be very careful; the wind blows hard on the break-water. Turn your back to the wind and look south and you'll have a good view of the marina. It's a busy place, with boats coming and going almost constantly during the too-short summer; in the winter it seems eerily abandoned, and the only noise coming from the water will be the screeches and whistles of gulls.

As you return west along the concrete breakwater, you'll notice that the rocks stuck into the side of the breakwater have strange, weather-beaten faces. Lean over the edge a bit to peer in the water, where you can see freshwater clam and zebra mussel shells.

From the western end of the breakwater, follow the paved path, which heads left (south) along the eastern edge of the park's other parking lot. The path soon bends right and heads west again, past Washington hawthorn trees full of bright red berries much of the year. The path connects at the triangle just east of the beach, and from there, it converges with a rocky path. Follow the rocky trail—not the paved path—straight ahead.

Here, you'll walk under the shade of deciduous trees and then follow a staircase up and over a large drain culvert. Continue along the path, heading west. You'll get an entirely different perspective on the shore from this lower trail, which extends almost all the way to the overlook. Scenic? Without a doubt. Before you go, take the steps at the far western end of the park about 30 feet down to the beach for one last look at Lake Erie and the Cleveland skyline.

NEARBY ACTIVITIES

Downtown Cleveland beckons! See page 25. Or just stick around Edgewater—park naturalists host activities, from stargazing and scavenger hunts to kayaking and beach parties, year-round. Find a calendar of events at **clevelandlakefront.org.**

Special thanks to naturalist Carol Ward of Cleveland Lakefront State Park for keeping lakefront activities going strong and for encouraging many a new hiker to explore the scenic north coast.

06 FORT HILL EARTHWORKS

KEY AT-A-GLANCE INFORMATION

LENGTH: 1.5 miles

CONFIGURATION: Loop

DIFFICULTY: Moderately difficult, with lots of stairs to climb

SCENERY: River views, earthworks

EXPOSURE: Mostly shaded

TRAFFIC: Can be busy, especially on warm weekends

TRAIL SURFACE: Dirt trail, wooden boardwalk, and stairs

HIKING TIME: 45 minutes

DRIVING DISTANCE: 15 miles from I-77/I-480 exchange

ACCESS: Daily, 6 a.m.–11 p.m. Nature center: Daily, 9:30 a.m.– 5 p.m. Note that the steps leading to the Fort Hill Earthworks are closed when icy; if in doubt, call ahead to check on weather conditions.

WHEELCHAIR TRAVERSABLE: No

MAPS: USGS North Olmsted; also available inside nature center and at clevelandmetroparks.com

FACILITIES: Restroom, pay phone, and water inside nature center

CONTACT INFORMATION: Call (440) 734-6660 or visit clevelandmetroparks.com.

IN BRIEF

While the initial climb might make your legs wobble, this hike provides spectacular views of the Rocky River that will leave you breathless. There's plenty for natural history fans too—a nature center, a "terrible fish," and ancient Native American ceremonial grounds. This hike is not recommended for those with a fear of heights. Others will find it gorgeous, a trip not to be missed.

DESCRIPTION

The earthworks on the Fort Hill Loop Trail are considerably less impressive than the better-known mounds of southern Ohio. But what these ridges lack in size, they make up for in location. To reach the earthworks, you'll have to do some climbing—130 steps of climbing, to be precise. The view is worth it. From the top of the stairway, you'll look upon the east branch of the Rocky River, more than 100 feet below, where it bends like a fishhook and snatches the breath from your mouth.

However, before experiencing the climb and the view, you might find yourself a bit breathless in front of the nature center. There, approximately where a welcome mat should be, you'll be greeted by the terrible fish known as *Dunkleosteus*. The huge hunter

GPS Trailhead Coordinates

Latitude 41° 24.557877'

Longitude 81° 53.050683'

Directions

From I-77/I-480 travel I-480 West and take Exit 7/Clague Road. Turn left off the ramp and follow Clague south until it ends at Mastick Road. Turn right, heading west about 4 miles to Rocky River Reservation. Turn left onto Shepherd Lane; follow it to Valley Parkway. Turn right on Valley Parkway and park in the nature center lot, located on the right at 24000 Valley Parkway.

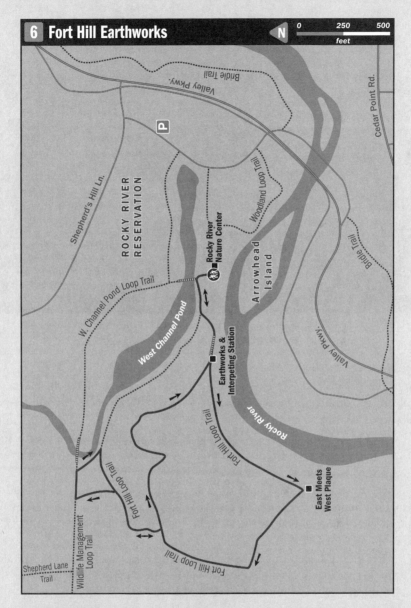

N

0   250   500

feet

Valley Pkwy.
Bridle Trail

Cedar Point Rd.

P

Shepherd's Hill Ln.

ROCKY RIVER
RESERVATION

Woodland Loop Trail

Bridle Trail

Rocky River
Nature Center

A r r o w h e a d
I s l a n d

Valley Pkwy.

W. Channel Pond Loop Trail

West Channel Pond

Earthworks &
Interpeting Station

Fort Hill Loop Trail

Rocky River

Fort Hill Loop Trail

East Meets
West Plaque

Wildlife Management
Loop Trail

Fort Hill Loop Trail

Shepherd Lane
Trail

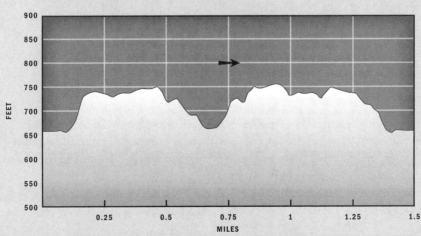

900						
850						
800			➔			
750						
700						
650						
600						
550						
500						

FEET

0.25   0.5   0.75   1   1.25   1.5

MILES

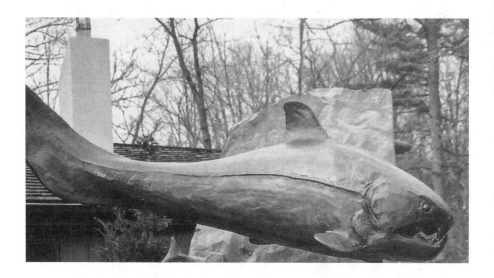

Dunkleosteus doesn't swim here ... anymore.

swam the oceans that covered Ohio millions of years ago, eating sharks and probably terrorizing other ancient sea critters. The well-preserved specimen was discovered nearby, in the shale cliffs above the riverbed, making it difficult to retrieve. The fossil remains were moved to the Cleveland Museum of Natural History, but you'll find a replica and an informational display about the beast inside the nature center.

Before beginning your hike from the back of the nature center, you can relax for a moment by watching for birds in the feeding area to your left and around West Channel Pond on your right. Now take a deep breath and head up the stairs on your left.

After you've scaled this steep section of the trail, you'll find yourself about 100 feet higher, likely taking another deep breath. There at the top of the trail, you'll notice a sign explaining what researchers understand about the earthworks in front of you.

The earthworks' ridges lie like mussed-up blankets under the shade of pin oaks. More than 1,000 years ago, Native Americans formed these earthworks, probably for ceremonial purposes. The mounds they left here are small, but the mystery is great: who were these people? What, besides the view, was so special about this spot? Inside the nature center, you can learn more about these Native Americans and the earthworks they left behind.

Here, an alternate, slightly shorter trail allows you to walk on both sides of the earthworks; however, following it will cheat you out of more breathtaking views of the river below. Continue on the main trail instead, following the bright yellow markers of the Fort Hill Loop Trail.

About 0.6 miles into your trek, you'll find an interpretive sign titled WHERE EAST MEETS WEST describing how the river has changed, and continues to change, the landscape. Approximately 360 million years ago, all but the southeast portion of Ohio was under ocean. While the ocean is long gone, the Rocky River continues to cut away at the land. It's obvious as you look at the trees clinging to the cliff sides, the soil that once supported them having eroded and washed into the river below. The soil and other sediment has formed islands in the river, and the trees that grow there—sycamores, cottonwoods, and willows—are ones that can survive the silt and changing water levels. The story told on the WHERE EAST MEETS WEST sign is a compelling one about the power of nature. It's worth reading, although the dizzying view may distract you from the text. Try to appreciate the magic of both before continuing along the trail.

The dirt path leaves the ridge and curves clockwise, descending slowly into thick woods. Wildflowers and a variety of trees, including hemlocks, are sprinkled along this portion of the trail.

As you bottom out near the northern edge of West Channel Pond, you'll find an interpretive station explaining the rusty red color in the groundwater. When Ohio was covered with seawater, minerals such as iron pyrite were trapped in the silt. Gradually, the rust sediments formed a new rock known as bog iron. It was mined extensively in the 1800s, and several large pig iron furnaces were constructed between Toledo and Cleveland. (One of the largest was in nearby Westlake.)

As you head back to the nature center, the trail is mostly boardwalk. You'll complete the clockwise loop by West Channel Pond, walking up a slight incline to return to the back of the nature center.

Before returning to the parking lot, stop in at the wildflower garden in front of the nature center. Even in the dead of winter, you'll find that you can identify some flowers—wild leek and wild ginger, for example—just by their stalks. A single dogwood stands in the center of the garden. A plaque there explains that there's more to the tree than its pretty spring blooms. In that way, it's rather like the earthworks here in the park—there's much more to both than meets the eye.

NEARBY ACTIVITIES

Don't leave the park without a good look around inside the nature center. There, children can wander through a tree-shaped activity center filled with fun, educational displays. Then explore the rest of the Rocky River Reservation—it offers more than a dozen hiking trails, plus bridle trails, a fitness trail, and the paved All Purpose Trail.

The Frostville Village Museum, also located inside Rocky River Reservation, honors the history of the local area from the 1800s. Restored buildings include a church, barn, several homes, a general store, and an outhouse. The museum building is located at the corner of Cedar Point and Lewis roads. For more information about the museum, see **olmstedhistoricalsociety.org** or call (440) 779-0280.

07 GARFIELD PARK RESERVATION

KEY AT-A-GLANCE INFORMATION

LENGTH: 2 miles

CONFIGURATION: Teardrop loop

DIFFICULTY: Easy, with two steep sections

SCENERY: Natural and historical stonework, waterfall, ravines

EXPOSURE: Mostly shaded

TRAFFIC: Moderate–heavy

TRAIL SURFACE: Crushed gravel and asphalt

HIKING TIME: Allow 1 hour to visit nature center and/or north end of the park

DRIVING DISTANCE: 7 miles from I-77/I-480 exchange

ACCESS: Daily, 6 a.m.–11 p.m. except where otherwise posted

WHEELCHAIR TRAVERSABLE: Yes, though steep sections may be difficult

MAPS: USGS Shaker Heights; also at nature center or clemetparks.com

FACILITIES: Emergency phones throughout park; water and restrooms inside nature center; grills, water, and restrooms at picnic areas

CONTACT INFORMATION: Call the Garfield Park Nature Center at (216) 341-3152 or see clevelandmetroparks.com for more information.

IN BRIEF

Garfield Park Reservation is rich in both history and features. The nature center on the park's eastern side offers a wide variety of educational programs for visitors of all ages; a paved trail encircling the park offers two heart-pounding hills for joggers and in-line skaters. Look closely and you may catch glimpses of the park's former life—in the middle of it all, there are remnants of the original stonework and bridges dating back nearly a century.

DESCRIPTION

Garfield Park opened in 1895 under the name Newburg Park. In 1896 Cleveland officials called it "an ideal place in the country to get away from it all," and area residents traveled miles to reach the park's tennis, fishing, and boating facilities. It became a part of the Cleveland Metroparks system in 1986. Start your stroll inside the historical park at Trolley Turn Trailhead, immediately south of Garfield Park Boulevard.

Follow the (paved) All Purpose Trail as it takes you uphill before looping around and taking you to the east, where you'll see a forest of maples, beeches, and elms on your left. Heading downhill along the southern end of the loop and curving left again, you'll notice

GPS Trailhead Coordinates

Latitude   41° 25.786078'

Longitude   81° 36.600959'

Directions ——————————→

From I-77/I-480, follow I-480 East and take Exit 23/OH 14/Broadway Avenue. Turn right and go north on Broadway, turning left onto Wolf Creek Lane just north of the Henry Street intersection. Turn left again onto Mill Creek Lane to reach the nature center. Follow Wolf Creek west to the Trolley Turn Picnic Area, approximately 1 mile west of the Broadway Avenue entrance, to start your hike.

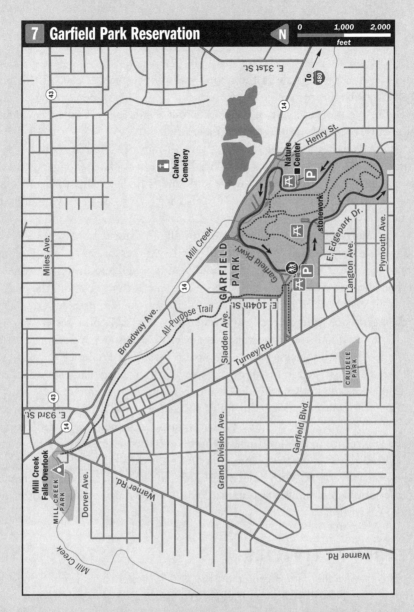

N

0   1,000   2,000
feet

To 480

E. 31st St.

Henry St.

Nature Center

Calvary Cemetery

43

14

stonework

E. Edgepark Dr.

Langton Ave.

Plymouth Ave.

Mill Creek

GARFIELD PARK

Garfield Pkwy.

Broadway Ave.

All-Purpose Trail

Sladden Ave.

E. 104th St.

Turney Rd.

CRUDELE PARK

14

43

14

E. 93rd St.

Mill Creek Falls Overlook

MILL CREEK PARK

Dorver Ave.

Warner Rd.

Grand Division Ave.

Garfield Blvd.

Warner Rd.

Mill Creek

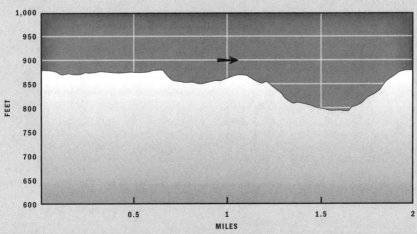

1,000
950
900
850
800
750
700
650
600

FEET

0.5   1   1.5   2

MILES

the lines of Bedford shale in the ravine walls above Wolf Creek. At this point, Wolf Creek begins to tumble over a series of stone ledges, descending nearly 70 feet. (On the northern side of the park about a mile away, Wolf Creek empties into Mill Creek and eventually into Lake Erie.)

On the eastern side of the park, the All Purpose Trail is actually the old park roadway. As such, it gives wide berth to strollers, bikers, joggers, and skaters. Happily, hikers can find a narrow and slightly higher footpath just inside the loop of the All Purpose Trail that affords better views of the ravine and creek so far below.

Just north of Red Oak Picnic Area, you'll see a stone staircase leading to an old trail that may be redeveloped in the future. At present, you can only glimpse from the top of the stairs part of the old boating pond and beautiful stonework that remains from the park's early days. (You can learn more about the park and the area's history at Mill Creek History Center, on the far north edge of Garfield Park Reservation where Broadway Avenue and Warner Road intersect.)

The pond and the stonework were part of a master park plan, developed in the 1890s, with the assistance of landscape architect Frederick Law Olmsted. (Olmsted also assisted in the design of New York's Central Park; he was the son and the namesake of America's great pioneer landscape architect.)

As you continue along the hilly, paved trail, you'll no doubt appreciate nature's stonework, which quite probably inspired some of Olmsted's designs. When you return to Trolley Turn, if you're interested in following a more rustic trail, head north from the picnic area along the 1.5-mile trail leading to Mill Creek Falls Overlook. With a nearly 50-foot-tall waterfall, this area offers plenty of inspiration. Also known as Cataract Falls, it is the only waterfall located in the city of Cleveland.

NEARBY ACTIVITIES

Be sure to visit the nature center on the park's eastern side, where educational programs are held all year long. Call (216) 341-3152 for program information or check **clemetparks.com.**

HUNTINGTON BEACH/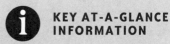
HUNTINGTON RESERVATION

IN BRIEF

Crawl through a hollow log, visit the stars, and hit the beach—all in the span of a mile.

DESCRIPTION

Huntington is one of the oldest of the Cleveland Metroparks reservations. It gets its name from English immigrant John Huntington, who purchased the land in 1881. He built a distinctive tower used to pump water from Lake Erie to irrigate his grape fields. The water tower still stands; today it is an ice cream shop, much appreciated by picnickers and beachgoers. A plaque on the side of the ice cream shop relates the park's history and illustrates some of the improvements made by the Cleveland Metroparks after purchasing the land in 1926.

Start your hike by wandering through the Lake Erie Nature & Science Center (LENSC). It is brimming with life, from turtles and tarantulas to pythons and piranha. Large aquariums full of critters fascinate folks of all ages. Nimble visitors can crawl through a 15-foot-long hollow tree that lies just inside the center's front door. LENSC also houses the Schuele Planetarium, which offers regular presentations on weekends. Outside, the center's lovely "backyard" is great for bird-watching and for relaxing.

KEY AT-A-GLANCE INFORMATION

LENGTH: 1.3 miles

CONFIGURATION: Out-and-back combined with loop

DIFFICULTY: Easy

SCENERY: A little creek, a Great Lake, Lake Erie Nature & Science Center (LENSC)

EXPOSURE: Mostly exposed

TRAFFIC: Path lightly traveled; beach very busy during summer

TRAIL SURFACE: Asphalt, dirt, sand

HIKING TIME: 40 minutes, plus playtime at the beach and LENSC

DRIVING DISTANCE: 20 miles from I-77/I-480 exchange

ACCESS: Daily, 6 a.m.–11 p.m. except where otherwise posted; LENSC: Daily, 10 a.m.–5 p.m. No pets are allowed on the beach.

WHEELCHAIR TRAVERSABLE: LENSC, yes; trails, no

MAPS: USGS North Olmsted; also at LENSC and clevelandmetroparks.com

FACILITIES: Restrooms and water inside LENSC and on both sides of Lake Road

CONTACT INFORMATION: Call (216) 635-3200 or visit clemetparks.com. Call LENSC at (440) 871-2900. For swimming conditions, call (216) 635-3383.

Directions

Take I-480 West to Exit 7/Clague Road to Westlake/Fairview Park. Turn right onto Clague and then left onto Center Ridge Road. Less than 2 miles later, you'll turn right onto Columbia Road and then left onto Wolf Road, where you'll see the entrance to Lake Erie Nature & Science Center (LENSC).

GPS Trailhead Coordinates

Latitude   41° 29.159338'

Longitude 81° 56.252761'

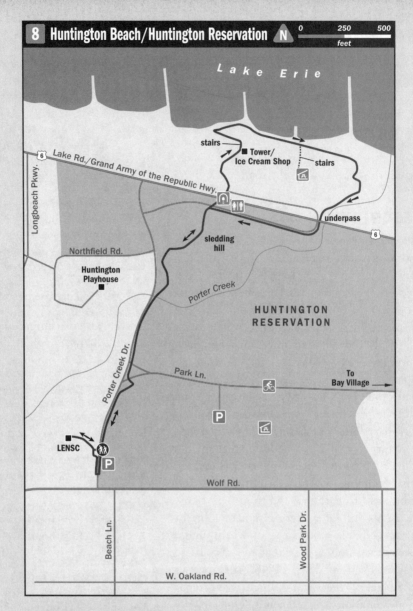

N

0   250   500
feet

L a k e   E r i e

stairs

■ Tower/
Ice Cream Shop

stairs

6

Lake Rd./Grand Army of the Republic Hwy.

Longbeach Pkwy.

underpass

6

Northfield Rd.

sledding
hill

**Huntington
Playhouse** ■

Porter Creek

**HUNTINGTON
RESERVATION**

Porter Creek Dr.

Park Ln.

To
Bay Village

P

■ **LENSC**

P

Wolf Rd.

Beach Ln.

Wood Park Dr.

W. Oakland Rd.

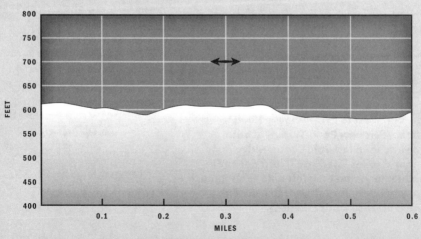

800
750
700
650
600
550
500
450
400

FEET

0.1   0.2   0.3   0.4   0.5   0.6

MILES

Once you've soaked up the sights inside and around the nature center, head north on the all-purpose path to the lake. You'll follow the paved trail past the Wolf Picnic Area (about 0.1 mile) down a slight incline and across a small bridge over Porter Creek. You'll share the way with light car traffic, so stay on the trail as you make your way back up the hill.

Just over the bridge, there's a lovely view of Porter Creek as it heads east before making its final turn to drop into Lake Erie. You'll lose sight of the creek as you climb up a small hill that serves as a sledding hill when conditions are right. There, on your left (western side of the trail), you'll see the Huntington Playhouse.

You can see the lake from here, but don't cross busy Lake Road to get there. Instead, turn right and follow signs to the pedestrian tunnel underpass. (Restrooms and pay phones are located near the tunnel's entrance.)

Emerging on the north side of the park, you'll find a shady playground area, a large picnic shelter, and the distinctive tower. Next to the tower (ice cream shop), follow the steep stairs—about 50 of them—down to the shore. During the too-short summer season, the beach is often crowded. But on a windy late fall day, you may even find solitude along the breakwater—on such days, the lake seems more green than blue, and the gulls are the only ones playing in the waves.

Walk east along the shore about 0.2 miles, where you'll find another set of stairs that lead up to the picnic shelter. If you continue walking east on the beach, however, you'll soon find a path that curves to the right and stays low. This narrow path along Porter Creek takes you south through the underpass—not the tunnel—under Lake Road.

Follow the dirt path along the side of the road as it curves west, toward the sledding hill and back to the all-purpose trail. From here, turn left to retrace your steps back to the LENSC.

NEARBY ACTIVITIES

Huntington Beach is open during the swimming season 11 a.m.–9 p.m.; fishing is permitted year-round.

You can catch a star-studded show at the Schuele Planetarium at LENSC each weekend. Call (440) 871-2900 or visit **lensc.org** for a schedule or for information about other programs at the LENSC.

Huntington Playhouse, 28601 Lake Road, is a popular community theater offering live productions for children and adults. To find out about the current season's shows, call (440) 871-8333 or see **huntingtonplayhouse.com.**

09 LAKE VIEW CEMETERY AND LITTLE ITALY

KEY AT-A-GLANCE INFORMATION

LENGTH: 3 miles

CONFIGURATION: Loop with out-and-back

DIFFICULTY: Easy

SCENERY: Splendid architecture, views of Downtown and Lake Erie

EXPOSURE: Half exposed

TRAFFIC: Moderate

TRAIL SURFACE: Dirt, grass, stone steps, and city sidewalks

HIKING TIME: 1–3 hours, depending on interest and stamina

DRIVING DISTANCE: 13 miles from I-77/I-480 exchange

ACCESS: Cemetery: Daily, 7:30 a.m.– 5:30 p.m. Do not walk in areas where there will be a burial and be respectful of families who are burying or mourning a loved one.

WHEELCHAIR TRAVERSABLE: Cemetery, no; Little Italy, yes

MAPS: USGS East Cleveland; also at Euclid Ave. office and mausoleum

FACILITIES: Restrooms in the cemetery office, Community Mausoleum, and the Garfield Monument

CONTACT INFORMATION: Stop in or call (216) 421-2665 for information about the burial schedule. Events are posted at lakeviewcemetery.com.

IN BRIEF

A cemetery is an unlikely tourist attraction, but Lake View's history and incredible beauty draw thousands each year. Lake View was designed after the garden cemeteries of Victorian England and France. Adding to its European appeal, it lies next to Little Italy, one of Cleveland's tastiest neighborhoods.

DESCRIPTION

Hiking through a cemetery strikes some people as rather strange. But Lake View Cemetery encourages visitors—tourists, even—and throughout the year offers tours highlighting its unique architecture, geology, history, and horticulture. If you choose to stroll through sans guide, call or stop in at the office for the day's burial schedule, so you won't walk near a burial or where a family is mourning.

Established in 1869, Lake View Cemetery is a Cleveland landmark. President James A. Garfield and industrialist John D. Rockefeller are both buried here. A tour booklet available in the cemetery administration office identifies the gravesites of The Early Settlers Association Hall of Fame members who are buried at Lake View. This description highlights only a few of the famous folks buried here and offers a basic introduction to some

GPS Trailhead Coordinates

Latitude   41° 30.595322'

Longitude 81° 35.495460'

Directions

From I-77 North, take Exit 163/I-90 East and then Exit 173A/Chester Avenue. Turn right onto Chester, going about 3 miles before turning left onto Euclid Avenue. The Lake View Cemetery entrance is on the right, at 12316 Euclid Avenue.

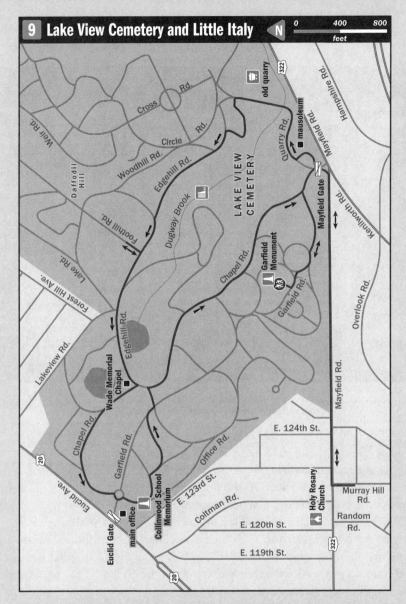

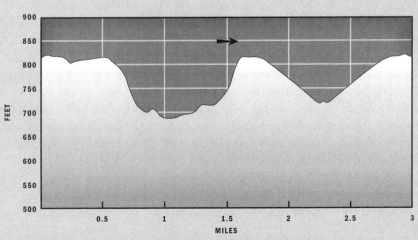

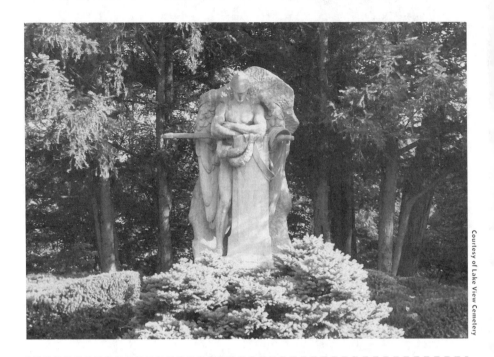

Courtesy of Lake View Cemetery

The Archangel Michael stands over John Hay's gravesite.

of Lake View's treasures. When you visit, you will discover many more.

Begin at the Garfield Monument, built in 1890, where you'll enjoy views of Cleveland and the lake. On the north side of the impressive monument is a terra-cotta plate showing Garfield in action, teaching geology and other sciences. A professor, Garfield also taught ancient languages at Hiram College. The monument is open April to mid-November. Inside you'll find 12 stained-glass windows and four windowlike panels, representing the 13 original states, Ohio, and war and peace. Garfield's statue stands in the middle of the monument; his and his wife's crypt are in the lower level.

From the Garfield Monument, head south on Garfield Road to the Mayfield Gate. Turn left onto Quarry Road. Along the way, you'll pass beautiful Japanese threadleaf maples on your left and the Mayfield Gate and mausoleum on your right. After crossing little Dugway Brook, you'll notice an old dirt road, closed to the public. It was once used for traffic coming and going from the quarry. In operation from the 1870s through the 1940s, the quarry's contents were never wasted. Dust from the quarry was used as the base for many of the headstones placed here; rocks from this quarry form the massive cemetery wall that stretches west from the Mayfield Gate to East 123rd Street and were incorporated in many of the cemetery's buildings.

(Visitors usually see the quarry on the cemetery's guided Geology Tour. See the website or inquire at the office about the tour schedule.) Continuing, you'll soon reach a traffic island splitting the road. Follow the road left and walk toward section 30, where the Van Sweringen brothers are buried. The Van Sweringens built Cleveland's rapid transit system and Terminal Tower. You can cross Circle Road to visit their gravesite (no. 117), or continue bearing left to pick up Edgehill Road, passing section 35 on your right and the ravine on your left. You'll soon reach the dam, standing 60 feet high and 500 feet across. It can impound 80 million gallons of water. When it was built in 1978, it was the largest concrete-poured dam east of the Mississippi. That it only has to hold back mild-mannered Dugway Brook seems odd, but suffice to say the waters here are well under control.

Proceed northeast along Edgehill to Summit Road. Just after Summit, turn right into section 3 to find the monument of Jeptha Wade (no. 4), founder of Western Union Telegraph Company and first president of The Lake View Cemetery Association. Just east of his monument is Daffodil Hill. Each spring, more than 100,000 daffodil blooms burst with color.

Return to Edgehill and head northwest until the road intersects Lake Road. Turn left and follow Lake Road as it passes between two scenic lakes. Just past the lakes, on the south side of Lake Road, is a memorial to Eliot Ness. After bringing down Al Capone in Chicago, Ness served as Cleveland's safety director from 1935 to 1942. He modernized the police department, developed an emergency medical system, and improved Cleveland's traffic fatality record from worst in the nation to twice winning the National Safety Council's award for greatest reduction of traffic deaths. When Ness died in 1957, he was cremated, and his ashes remained with his family for 40 years. In 1997 he was honored with a memorial service and this memorial stone. The grassy area by the lakes is graced with several pieces of sculpture, creating a good spot to sit, sip some water, and enjoy your surroundings.

When you're ready to continue on Lake Road, turn right at the intersection to follow Chapel Road as it goes north. On your right is Wade Chapel. Stop to admire the windows, designed by Louis Comfort Tiffany. When the chapel is open, you can go in to appreciate the interior. Also on your right, in section 5-C, are the remains of Carl Burton Stokes, the first African American mayor of a major U.S. city and the first African American Ohio state legislator.

Continue heading north on Chapel Road to the Euclid Gate. Cross Garfield Road and then follow Maple Road past the cemetery office. You'll reach Hatch Road, which bears to the right, but keep on Maple as it bears left and circles around section 26. Look for a road/path that leads right and cut across section 25 to Garfield Road. In this section, you'll find the Collinwood School fire memorial.

When an elementary school in Collinwood caught fire in 1908, 174 students and two teachers died inside. The tragedy caused numerous school inspections nationwide and spurred new, stricter building codes.

At Garfield Road, turn right (south). At the next intersection, turn left and then take an immediate right to pick up Chapel Road. Follow Chapel south to section 10, where John D. Rockefeller, founder of Standard Oil Company, is laid to rest. Other notable people in this section include Dr. Harvey William Cushing (no. 57), who pioneered brain surgery techniques, and John Hay (no. 73), President Lincoln's personal secretary during the Civil War and Secretary of State to President McKinley.

Heading back toward the Garfield Monument and to the Mayfield Gate, you'll appreciate the intricate gardening work and incredible planning for which Lake View is known. In the late 1800s, many Italian stonecutters and gardeners migrated to Cleveland for employment at the cemetery. When you leave the cemetery through the Mayfield Gate, turn right and walk west to the neighborhood they built.

As you amble downhill on the north side of Mayfield Road, you'll appreciate the craftsmanship on the impressive wall of Berea sandstone that runs west toward Little Italy. You'll know you've arrived when you see signs for *ristorantes* such as Primo Vino, Dino's, and Angelo's. Little Italy offers a wealth of Italian food and culture. Sample some locally made doughnuts, pizza, or Italian ice. You can walk off a few of those calories by climbing Murray Hill Road.

For a few days every August, part of Murray Hill and Mayfield roads are closed to car traffic for the Feast of the Assumption. The Italian-Catholic festival is celebrated with Masses at the church and with games, music, and dancing. Like an Italian Mardi Gras, the party happens as much on the street as inside the neighborhood's shops and eateries.

Before you say "ciao" to Little Italy, stop at Holy Rosary Church, 12021 Mayfield Road. Built in 1895, the grand redbrick building is the heart of the neighborhood and of the feast. As you head back up the hill, east to the cemetery, you're likely to have a belly full of Italian food and a new appreciation for Cleveland's history.

NEARBY ACTIVITIES

Lake View offers an almost constant schedule of tours and special events; check the website or call the office for details. For more information about happenings in Cleveland's Little Italy neighborhood, visit **littleitalycleveland.com.**

Special thanks to Mary Krohmer, director of community relations at Lake View Cemetery Association, for reviewing this section.

THE NATURE CENTER AT SHAKER LAKES

10

IN BRIEF

Located amid Shaker and Cleveland Heights, this preserved wilderness was nearly wiped out in the 1960s by a proposed freeway. Now dirt trails and boardwalks lead visitors past the nature center and its wildflower garden and around Ohio's oldest artificial lake.

DESCRIPTION

In the late 1800s, Cleveland city dwellers escaped to the relative "country" of the city's eastern side Heights area. In the 1960s, it seemed like a good place to run a freeway connecting the city and the eastern suburbs. That is, it seemed like a good idea to people who did not live in the Heights area. Residents were so opposed, in fact, that they hustled to establish a nature center and effectively prevented the freeway's placement. Good thing too—a few years later, the National Park Service named the center a National Environmental Education Landmark and a National Environmental Study Area. In short, coming here will probably make you smarter—and you'll have a good time too.

KEY AT-A-GLANCE INFORMATION

LENGTH: 1.5 miles with option to do shorter or longer loops

CONFIGURATION: Two loops, with a "sun ray" in the middle

DIFFICULTY: Easy

SCENERY: Birds; wetland, marsh, and lake views; wildflower and rain gardens

EXPOSURE: Mixed sun and shade

TRAFFIC: Rarely crowded

TRAIL SURFACE: Wooden boardwalk, dirt trails, and some asphalt

DRIVING DISTANCE: 13 miles from I-77/I-480 exchange

HIKING TIME: 1 hour, plus time for inside sightseeing and education

ACCESS: Trails: sunrise–sunset; nature center: Monday–Saturday, 10 a.m.–5 p.m. and Sunday 1–5 p.m. Foot traffic only—no bikes, blades, or pets permitted, though a bike trail does intersect hiking trail.

WHEELCHAIR TRAVERSABLE: Yes, nature center and one trail

MAPS: USGS Shaker Lakes; also at nature center

FACILITIES: Restrooms and water

CONTACT INFORMATION: Events offered year-round—visit shaker lakes.org or call (216) 321-5935.

Directions

The best way to get here is on the Rapid. Take the Shaker Green Line to the South Park stop; walk north about 0.3 miles. The nature center is on the left, at the bottom of the hill, at 2600 South Park Boulevard. By car, from the I-77/I-480 exchange, follow I-480 East to I-271 North. Take Exit 29/Chagrin Boulevard and then head west. Turn right on Richmond, going north to Shaker; turn left. Turn right onto South Park Boulevard. After going down a small hill, the road forks. Veer left; a sign and the driveway to the nature center will be on your left.

GPS Trailhead Coordinates

Latitude   41° 29.119020'

Longitude   81° 34.465921'

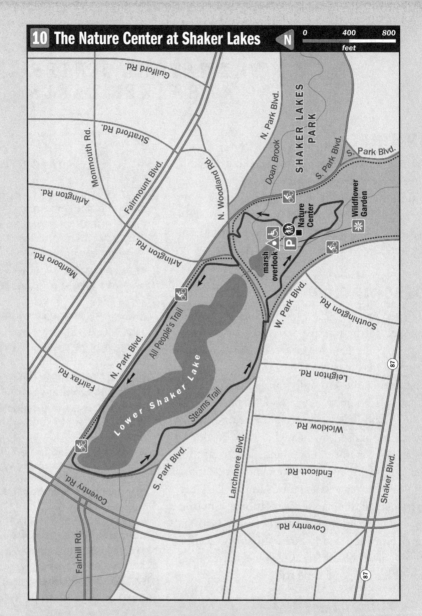

N

| 0 | 400 | 800 |

feet

SHAKER LAKES PARK

Guilford Rd.

Monmouth Rd.

Stratford Rd.

N. Park Blvd.

Doan Brook

S. Park Blvd.

S. Park Blvd.

Fairmount Blvd.

Arlington Rd.

N. Woodland Rd.

Wildflower Garden

Nature Center

Arlington Rd.

Marlboro Rd.

P

marsh overlook

All People's Trail

Southington Rd.

N. Park Blvd.

Lower Shaker Lake

W. Park Blvd.

Leighton Rd.

87

Fairfax Rd.

Stearns Trail

Wicklow Rd.

Larchmere Blvd.

S. Park Blvd.

Endicott Rd.

Shaker Blvd.

Coventry Rd.

Coventry Rd.

87

Fairhill Rd.

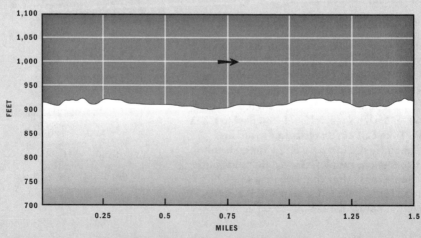

1,100						
1,050						
1,000						
950						
900						
850						
800						
750						
700						

FEET

0.25   0.5   0.75   1   1.25   1.5

MILES

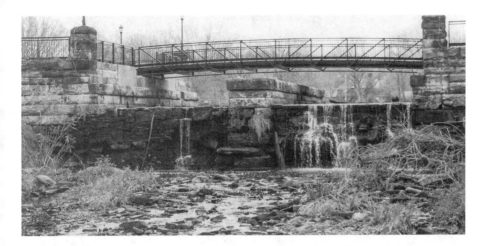

The view from the north end of Lower Lake

Start exploring on the short All People's Trail, a boardwalk featuring marsh and stream habitats and a small waterfall. You'll also get an interesting perspective on the park—from several spots on the All People's Trail, you're surrounded by natural beauty and, at the same time, you can hear the cars go by on North Woodland Road. That is the defining characteristic of this property: its preserved wildness is firmly entrenched in the densely populated, long-civilized cities of Shaker and Cleveland Heights.

From the north end of the parking lot, follow the All People's Trail north to a marsh overlook. Turn around and follow the trail clockwise. Looping around, you'll see a gate with a sign TRAIL TO LOWER LAKE. Obviously, that's your exit. Go through the gate, follow the wooden steps down to the dirt path, and follow it as it curves to the left, up a short hill, to cross North Woodland.

From the north side of Woodland, you can see most of Lower Shaker Lake. The bike trail splits off to the right; hikers should follow the stone steps down to a skinny dirt path along the lake. (If you aren't so sure-footed, take the high road, which in this case is the asphalt bike trail. It also offers lake views but from a wider, flatter trail several yards to the north.) About 0.2 miles north of Woodland, the bike path and walking trail merge into each other for a time and then round the northwest edge of the lake.

At the northernmost end of the lake, you'll have your choice of crossings: over a pretty wrought-iron bridge or via the smaller, older bridge just north of it. The older bridge, made mostly of wide, flat fieldstone, affords an interesting perspective on the lake as seen from under the wrought-iron bridge. Lower Shaker Lake is the oldest man-made lake in Ohio. It was formed from Doan Brook between 1826 and 1837. A few years later, Horseshoe Lake was formed, on the other end of the brook, to power the Shakers' mills. *Note:* After returning to the nature center, you may decide to walk down to Horseshoe Lake—see "Nearby Activities" on page 53.

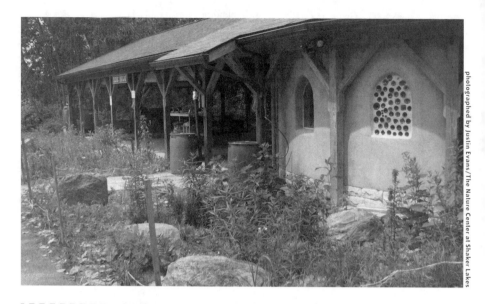

photographed by Justin Evans/The Nature Center at Shaker Lakes

Visit the rain garden along the Nature for All Trail.

As the path circles left and heads generally south, you'll parallel South Park Boulevard for a while before crossing Woodland again. As you head back to the nature center, the path is wider, part wood and part gravel.

Soon you'll be able to see Stearn's Trail, a series of boardwalks running alongside and over Doan Brook. At one point on the trail near the nature center building, under the shade of beech and oak trees, you'll pick up your feet to step over a tree root and realize that it joins two trees—one on either side of the trail. It begs some rather philosophical questions: Is this a root or a branch? Is this one tree or two? You may pick one of several park benches nearby from which to contemplate the answer . . . if there is one.

Where Stearn's Trail isn't boardwalk, it's hard-packed gravel. Looping and linking trails will take you back—when you're ready—to the nature center. Immediately southeast of the building, you'll find a small wildflower garden and some alarming news: some of these pretty flowers are intruders! Most of the flowers are planted natives for show, but purple loosestrife (which can actually be rather pinkish in color), Japanese knotweed, and spotted knapweed have more than unusual names in common. All three are rather pretty pests. They are invasive plants that crowd out native flowers and vegetation, harming animal habitats and increasing soil erosion in the process. But there's good news here too—by minding what we plant, or allow to grow, and working with our natural resources, we can minimize our footprint on the land.

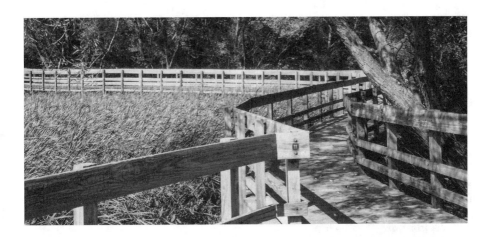

This urban park is an official Wildlife Habitat site and Audubon Important Bird Area.

Visitors to the nature center can pick up a good many ideas here, from the plant selection to the center's building design, which features rain barrels and swales to make wise use of water in the gardens, as well as compost bins that utilize organic waste rather than sending it to a landfill.

When you've learned all you can outside, go inside the nature center so your education, and fun, may continue.

NEARBY ACTIVITIES

Add 3 miles or more to your hike here by heading east from the nature center along either North Park or South Park Boulevard until you reach Horseshoe Lake. It's a popular trek for dog walkers, and the bike path that runs along North Park Boulevard is busy with cyclists as well.

Many thanks to Justin Evans, naturalist at the Nature Center at Shaker Lakes, for reviewing this hike description.

11 SQUAW ROCK

KEY AT-A-GLANCE INFORMATION

LENGTH: 2 miles

CONFIGURATION: Figure eight

DIFFICULTY: Moderate; steep, uneven stairs and uphill portions of All Purpose Trail are challenging

SCENERY: Curious old carvings, a waterfall, rapids along the Chagrin River, deep ravine overlooks

EXPOSURE: Almost entirely shaded

TRAFFIC: Moderate on Squaw Rock Loop Trail; heavy on the All Purpose Trail

TRAIL SURFACE: Dirt trail and stone steps on Squaw Rock Loop Trail; All Purpose Trail is paved.

HIKING TIME: 1 hour

DRIVING DISTANCE: 15 miles from I-77/I-480 exchange

ACCESS: Daily, 6 a.m.–11 p.m.; parking lots that close at sunset are clearly posted. Steps to Squaw Rock are closed when icy.

WHEELCHAIR TRAVERSABLE: No

MAPS: USGS Chagrin Falls; also available at clemetparks.com

FACILITIES: Restrooms at Squaw Rock parking area; public phone at the sledding hill parking lot south of Miles Road

CONTACT INFORMATION: Visit clemetparks.com or call (216) 351-6300.

IN BRIEF

A rocky ravine, gentle rapids, and a bit of a mystery are waiting for you in the Cleveland Metroparks South Chagrin Reservation. While you're there, you can enjoy a shady stretch of the Buckeye Trail and views of the scenic Chagrin River. Good hiking boots are highly recommended for this hike.

DESCRIPTION

Enter the trail at the eastern edge of the parking lot, where you'll see the blue blazes of the Buckeye Trail. The path veers right and then down 72 steep and uneven limestone steps to the banks of the river and a small waterfall. Although they are shallow, the falls can be rather boisterous after a rain. (And the steps can be quite slippery!) As you head south and upstream, the noise tapers off to a mere gurgle. Beautiful, picturesque rock formations rise 25–30 feet above you on the right. Continue south, hugging the skinny path about 12 feet above the Chagrin River.

You'll cross a stone footbridge at 0.1 mile and a wooden walkway just a few steps later, arriving at famous Squaw Rock at 0.2 miles. The rectangular sandstone rock is about 10 feet high. On its south face are several carvings, including a bundle of quivers, a tomahawk, a

GPS Trailhead Coordinates

Latitude   41° 24.986823'

Longitude 81° 24.911041'

Directions

Take I-480 East to Exit 26, follow US 422 East, and exit onto OH 91 (toward Solon). Turn right onto OH 91 South/SOM Center Road. Turn left onto Solon Road, following it about 2 miles to Hawthorn Parkway. Turn left, following Hawthorn east about 1.5 miles. The road ends at the bottom of the hill; Squaw Rock Picnic Area and parking is on your right.

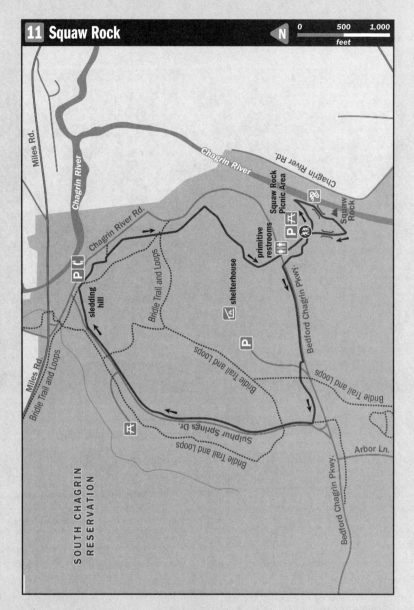

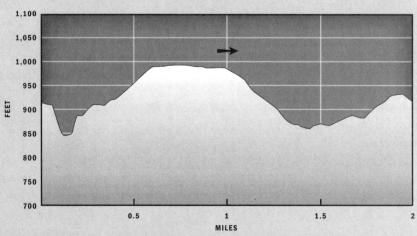

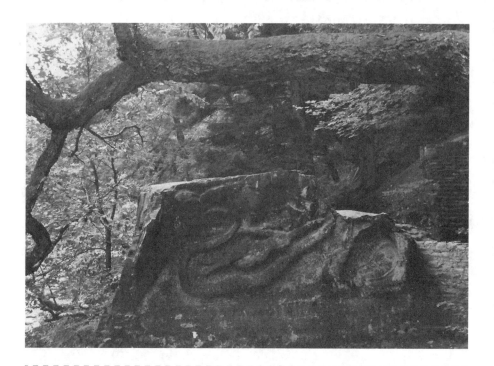

Henry Church carved images on this rock by lantern light.

Native American maiden, a rattlesnake, an infant, and a bird in flight.

Henry Church carved the images in 1885. Born and raised in Chagrin Falls about 2 miles east of here, Church was a blacksmith by trade. He also enjoyed painting and sculpting. Though his art was considered unusual at the time, in 1980 (64 years after his death) his work was featured in a special exhibit at the Whitney Museum of American Art in New York City.

Church reportedly walked from his home to Squaw Rock every night to carve by lantern light. He quit when his neighbors found out what he was doing. On the east face of the rock are unfinished carvings of a log cabin and the U.S. Capitol. What Church intended by the carvings is unknown. Some speculate that the collage is a celebration of American history; others believe that it was meant to be an artistic condemnation of our government's policies in the 1800s. This much we know: his work continues to lure many people to this trail.

Step back onto the path, again heading south. Climb up 63 stairs, where you'll see and hear a gentle waterfall about 12 feet high. If you're feeling adventurous, you can walk underneath it—but don't try unless you've got good balance and good boots. A bit farther south, you'll climb up another long set of stone stairs.

At the top, turn right. Though you may be winded from climbing the steps, you've only covered a little under 0.3 miles. Head north through a thick forest of hemlock, beech, and oak trees. You'll see an alternate path that heads west from here to Arbor Lane. Go straight instead to cross two sturdy wooden bridges. From either one, you can watch as thin tributaries bounce down to the river more than 50 feet below. The woods are thick here, so even with a faint wind, the rustling of leaves drowns out the river's sounds. Continuing north, you'll notice the blue blazes of the Buckeye Trail along this path before you return to the southeast corner of the parking lot.

(*Note:* The higher portion of this loop is flat and offers great views of the ravine. It makes a nice, easy stroll for those who aren't sure-footed enough to attempt the steps and lower trail. In dry weather, the surface is hard-packed enough for most strollers.)

Cross the parking lot, turning left from its northwest corner onto the All Purpose Trail that parallels Hawthorn Parkway. You'll notice that you're following the blue blazes of the Buckeye Trail as the path continues uphill for nearly a quarter of a mile. The hill will get your heart thumping just in time to cross the street at Shelterhouse Picnic Area, where you can try out the parcourse fitness trail, if you wish. Various exercise stations are positioned along the trail over the next 0.5 miles.

Follow the dirt-and-gravel trail west, then north as it bends right along Sulphur Springs Drive. The Buckeye Trail turns into the woods along with the Bridle Trail, but you'll stay on the now paved All Purpose Trail that parallels Sulphur Springs Drive. During the winter you're likely to hear howls of laughter coming from the sledding hill to your right.

Rounding the bottom of the hill, the trail curls to the east, past a small pond full of frogs and ringed with jewelweeds. The path rises gently and then crosses a wide stone bridge where you can peer into the river ravine again. You'll climb up just a few more feet before returning to the northeast corner of the parking lot where you began.

NEARBY ACTIVITIES

A sledding hill sits at the north end of Sulphur Springs Drive, and additional parking is available there. Fishing is allowed at Shadow Lake, located on Hawthorn Parkway about 2 miles southeast of OH 91. South Chagrin Reservation also offers seven picnic areas.

To visit Church's hometown, the quaint village of Chagrin Falls, travel about 2 miles east on Miles Road. There's a waterfall on the western side of Main Street, as well as several shops and restaurants that are worth a visit.

12 SQUIRE'S CASTLE AT NORTH CHAGRIN

KEY AT-A-GLANCE INFORMATION

LENGTH: 5.3 miles

CONFIGURATION: Loop

DIFFICULTY: Moderate, with difficult sections

SCENERY: Waterfall, deep ravine overlooks, beaver activity, historical country estate

EXPOSURE: Mostly shaded

TRAFFIC: Moderate–heavy

TRAIL SURFACE: All Purpose Trail is paved; bridle and hiking trails are hard-packed dirt

HIKING TIME: 2.5 hours

DRIVING DISTANCE: 24 miles from I-77/I-480 exchange

ACCESS: Daily, 6 a.m.–11 p.m.

WHEELCHAIR TRAVERSABLE: Sanctuary Marsh and All Purpose Trail, yes; other trails, no

MAPS: USGS Mayfield Heights; also available inside the nature center or at clemetparks.com

FACILITIES: Restrooms inside nature center; grills, water, and restrooms at each picnic area

CONTACT INFORMATION: Call the North Chagrin Nature Center at (440) 473-3370 or visit clemetparks.com.

IN BRIEF

North Chagrin Reservation has something for everyone. The nature center's exhibits are educational and fun for all ages; paved trails, bridle trails, and nature trails intersect throughout the reservation, leading visitors to a gentle waterfall, through fragrant ravines, and ultimately to a castle romantically set on a sloping hill.

DESCRIPTION

Start at the nature center, stepping onto the paved Sanctuary Marsh Loop Trail, which runs between Sunset Pond and Sanctuary Marsh. Sanctuary Marsh Loop Trail is perfect for strollers and wheelchairs; its boardwalk over the marsh affords a look at beaver habitat as well as a variety of waterfowl.

Head north on Sanctuary Marsh Loop Trail, connecting with Buttermilk Falls Loop Trail (blue trail signs). The falls overlook, on the western side of the parkway, is about 0.5 miles from your starting point. The pretty falls tumble over Cleveland shale, which tends to fracture at right angles. The stairsteps of Buttermilk Falls, therefore, look as if they were carved by a stonemason, but were in fact cut by natural forces.

Leave the waterfalls and head east (right), crossing the parkway, where you'll

-----

GPS Trailhead Coordinates

Latitude   41° 33.695998'

Longitude   81° 26.129580'

Directions

Exit I-271 at Exit 36/Wilson Mills Road. Head east about 0.5 miles, turning left (north) onto OH 91 (SOM Center Road). Go north about 2 miles to Sunset Lane and turn right (east) into the park. Turn right onto Buttermilk Falls Parkway and follow the signs south to the nature center.

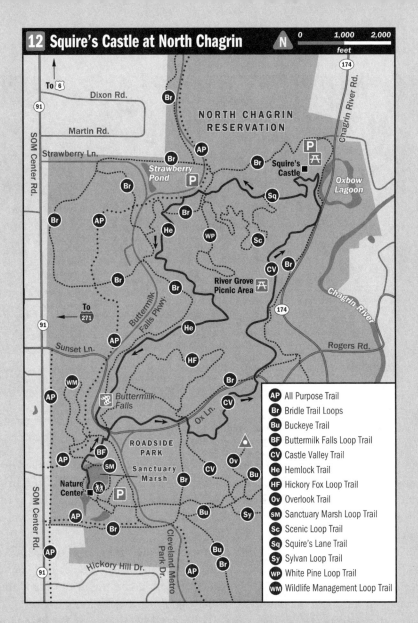

N

0   1,000   2,000
feet

To 6
Dixon Rd.
91
Martin Rd.
SOM Center Rd.
Strawberry Ln.

NORTH CHAGRIN RESERVATION

174
Chagrin River Rd.

Br
AP
Br
Br Squire's Castle
P

Br
Strawberry Pond
P
Br
Sq
Oxbow Lagoon

Br
AP
He
WP
Sc
CV Br

Br

River Grove Picnic Area

Chagrin River

Br
He

To 271
91
Buttermilk Falls Pkwy.
Sunset Ln.
AP
HF
174
Rogers Rd.

WM
Br
CV

AP
Buttermilk Falls
Ox Ln.
CV

ROADSIDE PARK
Ov

AP
BF
SM
Sanctuary Marsh
CV
Bu

Nature Center
P
Br

AP
Bu
Sy

AP
Br
Bu
Br

91
Hickory Hill Dr.
Cleveland Metro Park Dr.
AP

AP	All Purpose Trail
Br	Bridle Trail Loops
Bu	Buckeye Trail
BF	Buttermilk Falls Loop Trail
CV	Castle Valley Trail
He	Hemlock Trail
HF	Hickory Fox Loop Trail
Ov	Overlook Trail
SM	Sanctuary Marsh Loop Trail
Sc	Scenic Loop Trail
Sq	Squire's Lane Trail
Sy	Sylvan Loop Trail
WP	White Pine Loop Trail
WM	Wildlife Management Loop Trail

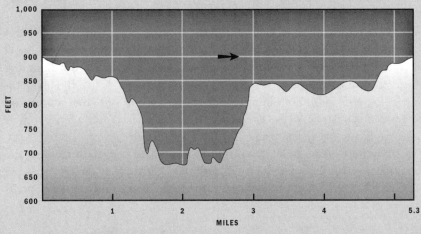

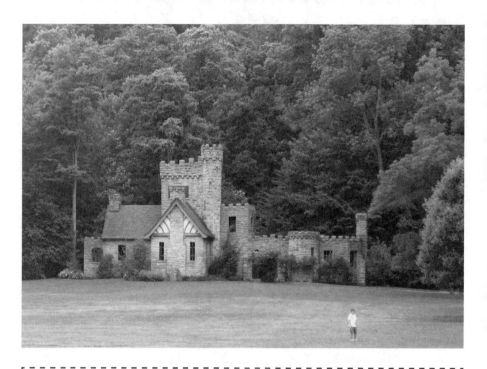

The former caretaker's cottage, better known as Squire's Castle

find a trailhead sign pointing to the Hickory Fox Loop Trail (marked by a squirrel symbol), the Hemlock Trail (marked by a bird symbol), and the Bridle Trail. Follow the Bridle Trail right, down a hill and heading east. The trail is hilly, rising up to parallel Ox Lane before intersecting with Castle Valley Trail (marked by a castle symbol).

From here you may choose to follow either the Bridle Trail or Castle Valley Trail to the castle. They cover approximately the same distance and connect several times. While a sturdy pair of sneakers will do on the Bridle Trail, you'll certainly want boots on the Castle Valley Trail, as it is rocky, narrow, and in places, quite steep. (*Note:* The wider, flatter Bridle Trail may be the best choice for runners; it is safer in wet or icy weather.)

For a bit of a challenge, head north (left) onto Castle Valley Trail. Hugging the side of the ravine, you'll take 38 steps down the valley and cross a little wooden footbridge into the woods. Poison ivy and jewelweeds grow along the trail here. Continue to drop down into the valley (you may notice the temperature dropping a bit too), bottoming out at about 1.8 miles to cross a creek on widely spaced sandstone steps. Rising up on the left (east) side of the trail is River Grove Picnic Area. The Bridle Trail is on your right.

Heading north from here, you'll spot at least three connector trails to the Bridle Trail, now running parallel to Chagrin River Road. As you approach the castle, Castle Valley Trail meanders over a ridge; the Bridle Trail runs about 10

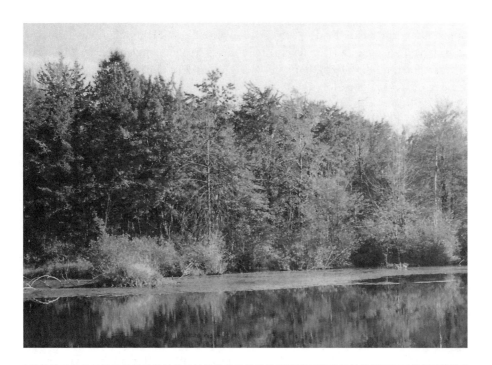

Sanctuary Marsh Loop Trail is ideal for strollers and wheelchairs.

feet below, level with the road.

Squire's Castle isn't really a castle, but it's pretty enough to earn the name. In fact, the building was a caretaker's cottage. Feargus B. Squire, a founder of the Standard Oil Company, owned 525 acres of land here, and he planned to build a vast estate. In the 1890s, he, his wife, and daughter summered in the cottage. As it happened, Mr. Squire never built his estate, and the Cleveland Metroparks purchased the land in 1925. To thwart vandals, the park filled in the basement of the cottage and gutted the inside of the castle. They could not, however, stop reports of Mrs. Squire's ghost. Although folks from the Metroparks explain repeatedly that no one has died in the castle, local legends abound, most of which feature Mrs. Squire carrying a red lantern through the cottage; some claim screaming can be heard along Chagrin River Road on cool, dark nights. What you believe is up to you, of course, but one way to avoid such encounters is to visit the castle in the sunshine.

No matter when you visit, you'll surely have company, as the castle and surrounding picnic area are quite popular with the area's living population.

After your tour of the "castle," exit through the back door, heading west on Squire's Lane Trail. The path rolls uphill as it leaves the castle behind. The trail is well marked, which is good, because it intersects several times with the Scenic Loop Trail and other trails—so mind the signs. At about 3.5 miles into the hike, Squire's Lane Trail ends. Follow the Hemlock Trail signs and travel south along the eastern side of the All Purpose Trail. Hemlock Trail is narrow and pretty, zigzagging over several tributaries to the Chagrin River. This trail offers amazing fall colors, thanks to a mighty mix of deciduous trees and evergreens. At least once along here, venture to the edge of the ravine and watch a leaf fall or a bird dive until you can no longer see it. The ravine is deep, fragrant, and peaceful. In my experience, Hemlock Trail is lightly traveled compared to the other trails here. Its beauty alone makes it worth the trip; stretches of solitude are a bonus.

Hemlock crosses the Bridle Trail before heading down steep railroad-tie steps to cross a wooden footbridge over another trickle of water. Go up, then down again, twice, and you'll meet the Bridle Trail again. Briefly plod along next to the Bridle Trail, passing Sunset Lane on your right. Hemlock winds down 16 railroad-tie steps for a final foray into and out of the valley. The path widens and levels out in time to return to the trailhead across from Buttermilk Falls. If you time your trip right, returning to Sanctuary Marsh at dusk, you may get to see some beavers at work.

NEARBY ACTIVITIES

Why leave? North Chagrin Reservation and the nature center offer programming for all ages and interests, from Stroller Science to Romantic Moonlight walks and the fun Fall in the Creek Hike. You can check the schedule online at **clemetparks .com** or call (440) 473-3370 for information.

Also nearby is one of Cleveland's prettiest golf courses, which sits at the north end of this Metroparks reservation. Call (440) 942-2500 to request a tee time at Manakiki. From North Chagrin Reservation, you're also about a 15-minute drive from Orchard Hills Park (see page 96), just over the border in Geauga County.

Poison ivy—in this case, leaves of two or three—let it be.

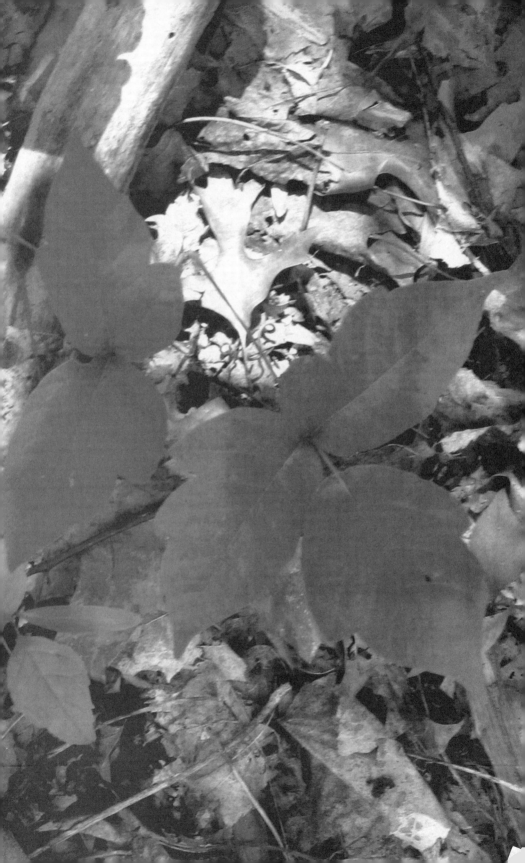

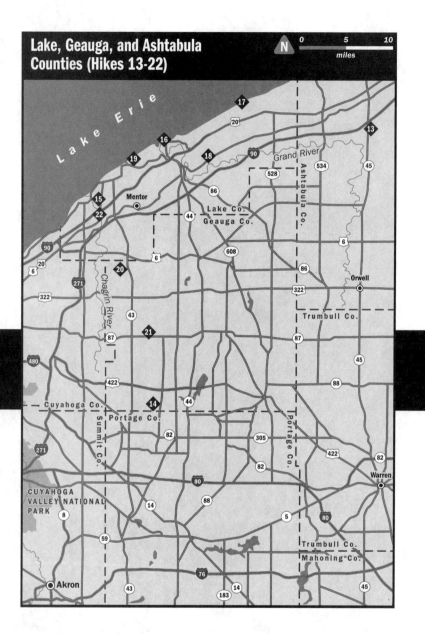

Lake, Geauga, and Ashtabula Counties (Hikes 13-22)

N

0   5   10
miles

Lake Erie

Grand River

Mentor

Lake Co.
Geauga Co.

Chagrin River

Orwell

Trumbull Co.

Cuyahoga Co.
Portage Co.

Summit Co.

Portage Co.

Warren

CUYAHOGA
VALLEY NATIONAL
PARK

Trumbull Co.
Mahoning Co.

Akron

LAKE, GEAUGA, AND ASHTABULA COUNTIES

13 | ASHTABULA: Underground Railroad and Covered Bridges

KEY AT-A-GLANCE INFORMATION

LENGTH: 1.5 miles (Harpersfield); 4.5 miles (Austinburg)

CONFIGURATION: Two loops

DIFFICULTY: Easy

SCENERY: UGRR sites, cemeteries, Ohio's longest covered bridge, river

EXPOSURE: Austinburg, exposed; Harpersfield, shaded

TRAFFIC: Both moderately busy

TRAIL SURFACE: Sidewalks, dirt

HIKING TIME: 1 hour plus in Austinburg; ¹/₂ hour plus at Harpersfield; 15 minutes driving between trails

DRIVING DISTANCE: 56 miles from I-77/I-480 exchange

ACCESS: Trails always open but Harpersfield parking may not be plowed November–March

WHEELCHAIR TRAVERSABLE: Austinburg, yes; Harpersfield, no

MAPS: USGS Ashtabula South; USGS East Trumbull; see website below

FACILITIES: Phone and restrooms at I-90/OH 45 exit; restrooms, concessions, and picnic shelters open April–October at Harpersfield

CONTACT INFORMATION: Reach Ashtabula County Metroparks at (440) 576-0717 or ashtabulacounty metroparks.org.

IN BRIEF

Ohio's largest county has a lot of secrets. Consider these two short hikes a teaser: the first introduces you to some of Austinburg's most notable Underground Railroad sites; the second takes you across Ohio's longest covered bridge.

DESCRIPTION

Travel light. On foot. At night. Leave behind your family, friends, and all that is familiar. Depend on the kindness of strangers to hide you from those who would capture you, beat you, and return you to a life of slavery.

Would you trust your life to an invisible thing called the Underground Railroad? The Underground Railroad (UGRR) operated from about 1816 until 1865. During that time, an estimated 40,000 freedom-seeking slaves passed through Ohio. Many were spirited through Austinburg along the UGRR, courtesy of the fervent abolitionists who lived here. This hike gives you a small taste of what they experienced.

Enter the Western Reserve Greenway Trail behind Austinburg Town Hall and follow it south about 1.5 miles. During warm weather you'll share the trail with bicyclists; if the trail is covered in snow, you may find yourself in

GPS Trailhead
Coordinates
Latitude   41° 46.336198'
Longitude 80° 51.131759'

Directions

Take I-90 East from Cleveland, and then go south on OH 45 (Exit 223). Follow OH 45 south about 1 mile to OH 307. Turn left to park at Town Hall, at the corner of OH 307 (River Road) and Miller Street; parking for the Western Reserve Greenway Trail is available off Lampson Road, about 0.5 miles south of OH 45. *Note:* Directions from Austinburg to Harpersfield are in the hike description.

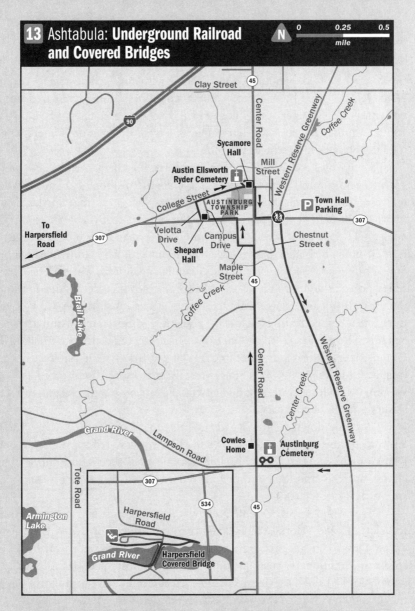

N

0   0.25   0.5
mile

Clay Street   45

90

Center Road

Coffee Creek

Sycamore Hall

Mill Street

Austin Ellsworth Ryder Cemetery

Western Reserve Greenway

College Street

AUSTINBURG TOWNSHIP PARK

Town Hall Parking

P

307

To Harpersfield Road

307

Velotta Drive

Campus Drive

Chestnut Street

Shepard Hall

Maple Street

Brail Lake

45

Coffee Creek

Center Road

Center Creek

Grand River

Lampson Road

Cowles Home

Austinburg Cemetery

Western Reserve Greenway

Tote Road

307

534

Armington Lake

Harpersfield Road

45

Grand River

Harpersfield Covered Bridge

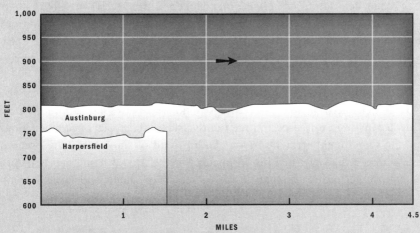

1,000

950

900

850

800

750

700

650

600

FEET

Austinburg

Harpersfield

1   2   3   4   4.5

MILES

the company of snowmobiles. Heed them, with this perspective: a run-in with either vehicle could be dangerous, but it would be nothing compared to meeting up with bounty hunters or your owner if you were a runaway slave in the mid-1800s. Admire the natural beauty along the trail, or imagine—where would you hide if you had to, to protect your life?

When you reach the Lampson Road Trailhead, turn right and follow the grassy berm along the north side of the road for about 0.5 miles, when you arrive at Austinburg Center Cemetery. Also known as the Cowles Cemetery, many of the burial plots here date to the first half of the 19th century. Look across OH 45 to see the Cowles family homestead. The northernmost house was the home of Betsey Mix Cowles, born in 1810. The family, headed by Giles Hooker Cowles, the minister at the Austinburg Church, was progressive for the times, to say the least. The Cowles family values included education and freedom for all (including women and African Americans). Betsey Cowles grew up to be a teacher, educating both black and white children in Austinburg's Sabbath Schools. She graduated from Oberlin College, served as the first female dean at Grand River Institute, and became one of the first female public school superintendents in the state. At a time when women were discouraged from public speaking, Cowles was nationally known for her very public presentations against slavery and discriminatory laws.

Continue down Center Road (OH 45) to Maple Street, where you'll turn left and follow it as it heads east and then veers north, past the First United Church in Austinburg. The church is recognized as the second-oldest Protestant church in Ohio, and the building, erected in 1874, is listed on the National Register of Historic Places.

When Maple meets OH 307, turn left (heading west) and follow the sidewalk to Velotta Drive. Velotta will lead you onto the campus of Grand River Academy, and you'll walk by Shepard Hall, where many abolitionists probably heard Cowles speak. In addition to hosting numerous abolitionist meetings, Shepard Hall—known on the UGRR as Main Hall—served as a safe house for fugitive slaves until they could be moved to the next location on their journey to freedom.

When Velotta meets College, turn right and head west—uphill a bit—past the Austin Ellsworth Ryder Cemetery, which dates to 1803. Many abolitionists from Austinburg and throughout Ashtabula County are buried there. Continue on College to find Sycamore Hall, which is enjoying a new life as a garden center and nursery.

If buildings could talk, Sycamore Hall would have much to divulge. Built by Eliphalet Austin in 1810, the expansive house features a secret compartment that the Austin family used to hide fugitive slaves. Historical accounts abound, and the secret compartment doesn't figure in all of those stories. Once, when a slave master had pursued his "property" to the Austin home and Mr. Austin reluctantly permitted the man inside to search the home, the master combed every room in the house. When he opened the door to one room and found

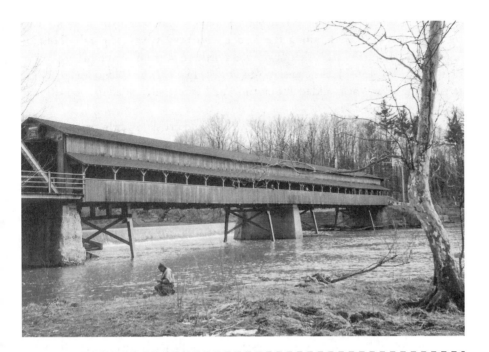

The Grand River runs beneath Ohio's longest covered bridge.

Mrs. Austin sleeping, he apologized for the intrusion. The master left, empty-handed. Once he left, the runaway slave slid out from under Mrs. Austin's bed and continued on his way north.

From Sycamore Hall, you can turn and head south on OH 45 to return to the Western Reserve Greenway Trail parking lot. From there you can drive to Harpersfield to discover a very different but notable spot in Ashtabula County.

Harpersfield Covered Bridge MetroPark is just about 4 miles west on OH 307. Drive past OH 534 and then turn left onto Harpersfield Road (County Road 154). Harpersfield Road winds down a steep hill and bottoms out at the small but popular county park.

Park in the lot at the bottom of the hill, where you can wander along the northern banks of the Grand River. The river, designated a Wild and Scenic River by the state of Ohio, bisects the small park and runs under the longest covered bridge in the state. The bridge measures 228 feet long and is just 1 of 16 covered bridges in the county. Ashtabula celebrates them all during the annual Covered Bridge Festival, held the second weekend of October.

From the parking lot on the north side of the park, you can walk east on a dirt-and-gravel path to the riverbanks and a boat launch, or walk west to find play equipment and picnic shelters. A seasonal kayak/canoe rental company does a brisk business here, and chances are that if you visit April–October, you'll see some of the small crafts heading down the river.

Cross the bridge on the cantilevered walkway and, when you emerge, read the historical marker detailing the bridge's history. It was originally built in 1868, but a 1913 flood washed away the northern section of the bridge. Later that year, a 140-foot steel extension was added; in 1992 the bridge was rehabilitated (the walkway was added at that time) and eventually added to the National Register of Historic Places.

The bridge is popular with photographers and artists, so bring your favorite tools to capture its likeness. Picnic tables abound, but perhaps the best spot from which to contemplate the bridge is a giant, flat rock planted on the riverbank, just southwest of the bridge. It's not the driest spot, but it offers great ambience.

Though the park's concessions and main parking lots are closed November–March, the river (and the park) is a popular year-round destination. It is also a good fishing spot; anglers here lure bass, trout, crappie, and bluegill onto their hooks.

NEARBY ACTIVITIES

The Western Reserve Greenway Trail is a paved, mixed-use trail running 43 miles from Ashtabula to Orwell. You can learn more about the Greenway Trail and other Ashtabula MetroPark projects at **ashtabulacountyparks.org** or by calling (440) 992-0717. The locally owned Raccoon Run Canoe Rental rents boats and organizes seasonal canoe trips. Call (440) 466-7414 or visit **canoeracconrun.com** for more information. For directions to all of Ashtabula's covered bridges (and many award-winning wineries too), visit the county visitors bureau website at **accvb.org**.

Special thanks to Meredith Miskowich and fellow historians at the Hubbard House Underground Railroad Museum in Ashtabula for reviewing this description and offering greater insight into the area and its role in history. To learn more about the museum, visit hubbardhouseugrrmuseum.org *or visit in person on weekends from Memorial Day through September. The museum is located in Ashtabula, about a 15-minute drive from Austinburg.*

BEARTOWN LAKES RESERVATION 14

IN BRIEF

Mature beech and maple forests, a small pine grove, and three lakes comprise this 149-acre park in southern Geauga County. Beavers, herons, hawks, and deer are prevalent. But will you see a bear?

DESCRIPTION

Bainbridge Township was settled in the early 1800s. At the time, the area was simply awash in bears. Local lore tells of a time when one of the McConoughey boys killed five bears in a single day. Not surprisingly, residents began calling the area Beartown.

In the 1960s and 1970s, three interconnecting lakes were constructed, and the surrounding land was operated as a private fishing club. In 1993 Geauga Park District purchased the land; Beartown Lakes Reservation was dedicated in 1996.

The park is a mixture of water (22 acres), wetlands (40 acres), and forest (70 acres). Three trails encircle the park. Each has distinct characteristics, and yet, like the wetlands, woods, and water they visit, all three are closely related. The trails also share a common trailhead area, under the shade of tall maples and oaks, just north of the parking lot.

KEY AT-A-GLANCE INFORMATION

LENGTH: 3 miles

CONFIGURATION: Three interconnecting loops

DIFFICULTY: Easy

SCENERY: Tall beech forests, three lakes, fish, wildlife; bear sightings unlikely!

EXPOSURE: Whitetail and Beechnut trails, mostly shaded; exposed by the lakes

TRAFFIC: Moderately busy, especially on warm weekend afternoons

TRAIL SURFACE: Lake Trail, paved; Whitetail, Beechnut, packed gravel

HIKING TIME: 1 hour

DRIVING DISTANCE: 23 miles from I-77/I-480 exchange

ACCESS: Daily, 6 a.m.–11 p.m.

WHEELCHAIR TRAVERSABLE: Lake Trail, yes; other trails, no

MAPS: USGS Mantua; trail guide usually posted at park welcome sign and at geaugaparkdistrict.org

FACILITIES: Restrooms and water at North Point Shelter in the middle of the park and at Minnow Pond Shelter on the east side of the park

CONTACT INFORMATION: Reach the Geauga County Park District at geaugaparkdistrict.org or call (440) 286-9516.

Directions

Follow I-480 East to Exit 26/US 422 east to OH 306. Turn right, following OH 306/Chillicothe Road south about 1.5 miles. Turn left (east) onto Taylor May Road; then turn right onto Quinn Road. Follow it south 1.4 miles to the park entrance, at 18870 Quinn Road.

GPS Trailhead Coordinates

Latitude 41° 21.298141'

Longitude 81° 17.777281'

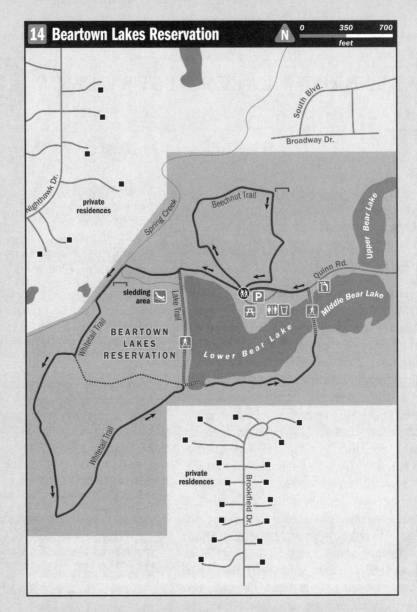

N

0   350   700
feet

South Blvd.

Broadway Dr.

Nighthawk Dr.

private
residences

Spring Creek

Beechnut Trail

Upper Bear Lake

Quinn Rd.

Middle Bear Lake

sledding
area

Lake Trail

P

Whitetail Trail

BEARTOWN
LAKES
RESERVATION

Lower Bear Lake

Whitetail Trail

private
residences

Brookfield Dr.

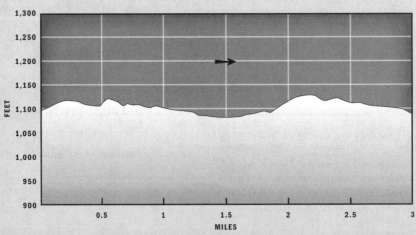

1,300

1,250

1,200

1,150

1,100

1,050

1,000

950

900

FEET

0.5   1   1.5   2   2.5   3

MILES

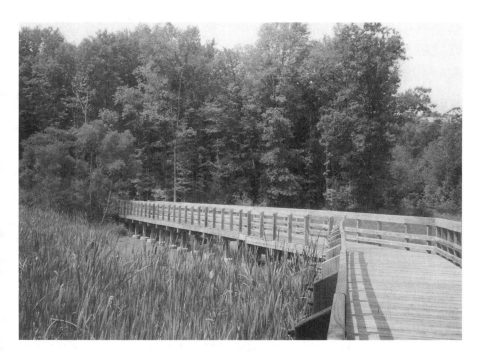

You'll see more fish than bears at Beartown Lakes.

LAKE TRAIL (a 0.7-mile, paved, all-purpose trail)

Lake Trail heads west from the trailhead and quickly bends left, crossing a wooden footbridge that overlooks the sledding hill. Lake Trail is exposed on the north-to-south stretch. As you head south, you'll be able to peer into Lower Bear Lake to catch a glimpse of a bluegill. They are easy to catch here, locals say, as long as you use short, live bait. (Any bait dangling off the end of your hook will be nibbled away; the fish is then free to go, having enjoyed a safe snack. It really is a game, isn't it?) In addition to the small bluegill, bass and northern pike are found in Lower Bear Lake. The park district encourages releasing all catches.

Cattails and duckweeds are plentiful at the south end of the lake. A boardwalk bridge runs across the corner of the lake; from it you'll head east through the woods. Avoid the unmarked paths that wander off from the south side of the Lake Trail, which lead to private residential areas.

Continue east until you reach the southeastern edge of Lower Bear Lake, where the woods open to reveal a boardwalk that spans the dam separating Middle and Lower Bear lakes. Turn left, crossing the boardwalk, where in the summertime you'll enjoy an amazing array of dancing dragonflies. From the north end of the walkway, turn left and follow the shoulder of the park roadway back to the parking lot.

BEECHNUT TRAIL (0.6 miles)

The Beechnut and Whitetail trails are not paved, and they run north together for a few yards before they split.

The Whitetail Trail veers to the left; follow the Beechnut (trail signs are marked by two beech leaves) to the right. The sandy dirt-and-gravel trail is flat, but it winds about as it leads you through the woods. You'll cross four small footbridges in the first quarter mile.

As you wind your way to the observation point at Upper Bear Lake, you might amuse yourself by watching for, or imagining you see, bears. Or maybe that's not so amusing. A bear—or two—seems to have made the rounds (and the local news) in Geauga as well as Portage County each year in recent memory. Black bears, typically young males in search of a territory, can and do wander in from Pennsylvania. Still, your chances of seeing a deer or a rabbit are much greater than that of seeing a bear.

Your chances of seeing a turtle, water snake, or frog from the observation deck at Upper Bear Lake are pretty good too. You can relax and watch on the western side of the lake before getting back on the path and heading south.

Before you leave the woods, you'll cross a fifth and final footbridge. The trail curves to the left and then goes up a short incline; its 5-foot rise is the only "climb" you'll have on this trail. The path ends at the park road, directly across from a fishing pier on Middle Bear Lake. Turn right, following the road back to the parking lot (the same return path as you follow for Lake Trail).

WHITETAIL TRAIL (1.5 miles)

From the Beechnut and Whitetail Trailhead, head west with the sledding hill on your left, following the trail to the edge of Spring Creek. The water here is quite clear and pretty, but remember: no matter how good a stream looks, the only water safe to drink is the stuff you brought from home, in your own bottle.

Crossing the creek is easy; relatively stable rocks lead the way. Even if you slip in, you'll find yourself in only 2–4 inches of water. Trudge uphill a few steps from the creek, where you'll come to a park bench, a great place to watch and listen for woodpeckers. Soon, the trail bends to the left. Whitetail Trail is the only one of the three trails designated for horseback riding, and you're likely to encounter a rider or two through here.

About 0.5 miles into the hike, you'll cross a small tributary where you may spot some spring peepers. Enjoy the fragrant pines as you go up a little hill and follow the trail as it bends left again. From here you can see some private farmland. Enjoy it while it lasts. Subdivisions abut the park on all other sides.

Heading east as you pass the farmland, the trail meanders through an old sugar bush (a narrow strip of sugar maples) and then heads northeast. At about 1 mile, Whitetail approaches the southwest corner of Lower Bear Lake. From here, you can follow the trail left, through the prairie, as Whitetail circles back onto itself, or you can jump onto Lake Trail and finish your hike on its paved path.

NEARBY ACTIVITIES

The park's picnic areas can be reserved through the park office at **geaugaparkdistrict .org** or by calling (440) 286-9516. Much of Middle and Lower Bear lakes are open to fishing, and several piers make it easy to get a line in the deep-water areas.

The small sledding hill north of Lower Bear Lake provides young children a gentle introduction to the downhill sport. (Groaning grown-ups will appreciate the steps on the side of the hill!) Geauga Park District offers year-round educational programming. Call for a schedule of activities or view the calendar online at **geaugaparkdistrict.org**.

Special thanks to the naturalists and other staff from Geauga Park District who reviewed this hike description.

15 CHAGRIN RIVER PARK

KEY AT-A-GLANCE INFORMATION

LENGTH: 1.5 miles

CONFIGURATION: Loop

DIFFICULTY: Easy

SCENERY: Deer and a wide variety of wading birds, woodland wildflowers, and a wide, curvy stretch of the Chagrin River

EXPOSURE: Mostly shaded

TRAFFIC: Moderate–heavy

TRAIL SURFACE: Paved, dirt, and gravel trails—all flat

HIKING TIME: 40 minutes

DRIVING DISTANCE: 27 miles from I-77/I-480 exchange

ACCESS: Daily, sunrise–half hour after sunset

WHEELCHAIR TRAVERSABLE: No

MAPS: USGS Eastlake; posted at trailhead kiosk and available at lakemetroparks.com

FACILITIES: Restrooms, water, public phone, reservable shelters, canoe launch

CONTACT INFORMATION: Visit lakemetroparks.com or call (440) 639-7275.

GPS Trailhead
Coordinates
Latitude   41° 39.523559'
Longitude   81° 24.422157'

IN BRIEF

The crooked Chagrin River runs wide through here, and this park takes full advantage of the river that serves as its southern boundary. A river access area near the park's entrance provides a shallow wading area. On dry land, a playground satisfies active little ones; grown-ups who want to play will enjoy the volleyball court. Seasonal wetlands on the park's north side attract a wide variety of birds, and therefore bird-watchers, to the park.

DESCRIPTION

From the south side of the parking lot, a wood-chip path leads to Riverwood Loop Trail. Turn left at the intersection and follow the trail northeast about 0.2 miles to greet the river. Wooden steps lead down to the river overlook, which serves as entry to a pleasant

----

Directions ⟶

Take I-77 or I-271 to I-90, following it east to Exit 193/OH 306, which merges into OH 2, and then exit at Lost Nation Road. Take Lost Nation north to Reeves Road. Turn left (west) onto Reeves and left again to enter the park on the south side of the road. Follow the park road west 0.2 miles to the main parking area, by a playground and picnic shelter. (Other entrances to the park can be found off Erie Drive in Willoughby and Rural Road in Eastlake.)

Lost Nation Road may be closed due to construction. Check willoughbyohio.com for updates. If the road is closed, turn right at OH 91/SOM Center Road; then turn right to merge onto OH 2 East toward Painesville. Exit onto OH 640 West/Vine Street West; turn right onto OH 91/SOM Center Road. Turn right onto Lakeshore Boulevard and then right onto Reeves Road. Follow the directions above from Reeves to the main parking area.

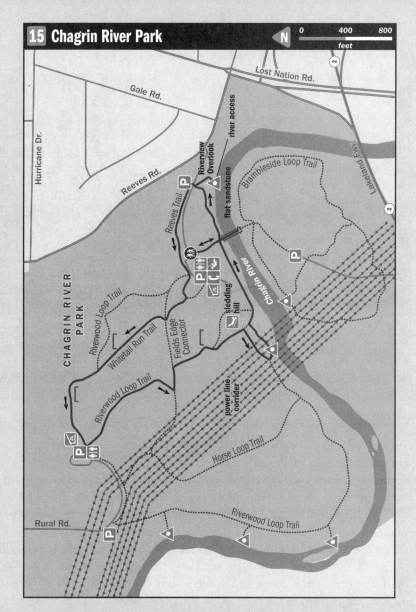

15 Chagrin River Park

N

0   400   800
feet

Lost Nation Rd.

2

Gale Rd.

Lakeland Fwy.

Hurricane Dr.

2

Reeves Rd.

Reeves Trail

Riverview Overlook

river access

flat sandstone

Brambleside Loop Trail

P

Chagrin River

P

P

Riverwood Loop Trail

CHAGRIN RIVER PARK

Whitetail Run Trail

Fields Edge Connector

Sledding hill

Riverwood Loop Trail

power line corridor

Horse Loop Trail

P

Rural Rd.

P

Riverwood Loop Trail

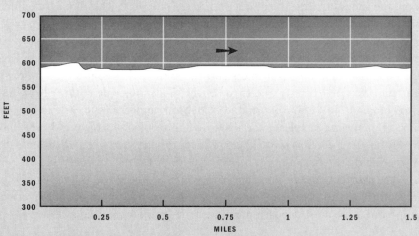

FEET						
700						
650						
600						
550						
500						
450						
400						
350						
300						
	0.25	0.5	0.75	1	1.25	1.5

MILES

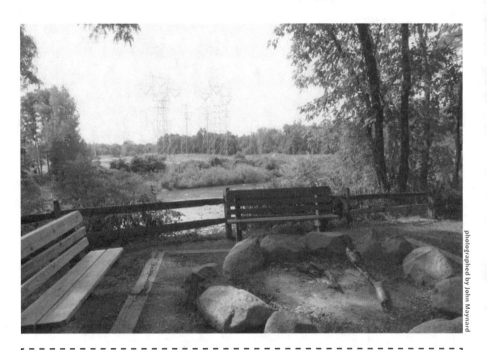

photographed by John Maynard

Next stop, relaxation: This park is so metro that the city bus stops here.

wading area. The Chagrin River is shallow here, and a flat sandstone area in the middle of the river serves as a good gathering spot. Kids like it because they can wade out to their own space and sit in the middle of the river, within sight (but out of earshot) of adults, who might prefer to stay dry on the river's edge.

From the top of the steps, cross the park road and turn left onto the paved Reeves Trail. Several memorial trees have been planted here, among them Cimarron ash and celebration maples. When you return to the main parking lot and playground area, join the Riverwood Loop Trail again briefly, following part of the 1.6-mile trail past dense shrubs and woods that are as heavily populated with birds as the playground is with children. As you walk along on a summer afternoon, the songs of birds, the drone of insects, and the squeals of playful children mix together in a surprisingly loud but delightful way.

About 0.5 miles into your hike, the Fields Edge Connector Trail heads toward the center of the park. Turn left and follow it until it ends; there Riverside Loop Shortcut juts off to the right. Leave the field's edge as you follow the shortcut past tangled trees and shrubs. Deer beds are evident along here; angel wings bloom in July and August, and goldenrods appear in the early fall to make some of us sneeze. Maples and oaks grow tall on this shortcut, and their fallen friends lie alongside the trail. The park department leaves the fallen limbs here so woodland critters can make their homes in or eat the rotting trees.

The shortcut does its job, delivering you back to the "real" Riverwood Loop Trail. Turn left to continue your trek southwest. This part of the Riverwood Loop Trail is the most exposed portion of the gravel trails. In the relatively open area just north of the trail intersection, a few lonely corn stalks grow. No doubt they were planted by a fly-by farmer, perhaps a jay, who dropped a few kernels he stole from a nearby cornfield.

Stay on Riverwood as the trail veers left, where it grows considerably shadier. Inside the horseshoe of the turn, a park bench is positioned so that you'll sit with your back to the trail, facing a thicket of tall bushes and weeds. This is an absolute haven for birds, and therefore, it's inviting to bird fanciers too. In fact, Audubon Ohio recognizes this park as an important birding area.

At this point, you've logged about 1.1 miles. The sledding hill in front of you presents a choice: will you climb over it for an aerobic challenge or stay on the trail as it wraps around the south side of the hill? Either way, don't miss the narrow, grassy trails heading from the south side of the trail to the river. While the footpaths obviously provide more river access, the park (like most) discourages use of these unofficial trails.

Follow the skinny trail through a field of tall grass for less than 0.1 mile to reach a wide and quiet stretch of the Chagrin River. The tawny heads of bull thistles grow in the clearing along the river. At this point, some hikers step down a couple of feet from the sandy banks and wade in. Follow this loop trail back onto Riverwood, and turn right to return to the parking lot.

When you visit Chagrin River Park, you'll see that it's one of the Lake Metroparks that truly embodies the "metro" part of its name. For one thing, the park is on the bus line. A habitat management area in the middle of the park spans several acres and sits below power lines. The deer here are so accustomed to their human neighbors that they often stand by the trail instead of bounding away when you walk by. It's eerie, like passing mannequins that are a little too lifelike.

Of course, this strip of land by a bend in the river has been part of a metro area for countless generations. Several archeological excavations here have uncovered a number of artifacts from the Whittlesey culture; many of those are displayed at the Indian Museum of Lake County. While it may be tempting to leave a clue about our culture for future generations, please don't. Be a good hiker and pack out your trash and any other "artifacts" you may have brought in.

NEARBY ACTIVITIES

A volleyball court and large playground by the main parking lot can occupy kids of all ages. If it's more hiking you want, you can find it here—more than 3 miles of trails wind through this park. Or, having hiked by the river, if you'd like to walk on the lakeshore, head north on OH 2 to Mentor Lagoons (see page 92), which is about a 15-minute drive from here.

To learn a little bit about the Whittlesey culture and other early inhabitants of Lake County, visit the Indian Museum of Lake County on Willoughby's Public Square. For hours and more information, call (440) 951-3813 or visit **indianmuseumoflakecounty.org.**

16 FAIRPORT HARBOR

KEY AT-A-GLANCE INFORMATION

LENGTH: 1.3 miles

CONFIGURATION: Two loops and out-and-backs

DIFFICULTY: Easy beach stroll; lighthouse requires some climbing

SCENERY: Lake Erie, lighthouse, beach, stacks of nuclear power plant

EXPOSURE: Almost entirely exposed, except in lighthouse and museum

TRAFFIC: Moderately heavy, especially on warm weekends

TRAIL SURFACE: Pavement, beach

HIKING TIME: 45–50 minutes

DRIVING DISTANCE: 39 miles from I-77/I-480 exchange

ACCESS: Lighthouse and museum: Open seasonally; admission applies. Park: Daily, sunrise–half hour after sunset; $3 parking fee ($2 for Lake County residents).

WHEELCHAIR TRAVERSABLE: No; surf chair available at the beach

MAPS: USGS Mentor OE N; also posted at county park entrance

FACILITIES: Restrooms, water fountains, concessions at park

CONTACT INFORMATION: Reach Lake Metroparks at (440) 639-9972 or lakemetroparks.com; for area attractions, visit fairportharbor.org or fairportlighthouse.com.

IN BRIEF

Summer is too precious in northeastern Ohio— just in case you're not convinced, a visit to Fairport Harbor will do the trick.

DESCRIPTION

At the top of the town stands a small stone lighthouse, originally built in 1825. Behind the lighthouse sits the keeper's house, now a marine museum, packed with nautical exhibits as well as a mummified cat. But of course there's more to that tail. Er, tale.

In fact, the lighthouse harbors many tales. Step inside the museum (open seasonally) to begin your hike, tour, and history lesson.

Samuel Butler was the first lighthouse keeper and an abolitionist. Under his watch, the lighthouse was a stop on the Underground Railroad, offering a new life for many escaped slaves who were able to reach Canada via Lake Erie. Later, Civil War veteran Joseph Babcock became keeper of the lighthouse, newly rebuilt in 1871. He and his wife, Mary, had several children, two of whom were born in the keeper's house. Unfortunately, their youngest son, Robbie, died of illness at the age of five, and Mary spent several years afterward in bed— sick, depressed, or both.

Reportedly, Mary loved cats and had

GPS Trailhead Coordinates

Latitude   41° 45.4o9677'

Longitude 81° 16.633322'

Directions

Take I-77 North to I-90 East (Exit 163), following signs to Erie, PA. Merge left onto OH 2 and follow signs to Painesville, exiting at OH 283/OH 535 Richmond Street toward Fairport Harbor. Continue west on Richmond and then High Street. The lighthouse is at the corner of High and Second streets; the park is down the hill, where High Street becomes Huntington Beach Drive.

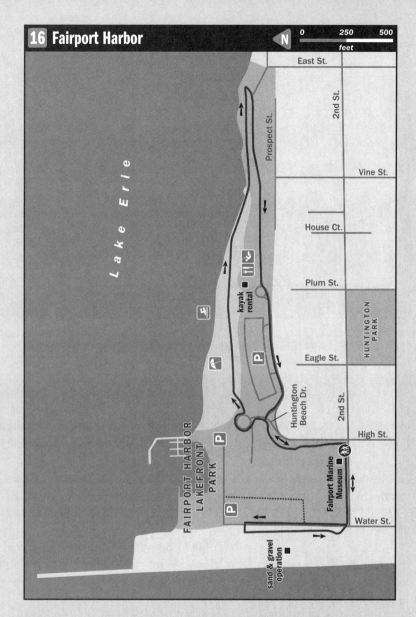

N

0   250   500
feet

East St.

2nd St.

Prospect St.

Vine St.

House Ct.

Plum St.

kayak rental

HUNTINGTON PARK

Eagle St.

P

Huntington Beach Dr.

2nd St.

High St.

P

FAIRPORT HARBOR LAKEFRONT PARK

P

Fairport Marine Museum

Water St.

sand & gravel operation

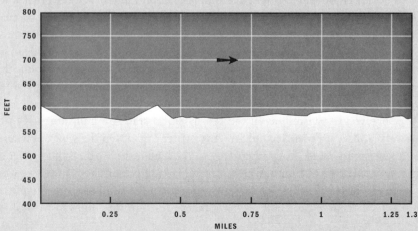

800
750
700
650
600
550
500
450
400

FEET

0.25   0.5   0.75   1   1.25 1.3

MILES

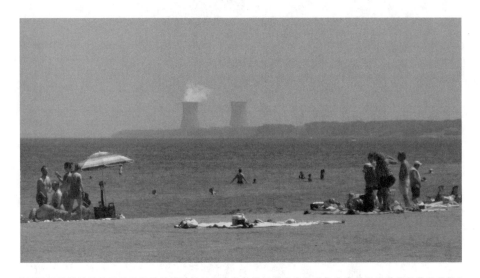

The Perry Nuclear Power Plant, seen in the distance, opened in 1986.

several, including a gray one. After Mary died (also in bed in the keeper's house), numerous people have reported seeing a ghost cat playing in the kitchen and elsewhere on the grounds. When HVAC repair workers found the mummified body of a cat inside a crawl space, it seemed to confirm the stories, and tales of the feline apparition live on.

After a new lighthouse was constructed in Lake Erie in 1925, the original lighthouse was ordered demolished. But local residents and the historical society managed to save it; today volunteers continue to maintain the lighthouse and operate the popular museum.

If you come here during the summer on a day the lighthouse is open, pay the small fee that grants access to climb the 69 steps to the top of the light and look upon Lake Erie, where you will see the new light, Fairport Harbor West Breakwater Light.

The newer, oft-photographed red-and-white building sits on the breakwater, where it is still operated by the U.S. Coast Guard. (*Note:* Sale of the property was pending as of this book's publication date.) Under the lake's choppy waves, a busy salt mining operation provides the road salt that drivers are so dependent on during the winter months. In the summertime, it's easy to forget about that, especially as you watch boaters zipping along on the surface, enjoying the too-short summer season on the lake.

Once you've twisted down the skinny spiral staircase and returned to the sidewalk, follow it down Second Street to Water Street. On the way you'll surely see a few yachts cruise by on their way to the club just past the sand and gravel operations. Turn right onto Water Street, passing a bait shop and—on warm afternoons, at least—a line of cars awaiting entry (or admission) to the port. A launch fee is charged for boaters here, but pedestrians are allowed to walk out onto the breakwater, although the public is not permitted to access the newer lighthouse. When you've appreciated the beauty, industry, and recreation this great lake offers residents of Fairport Harbor, turn and retrace your steps to the original lighthouse site.

Once back at the historical marker, look northeast and down the hill toward Fairport Harbor Lakefront Park, which sits like a beacon for summer-lovers of all ages. Follow the sidewalk as it curves down to the right, and you'll probably spot beach umbrellas and families enjoying the lake well before you reach the park's entrance.

Before heading to the beach, you should know that while there's no admission fee for visitors walking on the beach, a nominal parking fee is charged. Lake Metroparks makes available a surf chair, an all-terrain wheelchair for visitors with physical disabilities. (Call [440] 639-9972 for more information.) Dogs are allowed only on the paved parking lot and in the designated dog swim area, and all dogs must be leashed.

Stroll on the sand or take off your shoes and wade into the shallowest of the Great Lakes. The park offers very little shade, but the beach is dotted with all the amenities that make a visit, well, a day on the beach. Two small playgrounds, food concessions, kayak rentals, volleyball courts, and several picnic tables are sprinkled on the south side of the park.

You can walk about a third of a mile along the beach before you reach the end of the park, all the while eyeing the two thick, silent stacks of the Perry Nuclear Power Plant perched on the horizon. As oddly out of place as the stacks may seem in this otherwise picturesque landscape, they're quiet and easy to ignore—but hard to resist snapping with your camera.

Once you've soaked up some sun and stored a few images in your mind, camera, or both, return to the top of the village of Fairport Harbor, where your visit began.

NEARBY ACTIVITIES

During the summer months, there's plenty to do right here. Besides swimming, active visitors can rent kayaks at the park to enjoy Lake Erie's waves. Folks who like fish and fish stories will enjoy the annual Perchfest, held the weekend after Labor Day, and history buffs can visit the Finnish Heritage Museum, just down the street from the lighthouse (**finnishheritagemuseum.com**; [440] 352-8301). Guided walking tours of Fairport Harbor can be arranged by calling (440) 358-9294. Or enjoy another (usually less crowded) look at Lake Erie from Mentor Lagoons (see page 92), less than 10 miles from Fairport Harbor.

17   LAKESHORE RESERVATION

KEY AT-A-GLANCE INFORMATION

LENGTH: 1.5 miles

CONFIGURATION: Two loops

DIFFICULTY: Easy

SCENERY: Lake Erie's shore, a variety of native and ornamental trees and shrubs, sculpture garden

EXPOSURE: Mostly exposed

TRAFFIC: Moderate

TRAIL SURFACE: Asphalt, sand, and dirt

HIKING TIME: 45 minutes

DRIVING DISTANCE: 46 miles from I-77/I-480 exchange

ACCESS: Daily, sunrise–half hour after sunset

WHEELCHAIR TRAVERSABLE: Yes, three of the four trails are paved; Birdwatcher's Trail is hard-packed grass and dirt.

MAPS: USGS Perry; also available at the park trailhead and lakemetroparks.com

FACILITIES: Restrooms, water, two picnic shelters with grills

CONTACT INFORMATION: Lake Metroparks can be reached by phone at (440) 354-3434 or online at lakemetroparks.com.

IN BRIEF

Hike in the company of various shorebirds, gaze over Lake Erie, and enjoy the work of Charles Irish, a Lake County arborist whose use of rhododendrons and other nonnative plants are still visible today, as well as modern stone sculptures by Lake County artist Carl Floyd.

DESCRIPTION

Prior to becoming a park in 1968, Lakeshore Reservation was owned by a group of individuals who built summer cottages along Lake Erie. Arborist Charles Irish owned the largest of these properties. His work—placing ornamental trees among the native species and planting a large group of rhododendrons along the eastern boundary of the park—is still apparent.

The property may have appealed to the park system because Irish had laid this groundwork. However, the park was ultimately acquired because of its naturally stable beach condition and mature stand of trees—the largest such property along Lake Erie in the county.

Adding to the park's natural beauty, an interesting sculpture garden graces Lakeshore Reservation's east side. It was dedicated in 1978 and includes work by the nationally known Lake County sculptor Carl Floyd. Sculpture

GPS Trailhead
Coordinates

Latitude   41° 48.732119'

Longitude   81° 7.080238'

Directions

Take I-77 North to Exit 163/I-90 East. Follow I-90 East and merge onto OH 2 East (toward Painesville). Follow OH 2 as it becomes US 20 East/North Ridge Road. Turn left onto Antioch Road. Enter the park and turn right, proceeding to the easternmost parking lot and trailhead.

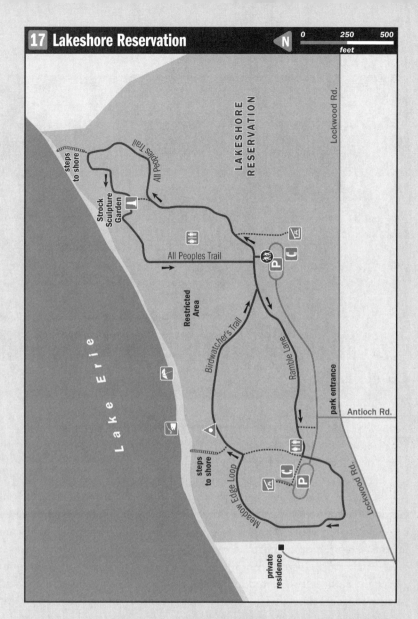

N

| 0 | 250 | 500 |

feet

LAKESHORE RESERVATION

Lockwood Rd.

steps to shore

All Peoples Trail

Strock Sculpture Garden

All Peoples Trail

Restricted Area

L a k e   E r i e

Birdwatcher's Trail

Ramble Lane

park entrance

Antioch Rd.

Lockwood Rd.

steps to shore

Meadow Edge Loop

private residence

P

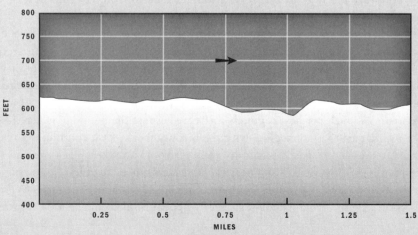

FEET

800
750
700
650
600
550
500
450
400

0.25   0.5   0.75   1   1.25   1.5

MILES

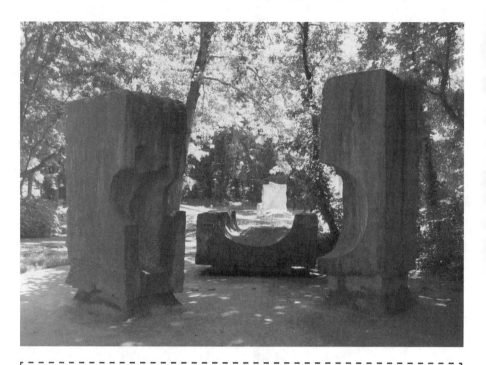

Sculptures add interest along the trail.

pieces here include a sundial and a cable bridge.

Begin your hike from the easternmost of the two parking areas. Take the All Peoples Trail as it heads northeast 0.2 miles to reach the Strock Sculpture Garden. As soon as you can see the sculptures, you'll want to go in and have a closer look, but wait—you'll return here soon. Follow the path as it continues northeast a bit, looping north to reach a set of steep and shady steps that lead to Lake Erie's shore. Instead of walking on the beach now, give in to temptation to go see the stone artwork and follow the trail back to the center of the sculpture garden to appreciate the unusual pieces. Wander through the large, interesting sculpture pieces (worth the wait, weren't they?) before heading west on the paved trail. Soon it turns left and heads south back to the parking lot.

When you arrive at the intersection with Ramble Lane, you will have covered about 0.5 miles. Turn right to follow paved Ramble Lane. Along this section you will have a good picture of the property as it once was—a string of private residences, blissfully situated overlooking the lake. One private home remains here; it is clearly marked and landscaped to blend into the park and afford its residents as much privacy as possible. (Please respect the boundaries here.)

Walk past the intersection with the Birdwatcher's Trail, continuing to head west. You'll venture past a picnic area and restroom and then reach the intersection with Meadow Edge Loop near the park's entrance. Turn left, following the still-paved trail as it ventures south and then loops to the right to pass by hemlocks and pretty ornamentals that clearly appeal to birds in the area. The trail straightens out and then once more curves to the right, moving into denser woods, before reaching another set of steps to the shore. The paving ends just past the steps, and Birdwatcher's Trail begins. At this point, you will have hiked about 1 mile.

Birdwatcher's Trail is graceful, narrow, and grassy. Soon after you step onto it, you're invited to step off again, onto a wooden platform deck overlooking the lake. As the woods, water, and shore converge here, so do the jays, ducks, and gulls. A bench on the overlook invites you to watch and listen to them argue over food and territory.

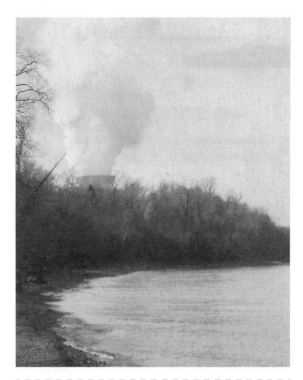

Here, you can walk along Erie's shore in almost every season.

From the Lakeview Overlook, step back onto the trail and turn left, heading east again. Follow the narrow, hard-packed dirt trail through young woods around the home in the middle of the park, where it merges with Ramble Lane and returns you to the parking lot.

If you didn't walk along the beach before, consider it now. On your way to the beach, notice the tall, reedlike grasses that help hold down the sand here. When you reach the beach and look west, you can't help but notice the Perry Nuclear Power Plant. Of the 103 nuclear power plants in the United States, two sit on the Lake Erie shore—Perry, here, and Davis-Besse, in Port Clinton. Like the sculptures you saw earlier, the giant stacks are an awesome, if unnatural, site along the shore, adding interest and beauty to the entire picture.

NEARBY ACTIVITIES

Perry, perhaps even more than other parts of Lake County, is dotted with nurseries and greenhouses. If you're looking for a specific tree or plant, or advice on growing almost anything, you're likely to find what you're looking for within a mile or two of Lakeshore Reservation.

Heading home along OH 2? You're about 12 miles from Fairport Harbor (see page 80). Why not stop and get a look at the lighthouse there?

18   MASON'S LANDING

KEY AT-A-GLANCE INFORMATION

LENGTH: 1.2 miles

CONFIGURATION: Out-and-back

DIFFICULTY: Easy

SCENERY: Grand River, good bird-watching along the trail

EXPOSURE: About half shaded

TRAFFIC: Light

TRAIL SURFACE: Dirt and sand

HIKING TIME: 35 minutes

DRIVING DISTANCE: 39 miles from I-77/I-480 exchange

ACCESS: Daily, sunrise–sunset

MAPS: USGS Painesville; also available at park kiosk and at lakemetroparks.com

WHEELCHAIR TRAVERSABLE: No

FACILITIES: Restrooms, small picnic area with grills, playground, canoe launch

CONTACT INFORMATION: Reach a park ranger at (440) 354-3434 or visit lakemetroparks.com for more information.

IN BRIEF

This short hike meanders along the banks of the Grand State Wild and Scenic River. The trail, wisely, lets the river be its guide.

DESCRIPTION

From the parking lot, head west up a slight hill on a sandy dirt trail. The path snakes along the north bank of the river and offers shade and good bird-watching opportunities. Be sure to notice along the trail, and high above your head, the large bird boxes available to sleepy owls. The trail rises and falls and wiggles and bumps over several hills, each 5–7 feet tall. Turn south to pass within a few feet of the riverbank, and then turn north, running 20 feet or more into the woods. As a result of the trail's wending and winding, your perspective of the river changes almost constantly.

If you veer off the main trail, you can follow a fishermen's trail that runs much closer to the water. On a sunny day, you can expect to find a snake or two soaking up the rays' warmth along the sandy riverbank.

About 0.5 miles west of the starting point, a park bench waits for you. Rivers Edge Trail ends just a few feet beyond the bench. From the bench, you can watch the river as it heads south or look east to the bridge. In between,

GPS Trailhead Coordinates

Latitude   41° 43.599901'

Longitude   81° 11.114037'

Directions

Follow I-480 East to I-271 North. Take I-90 East to Exit 205 and turn left onto Vrooman Road. Follow Vrooman north about 1.5 miles. Mason's Landing Park is located on Vrooman Road, just south of OH 84, on the west side of the road.

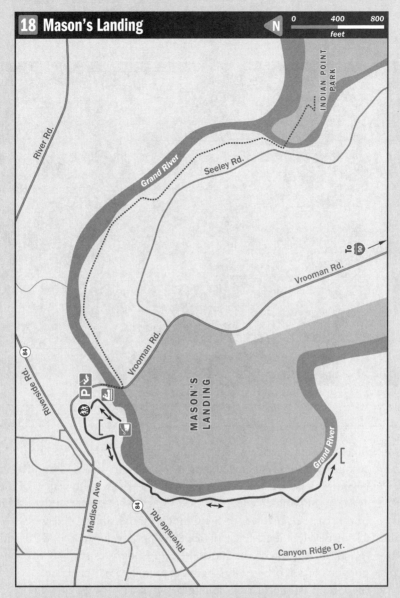

N

0   400   800
feet

River Rd.

Grand River

Seeley Rd.

INDIAN POINT PARK

To 90

Vrooman Rd.

Vrooman Rd.

84

Riverside Rd.

MASON'S LANDING

Grand River

Madison Ave.

84

Riverside Rd.

Canyon Ridge Dr.

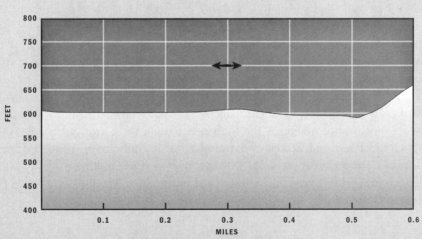

FEET

800
750
700
650
600
550
500
450
400

0.1   0.2   0.3   0.4   0.5   0.6

MILES

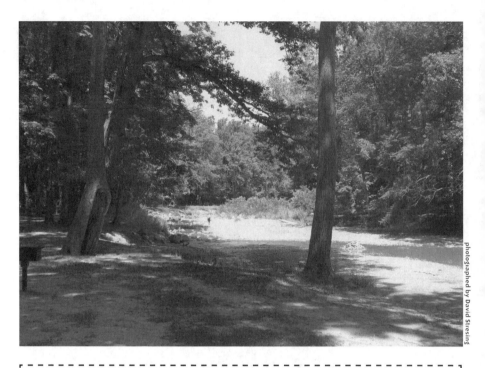

photographed by David Stresing

Bring your canoe.

you're likely to see someone wading in, pole in hand, angling for one of the river's many residents. Fishing is allowed, and it is good here in the Grand River.

As you walk beside and contemplate the relatively calm waters of the Grand River, you might wonder what's "wild" about it—there certainly are no rapids here. In this case, *wild* refers to the Grand's inaccessibility (except by foot trail) and lack of development. Back in 1968, Ohio developed the Wild and Scenic River program to protect the natural beauty of rivers such as this one. Since then, portions of ten other rivers have been designated scenic.

The Grand is one of two double designees (Little Beaver Creek is Ohio's other State Wild and Scenic River), due in part to it being home to more than 60 species of fish and at least 25 unique plant species. Bestowing the title in 1974, the state proclaimed, "The Grand River, with its rugged topography and limited human impacts, represents one of the finest examples of a natural stream to be found in Ohio."

As you make your way back along the bumpy path, tread lightly and enjoy deeply. When you return to the parking lot, walk down to the canoe launch on the northwestern side of the bridge. A plaque there relates the history of the Grand River and describes its wandering, 102-mile path, which begins in Geauga County. It also explains that this river is more than its wild and scenic designations—the river and its watershed drain about 456,000 acres of northeastern Ohio before emptying into Lake Erie.

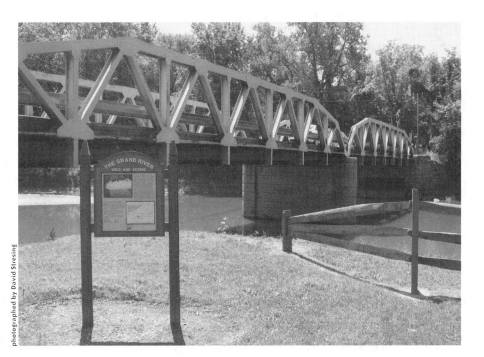

photographed by David Stresing

Good fishing makes for a Grand River.

NEARBY ACTIVITIES

If you have a canoe, bring it here—you can put in and paddle up the Grand River into Ashtabula County. If you prefer to stay on land, walk across the Vrooman Road bridge and follow another footpath east to Indian Point Park, about a mile from Mason's Landing. Indian Point is also a Grand River Reservation, and it is listed on the National Register of Historic Places. The park features two earthworks built by some of Ohio's earliest people—known as the Whittlesey culture, who lived here between AD 900–1650—and a totem pole carved by campers in the early 1900s.

19 MENTOR LAGOONS NATURE PRESERVE

 KEY AT-A-GLANCE INFORMATION

LENGTH: 3.7 miles

CONFIGURATION: Loop

DIFFICULTY: Easy

SCENERY: Lake Erie shore, riverine marshes, woodlands, wildflowers

EXPOSURE: Mostly exposed

TRAFFIC: Moderate

TRAIL SURFACE: All-purpose trail, hard-packed limestone; nature trails, hard dirt to soft sand

HIKING TIME: 1.5 hours for all trails

DRIVING DISTANCE: 33 miles from I-77/I-480 exchange

ACCESS: Daily, sunrise–sunset. Swimming prohibited. Pets permitted, on leash, on all trails except Marsh Rim and Lakefront. Bikes OK on Woods and Marina Overlook trails.

MAPS: USGS Mentor; also at trailhead and cityofmentor.com

WHEELCHAIR TRAVERSABLE: No, but electric carts available for those who have trouble walking; call (440) 205-3625 prior to visit for cart.

FACILITIES: Pay phone and portable restrooms by marina office

CONTACT INFORMATION: Contact the Parks, Recreation & Public Facilities Dept. at cityofmentor.com or (440) 974-5720.

IN BRIEF

This great preserve protects the largest unbroken bluff forest in northeast Ohio and one of the finest coastal dune communities in the state. Rare plants and more than 150 species of birds can be found here—along with some solitude.

DESCRIPTION

Purchased by the city of Mentor in 1998, the 450-acre Mentor Lagoons Nature Preserve protects one of the few riverine marshes still surviving along Lake Erie's shore. Even more land is preserved in the 644-acre Mentor Marsh State Nature Preserve, on the east side of Mentor Lagoons. On the west side of this city preserve is the city's marina, dedicated to recreation, not preservation, which isn't necessarily a bad thing—after all, enjoying our natural resources makes us more likely to want to protect them. With that in mind, head north from the trailhead parking lot and step onto Marsh Rim Trail. Follow the shady trail north about 0.5 miles. From there it heads east, skirting the border between this park and its neighbor, Mentor Marsh State Nature Preserve. In the summer, you'll hear the roar of outboard motors even here, in the deep of the woods. (Think of it as audible proof of enjoyment.) Tangles of grapevines along the trail offer

----

GPS Trailhead Coordinates

Latitude   41° 43.612261'

Longitude   81° 20.324221'

Directions ⟶

Take I-77 North to Exit 163/I-90 East. Merge onto OH 2 East and exit at OH 165/Center Street. Turn left and follow Center Street as it becomes Hopkins Road. Turn right onto Lakeshore Boulevard and then left onto Harbor Drive. Trailhead parking is to the east of the docks and marina office.

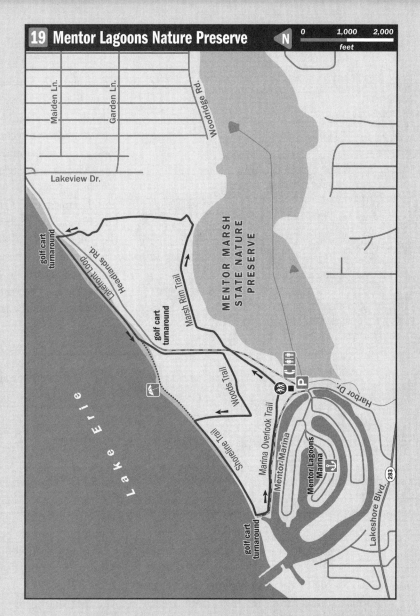

N

| 0 | 1,000 | 2,000 |

feet

Maiden Ln.

Garden Ln.

Woodridge Rd.

Lakeview Dr.

golf cart turnaround

Lakefront Loop

Headlands Rd.

Marsh Rim Trail

M E N T O R   M A R S H
S T A T E   N A T U R E
P R E S E R V E

golf cart turnaround

Woods Trail

L a k e   E r i e

Shoreline Trail

Marina Overlook Trail

Mentor Marina

Mentor Lagoons Marina

Harbor Dr.

Lakeshore Blvd.

283

golf cart turnaround

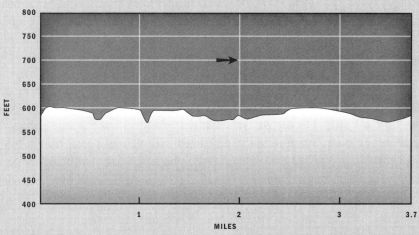

FEET	

800
750
700
650
600
550
500
450
400

1   2   3   3.7

MILES

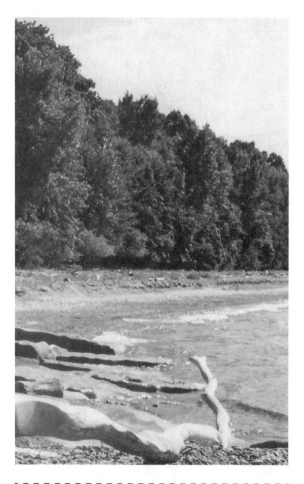

Keep it clean—pack out your trash.

atmosphere for you, as well as shelter for many small animals. Animals and bikes are not permitted on this or the Lakefront Loop trail.

After traipsing about 1 mile through the woods, you'll emerge to find a bench perched high above the lake. You'll also find your feet on the limestone of Lakefront Loop. If you turn right, the trail continues northeast to a gated residential area immediately west of Mentor Marsh. Instead, head west–southwest for about a mile along this completely exposed section of Lakefront Loop, walking high enough above the water to enjoy a great view of wildflowers growing amid tall marsh grasses. This is a great place for birdwatching, and because you're not far from Lost Nation Airport, don't be surprised if a big bird (a small plane) buzzes by too.

About 2 miles into your hike, you'll reach a cart turnaround. Here, by a rocky outcrop, a narrow unmarked path leads down to a very narrow beach, which is not much wider than a hiking boot. If you're willing to take the narrow path, walk down to the shore and follow along the beach for the next 0.5 miles. Otherwise, you can continue along Lakefront Loop, which eventually turns into Woods Trail and intersects Shoreline Loop.

The shore of Lake Erie is interesting. You'll probably spot a working rig or two on the lake; when you look east, you can see the east pier light near the Port of Cleveland. On the coarse sand, driftwood as smooth as a baby's skin rests among stones worn smooth and ringed with various pastel colors. Rather than the "sh-sssshh" of an ocean wave, these waves lap loudly, often with a bang and a crash. Rough-looking, rocky outcrops and ceaseless wind make the area seem especially wild; at times you can imagine that it is too big to be

tamed. Unfortunately, you cannot forget that you're surrounded by the civilization of a large industrial center, thanks to the eclectic collection of manufac-
tured items also found here on the beach. The odd pieces of debris mingle on
the beach next to the driftwood and sea oats. Gulls perch on antique machine
parts; castaway tires embedded in the sand hold back erosion. It's something of
a compromise, this use and abuse of our unique landscape.

As you continue south and west along the shore, about 2.5 miles from your
starting point, you'll see two sets of wooden stairs leading up to the Woods
Trail on your left. True to its name, the trail is entirely shaded. If you're looking
for a cooler, greener trail, head in. It will take you east, and back to the inland
portion of Lakeshore Loop, in just about 0.6 miles. If you prefer to continue on
the water's edge, you'll soon land on Shoreline Loop, which deposits you onto
Marina Overlook Trail.

Marina Overlook is a mix of sand and dirt with a bit of gravel here and
there. It takes you east, along the docks, under the shade of tall maples and oaks.
The trail leads you up a short hill and then flattens out into an S-curve before
returning past the marina office and back to the parking lot.

NEARBY ACTIVITIES

If you visit during the warmer months, you can rent kayaks, canoes, or bicycles to
explore the preserve from both sides of the shore. (Contact the parks and recreation
office in advance at [440] 255-1100 or **cityofmentor.com**.) For a look at a different
sort of shoreline habitat, plan a visit to the lagoon's next-door-neighbor, Mentor
Marsh State Nature Preserve. The entrance is at 5185 Corduroy Road in Mentor.

Looking for a smaller park with a playground? Try Veterans Park, located
on Harbor Drive, south of Mentor Lagoons.

20 ORCHARD HILLS PARK

KEY AT-A-GLANCE INFORMATION

LENGTH: 3.5 miles

CONFIGURATION: Several connected loops

DIFFICULTY: Moderate

SCENERY: Pine stands, pudding stones, orchard, meadows, wetlands, a glimpse of Lake Erie

EXPOSURE: Mostly exposed

TRAFFIC: Moderately heavy on weekends and evenings, particularly in the fall

TRAIL SURFACE: Most are paved

HIKING TIME: Allow an hour or more

DRIVING DISTANCE: 30 miles from I-77/I-480 exchange

ACCESS: Daily, 6 a.m.–11 p.m.

MAPS: USGS Chesterland; also posted at trailhead and at geaugaparkdistrict.org

WHEELCHAIR TRAVERSABLE: Yes, the paved trails are, though some are steep

FACILITIES: None

CONTACT INFORMATION: Visit Geauga Park District online at geaugaparkdistrict.org, or call (440) 286-9516.

IN BRIEF

Rolling over 237 acres, Orchard Hills Park is a unique park in Chester Township. Operated as a golf course until 2007, today the property situated immediately west of the Patterson Fruit Farm invites nature lovers to enjoy its splendid rock outcrops, dramatic hills, and a panoramic view of Lake Erie.

DESCRIPTION

Note: Orchard Hills was a very new park property when this book went to press, and the park district's resource and planning survey was underway. Because trails were under development at the time, this description and the accompanying map offer only an approximate guide. The best advice to really get to know this property is to head for the hills!

Mark Twain is credited with saying that golf is "a good walk spoiled." Whether you agree probably has something to do with your last game. Regardless, Orchard Hills has offered visitors a chance to walk for decades. Established in 1961 as a golf course, it saw its last tee time in 2007. The 18-hole, regulation course had a par of 72 and a slope rating of 126. The rating is but one measure of the sport's difficulty. The maximum rating is 155,

GPS Trailhead Coordinates

Latitude   41° 33.555901'

Longitude   81° 21.952500'

Directions

From the I-77/I-480 exchange, follow I-480 East to I-271 North. Continue north on I-271 to Exit 34/Mayfield Road/US 322. Travel east about 5 miles on Mayfield to Caves Road and turn left to go north. The park entrance is on the west side of Caves Road.

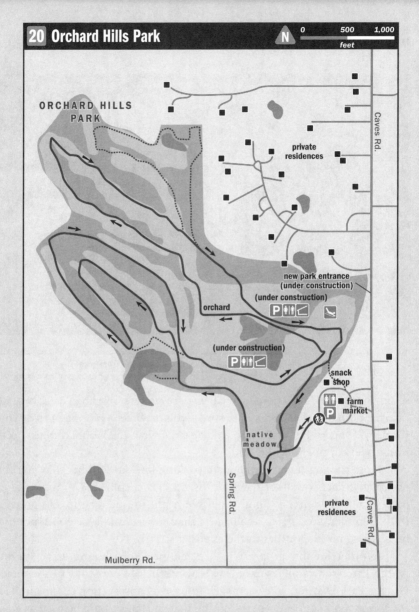

N

0   500   1,000
feet

ORCHARD HILLS
PARK

private
residences

new park entrance
(under construction)

(under construction)

orchard

(under construction)

snack
shop

farm
market

native
meadow

Spring Rd.

Caves Rd.

Caves Rd.

private
residences

Mulberry Rd.

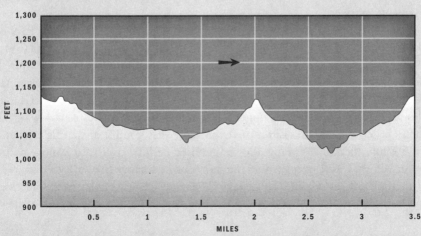

1,300
1,250
1,200
1,150
1,100
1,050
1,000
950
900

FEET

0.5   1   1.5   2   2.5   3   3.5

MILES

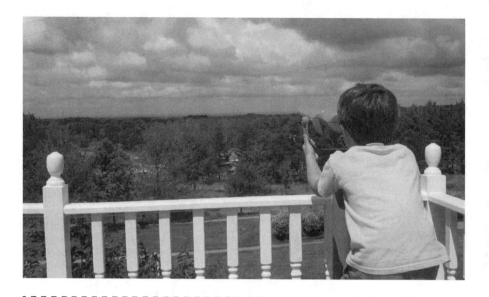

Even on a cloudy day, you can see Lake Erie from here.

so obviously these hills posed a challenge for golfers over the years. Now they're offering both a challenge and a reward—you may feel a bit of a burn as you walk the new "course," but you'll also enjoy a great view and wonderful perspective on many facets of this versatile land.

From the south end of the main parking lot, the trail beckons you through new, native meadows that the park district has encouraged to return along the now-abandoned fairway. Soon you'll veer right to find a petite but pretty pond. In the summer, noisy frogs and insects chatter here, and it's a good spot to watch butterflies and dragonflies in the exposed stretch.

In order for this property to become the idyllic hiking destination that it is, the Patterson family worked with Western Reserve Land Conservancy and Geauga Park District. They arranged to have a conservation easement placed on the former golf course property stating that the land would be used as a passive-use public park.

In this case, *passive* is a legal term; those who visit Orchard Hills Park can enjoy a variety of activities. The natural rolling hills in this part of Geauga County lend themselves to cross-country skiing, and several trails are designated for skiing when conditions are right. Because many of the trail sections were originally developed for golf cart traffic, visitors can enjoy much of the park on wheels (bicycles or strollers); however, it's important to remember that pedestrians always have the right of way, and all visitors are expected to use good trail-sharing etiquette.

While the land is being allowed (and helped) to return to a more natural state, you may still notice some remnants of its former life as a golf course in both the trail layout and landscape. The wide clearings that were necessary for long drives have also made this piece of land a favorite haunt of hawks

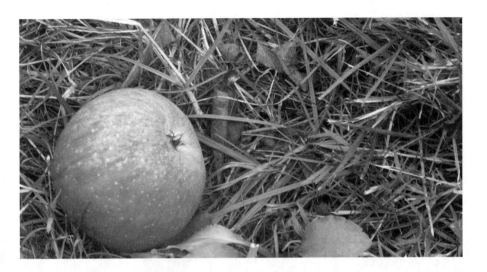

Don't pick the apples . . . but *do* pick up some from the farmer's market to take home.

and other birds of prey; you'll probably see quite a few of them as you wander Orchard Hills's paths.

Three connected loops extending northeast take you through lush meadows to visit pine stands, native forest, and wetlands. When the paths turn you back toward the parking area, you'll emerge from the shade of deciduous trees (with several apple varieties in the mix) to walk along the edge of an apple orchard. The orchard is a sweet reminder of the annual treasure to be found here. But it won't be the first reminder you'll have—throughout the property, it's almost impossible to miss apples, as the fruit and their seeds have been scattered here for years by a variety of critters. (*Note:* Please don't pick the apples! The orchard here is still maintained by the Patterson family.)

As you continue east (cross through the parking lot with care), you can stay in the park on one of several looping paved paths to appreciate numerous lovely outcrops of Sharon conglomerate. Park benches are strategically placed (for hikers now, rather than golfers) to consider the changes this land has seen in a relatively short span of time.

Before you leave, head up one of the steep paths that lead to the Patterson's farm market and snack shop. While you may want to look down to check your footing (especially when the trails are wet or snowy), remember to lift your eyes to enjoy a sweeping vista to the north. These hills offer a view of Lake Erie that's not available from most of Geauga County. Even on an overcast day, you can spot a layer of deep blue-gray on the horizon. That's the lake; the stacks to the far right belong to the Cleveland Electric Illuminating Company. While it's hard to tear yourself away from the view, the market and snack shop offer plenty of other tempting treats—and of course, you can return to the park to enjoy them, and the view. Satisfying, indeed.

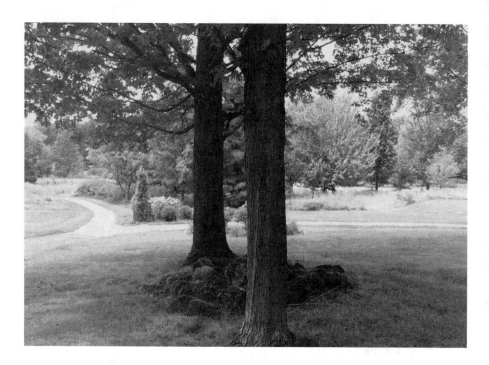

No more scorecards—just enjoy the trails and scenery on the former fairways.

NEARBY ACTIVITIES

Obviously, there's more to do right here. The farmer's market is open year-round, offering fresh produce and baked goods. Patterson's Family Fun Fest celebrates the apple harvest season September–October, when young visitors enjoy darting around haystacks, racing down a 50-foot-long slide, and finding their way though a corn maze. Group hayrides can be scheduled May–November; call (440) 729-1964 to discuss availability and rates.

Wetland restoration work undertaken by the park district during Orchard Hills's development meant that some dirt had to be relocated on the property and—voila!—a long sledding hill was created on the park's north side. Construction of a shelter at the bottom is planned to provide visitors with a nice place to warm up. Visit **geaugaparkdistrict.org** or call (440) 286-9516 for sledding condition updates.

If it's more hiking you want, head east on Chardon Road (OH 6) from here to find North Chagrin Reservation (see page 58).

Thanks to Paige Hosier for her careful review of this property, even as it was transforming into a Geauga County Park District property.

THE WEST WOODS 21

IN BRIEF

The West Woods, in Russell and Newbury townships, spans 900 acres and shelters several dwindling species. Learn how a small cave was shaped by the area's geology and how it played into the county's history.

DESCRIPTION

Start at Pioneer Bridle Trail, a wide dirt trail carpeted with pine needles that begins from the southwest end of the parking lot. As the trail dips and bends sharply to the right, it heads downhill, winding through the dense woods.

Where the trail runs parallel to OH 87, you'll notice lots of chain ferns. The path narrows as it heads west. For a short time, you walk very close to the road, but then the shady path widens and drops down a short, steep hill, below the traffic where it's a much quieter world. On your left is a small creek, and during the summer, the surrounding Joe-Pye weed, tall thistles, ragweed, and Queen Anne's lace create a haven for birds, butterflies, and a crowd of dragonflies.

Before you've logged a mile, you'll cross the creek and turn left (south), leaving OH 87 traffic behind for good to enter a sweet-smelling pine forest. The path can be muddy here, but where it is at its stickiest,

KEY AT-A-GLANCE INFORMATION

LENGTH: 4 miles
CONFIGURATION: Three loops
DIFFICULTY: Moderate
SCENERY: Forest, wildflowers, pristine Silver Creek, remarkable variety of bugs and butterflies
EXPOSURE: Mostly shaded
TRAFFIC: Light
TRAIL SURFACE: Hard-packed dirt, gravel
HIKING TIME: 1 hour and 40 minutes
DRIVING DISTANCE: 25 miles from I-77/I-480 exchange
ACCESS: Daily, 6 a.m.–11 p.m. Nature Center: Daily, 10 a.m.–5 p.m.
MAPS: USGS South Russell; also available inside nature center
WHEELCHAIR TRAVERSABLE: No
FACILITIES: Emergency phone, restrooms, and water at nature center; two picnic shelters
CONTACT INFORMATION: Reach the Geauga County Park District at geaugaparkdistrict.org or call (440) 286-9504.

Directions

Take I-480 East to Exit 26/Miles Road. Follow Miles Road north to OH 91/SOM Center Road and turn left. Follow SOM Center to South Woodland Road and turn right; turn left onto OH 87. The West Woods is on the south side of OH 87, 2 miles east of OH 306.

GPS Trailhead Coordinates

Latitude   41° 27.734041'
Longitude   81° 18.308280'

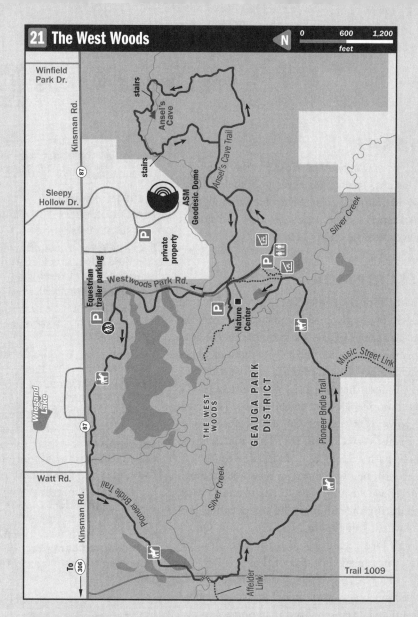

N

| 0 | 600 | 1,200 |

feet

Winfield
Park Dr.

Kinsman Rd.

87

Sleepy
Hollow Dr.

stairs

Ansel's
Cave

stairs

stairs

Ansel's Cave Trail

Silver Creek

ASM
Geodesic Dome

P

private
property

Equestrian
trailer parking

Westwoods Park Rd.

P

P

Nature
Center

P

Music Street Link

THE WEST
WOODS

GEAUGA PARK
DISTRICT

Pioneer Bridle Trail

Wiegand
Lake

87

Watt Rd.

Kinsman Rd.

Pioneer Bridle Trail

Silver Creek

To
306

Affelder
Link

Trail 1009

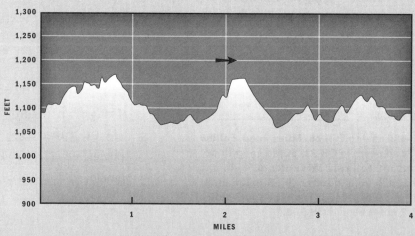

1,300							
1,250							
1,200							
1,150							
1,100							
1,050							
1,000							
950							
900							

FEET

1   2   3   4

MILES

walk-arounds have been worn for you. Remember that this is a bridle trail, so yield to those on horseback.

You'll soon reach the Affelder Link trail heading right (west) off the trail—it leads to OH 306 and does not loop back. Stay on the main path, eventually crossing a wide, wooden footbridge where the creek is wider than before.

As the trail wiggles through the forest, it continues to climb slowly. You move, gradually, from a thick stand of thin trees to an area of older growth. Under the taller trees, you'll find mulberry bushes, and in the summer you'll spot angel wings and jewel-weed along the way. Before you reach the back of the nature center, you'll roll up and then down a small hill, arriving at The West Woods

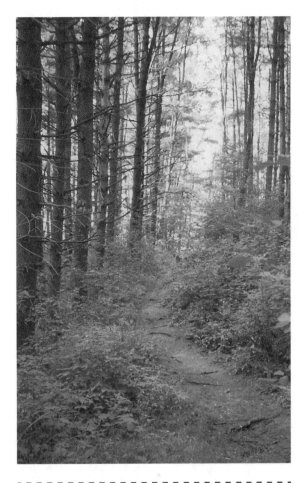

You can find solitude within a few miles of the city limits.

Nature Center and two picnic shelters. If you can, make time to visit inside the nature center for hands-on lessons about the geology, hydrology, and ecology of Geauga County.

From the nature center, you can continue north on a wide path, next to the park road, and return to the north parking area to complete the first loop of your hike. To continue, cross the road and follow the trail leading east to Ansel's Cave.

The hard-packed, dirt-and-gravel trail eases up a gentle rise; several benches along the way offer rest. Continuing along the edge of a 15- to 20-foot-deep ravine, you'll cross over a short wooden footbridge, passing increasingly larger outcrops of Sharon conglomerate sandstone infused with small, smooth pebbles.

The trail snakes a bit but heads generally east and up. After a few minutes of steady uphill action, you (and the path) will reach the top of a large shale formation. From here you'll have a good look at the ravine, now 20–25 feet

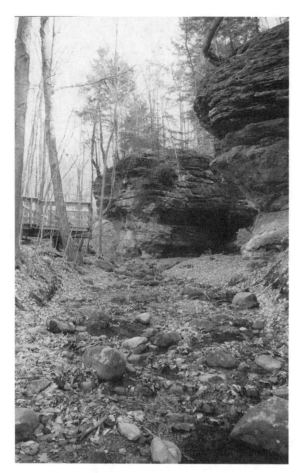

Entering what remains of Ansel's Cave

below. You're surrounded by maples and probably ready for a bit of a break. Ahead, you'll begin your descent with the aid of a wooden stairway, and then another. At the bottom of the second stairway, you'll see the rock formations for which the trail is named.

In the early 1800s, the cave—now more aptly described as a rock wall—was the home of Ansel Savage. Whether he was a hermit, as some rather romantic accounts contend, is not certain. What hermit pursues political office? Savage served as a clerk, treasurer, and trustee of Russell township between 1830 and 1833. Although he drops off the local historical records in 1834, lore about the cave continues. The cave was a wolf den for some time into the 1840s; it's also said that a band of counterfeiters both hid out and worked inside the cave.

But as you follow the boardwalk alongside a crooked creek bed, you may wonder, "What cave?" A waterfall and the feature popularly referred to as a cave stands about 75 feet off the trail to your right. Based on the best understanding we have of the area's geology now, there was no cave—regardless of its name, what we have here is actually an outcrop of Sharon conglomerate ledges. An assortment of graffiti remains here too, some of it dating back to 1877. (Read it, but please, don't add to it.)

Once you've had a good look around, turn and continue up the dirt trail. A series of S-shaped curves will lead you in a semicircle that loops back to the main trail under tall black walnut and white pines. But as you near the top of the rise, just west of the cave, you can't help but notice another striking formation: the Geodesic Dome at Materials Park.

Materials Park is the world headquarters of ASM International. ASM (formerly the American Society of Metals) is an international society for materials engineers and scientists. ASM's Geodesic Dome, the largest of its kind in the world, was designed by ASM member Buckminster Fuller. It is 103 feet high, 274 feet in diameter at its base, and contains 13 miles of aluminum tubing and rods; foundations for the dome pylons extend 77 feet below ground.

Gawk, but don't trespass: Materials Park is private property. With permission, you may be able to walk under the dome—during daylight hours. Contact ASM's executive offices at (440) 228-5151 to inquire about getting a closer look at the dome. With development obviously chewing up large portions of the county, visitors can take comfort in the fact that, to complete The West Woods, the Geauga Park District purchased more than 500 acres from ASM. Today, The West Woods' mature forests are home to barred owls, flycatchers, thrush, vireos, and several threatened plant species. Butternut trees, closed gentian, blunt mountain mint wildflowers, and tall manna grass all live here. The Ohio Department of Natural Resources Wildlife Division selected Silver Creek's tributaries as key spots to reintroduce the native brook trout, considered a threatened species. ASM's founder, William Hunt Eisenman, revered "big plans" and the magic they can contain. Obviously, The West Woods is a result of some big plans, and the park district has created some magic here, making wise use of donations of money, land, and volunteer hours.

The trail adjacent to ASM's headquarters loops back into itself before returning to the park road, where a wide, mulched trail skirts the road and leads you back to the north parking lot where you began.

NEARBY ACTIVITIES

The West Woods hosts a variety of activities, from concerts to photography exhibits to children's nature programs. The Rookery, just north of here, offers more trails, including the Interurban Trail for hikers and bicyclists. More hiking in Geauga County can also be found at Beartown Lakes Reservation (see page 71) to the south.

Special thanks to the Geauga Park District naturalists, staff, and volunteers who reviewed this hike description.

22 WILLOUGHBY HAUNTS

KEY AT-A-GLANCE INFORMATION

LENGTH: 2 miles

CONFIGURATION: Loop

DIFFICULTY: Easy

SCENERY: Historical Western Reserve architecture, Chagrin River, perhaps a spirit or two

EXPOSURE: Almost entirely exposed

TRAFFIC: Moderately heavy, especially on warm evenings and weekends

TRAIL SURFACE: City sidewalks

HIKING TIME: 45 minutes or more depending on stopping/shopping

DRIVING DISTANCE: 26 miles from I-77/I-480 exchange

ACCESS: Public sidewalks

WHEELCHAIR TRAVERSABLE: Yes

MAPS: USGS Eastlake

FACILITIES: Public restrooms available inside library

CONTACT INFORMATION: Reach the city at (440) 951-2800 or willoughbyohio.com; learn more about Willoughby's haunts by taking the Willoughby Ghost Walk ([440] 710-4140; willoughbyghostwalk.com).

IN BRIEF

Evidently, some find Willoughby such an interesting town that they can't leave. Ever. Discover Willoughby's rich history and some of its more spirited spots on this city tour.

DESCRIPTION

Magazine articles that include Willoughby on their list of best places usually mention the city's charming downtown, which is listed on the National Register of Historic Places. The local historical society touts Willoughby's role in developing the modern traffic light, and residents enjoy its location, perched on the bank of the pretty Chagrin River, not far from Erie's shore. But who likes to talk about cadaver parts? Stinky canine apparitions? That's Cathi Weber's job.

As the owner of Willoughby Ghost Walk, Weber leads tours and investigates paranormal activity in Willoughby and throughout northeastern Ohio. Whether you believe in ghosts hardly matters—learning a little about the town's history and its historical streets will give you an appreciation for how residents have left their marks here.

Public parking is available at city hall and on several surrounding blocks. Starting from the three-way intersection of River

GPS Trailhead Coordinates

Latitude   41° 38.387403'

Longitude   81° 24.410219'

Directions

Take I-77 North to I-90 East, following signs for Erie, PA; take Exit 163 and then veer right onto OH 2 East. Exit at OH 640 East/Vine Street East. About 1 mile east of the exit, look for the public parking lot along Erie Street and Public Square.

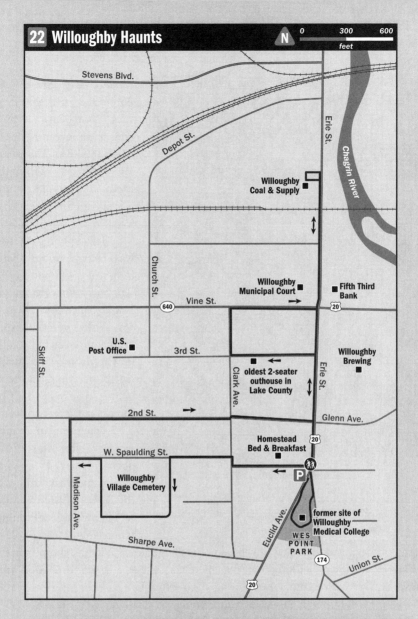

N

| 0 | 300 | 600 |

feet

Stevens Blvd.

Depot St.

Erie St.

Chagrin River

Willoughby
Coal & Supply

Church St.

Willoughby
Municipal Court

■ Fifth Third
Bank

640 Vine St. 20

Skiff St.

U.S.
Post Office

3rd St.

Willoughby
Brewing

Clark Ave.

oldest 2-seater
outhouse in
Lake County

Erie St.

2nd St.

Glenn Ave.

20

Homestead
Bed & Breakfast

W. Spaulding St.

Madison Ave.

Willoughby
Village Cemetery

P

Euclid Ave.

former site of
Willoughby
Medical College

WEST
POINT
PARK

Sharpe Ave.

174

Union St.

20

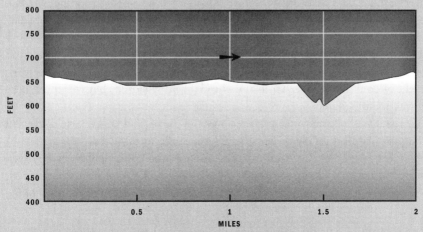

800				
750				
700				
650				
600				
550				
500				
450				
400				

FEET

0.5 1 1.5 2

MILES

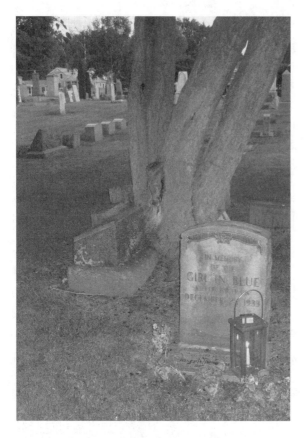

A pretty stranger was laid to rest by caring townspeople.

Street, Erie Street, and Public Square, you'll see Wes Point Park with its quaint bandstand. Behind it is the site of the former and infamous Willoughby Medical College, named for a doctor who never lived here.

To explain, the town was many things before it became known as Willoughby. First home to Native Americans, the town was settled in the 1750s by French pioneers who called it Charlton. The British called it Chagrin River, later Chagrin Mills, and then just Chagrin. Eventually, when the town postmaster (who was also a doctor) wanted to establish a medical college in town, he enlisted the help of Dr. Westel Willoughby Jr. of New York. To flatter the good doctor and entice him to support the medical college, the postmaster renamed the town Willoughby. The medical college got off to a good start; however, Dr. Willoughby never did move to Ohio.

After a few years, however, the school was plagued with rumors that the cadavers used by the students were a little *too* fresh. According to some oral histories, a widow was awakened one night by her dead husband, who was screaming that his grave had been robbed and he was being ripped limb from limb—a bad dream for the widow, and a public relations nightmare for the school. And unfortunately, some of the cadavers had been, uh, dug up from not so far away. The school couldn't recover from the scandal and it closed, but the town kept the good doctor's name.

Shake off the gruesome pictures in your head and cross Erie Street to Willoughby Public Library where the ghosts don't scream; they shush. Established in large part from an Andrew Carnegie grant in 1906, the library has been renovated at least twice in recent years. Each time seems to stir up some spirits, but reports suggest that they're all pretty congenial. Just east of the library along

Erie Street, turn left onto Spaulding Street.

The Homestead House Bed & Breakfast at 38111 West Spaulding Street was rebuilt after it was all but destroyed in a fire in 1883. A few of the charred beams in the basement remain, and evidently, so do some of its former residents. While the accommodations and hosts get high marks from all their guests, some also report hearing people on the stairs . . . when no other guests are inside. While sightings have been rare, those folks upstairs are usually dressed in Victorian-era clothing.

Continue west on Spaulding to the gates of Willoughby Village Cemetery, first opened in 1929. Among its occupants are nearly 100 Civil War veterans. While the vast majority of the cemetery plots here belong to people who lived in Willoughby for

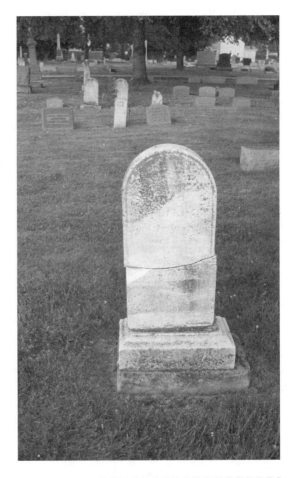

Is this cemetery haunted?

part or most of their lives, there's one very notable exception who—to everyone's understanding—spent just one night in this little town.

When the pretty young woman arrived by bus on December 23, 1933, she wore a blue hat, skirt, and sweater. Her reasons for visiting the town were somewhat mysterious and aren't fully understood today. She spent the night in a boarding house and, sadly, the next day she was killed by a train. Willoughby residents were distraught that not only had she died so young, and on Christmas Eve, but was also a stranger. A plot in the cemetery was donated, and her grave was well kept while townspeople made many attempts to learn who the stranger was. Almost five years passed before they were able to identify her. Today, her headstone lists both her given name (Josephine Klimczak) and The Girl in Blue. Visitors to the cemetery often report seeing a cloud of blue mist floating near her gravesite, and blue orbs sometimes appear in pictures of the spot.

When you leave the old cemetery, turn left onto Spaulding, and then right on Madison Avenue and right again on Second Street, following it back to Erie Street. As you venture farther north, turn left onto Third Street and try to locate the oldest home in Willoughby that's still standing: it's a beautifully restored burgundy-colored building on the north side of Third Street. Behind it you'll find the oldest *two-seat* outhouse in Lake County. And as if that doesn't make it unique enough, the odd but quaint little building is appointed with European stained-glass windows. Continue west to Clark Avenue, and then turn right again on Vine Street until you reach Erie Street (OH 20). Cross the street carefully so you can see The Willoughby Coal & Supply Co. at 3872 Erie Street.

The building began life in about 1890 as a flourmill; later it served as the town's first inn. Today it's an independently owned garden supply store and quite possibly still "home" to some of its former occupants. One, Don Norris, died in an accident (although no one's sure quite how) at the building's entrance; another, more recently departed than Mr. Norris, is a somewhat smelly but friendly dog named Yukon. He seems to just enjoy napping in the entryway.

Leave the furry spirit to get some rest as you turn around and stroll back along Vine Street, lined with at least two dozen unique restaurants and shops. Weber has interviewed many shop employees who have told her that they always feel like they have company in their stores—even when they are alone. Weber believes that it's quite possible spirits who had a very (ahem) spirited time in Willoughby during the Prohibition era may still be around—the basements of many of these shops housed speakeasies at that time.

Whatever spirit you're in when you visit, it's highly unlikely that you will find yourself alone in Willoughby, as the town is typically full of real, flesh-and-blood visitors enjoying the historical downtown.

NEARBY ACTIVITIES

Willoughby hosts many concerts and other events in its downtown area throughout the year. Call or check the city's website for upcoming events. Enjoy hiking along the river at Chagrin River Park (see page 76) or drive north to Fairport Harbor (see page 80) where you can visit a lighthouse that may be haunted by a cat.

Thanks to Cathi Weber, Willoughby's own ghost storyteller and founder of Willoughby Ghost Walk, for sharing her enthusiasm for the town and all of its residents—no matter what form they take.

The lighthouse at Fairport Harbor

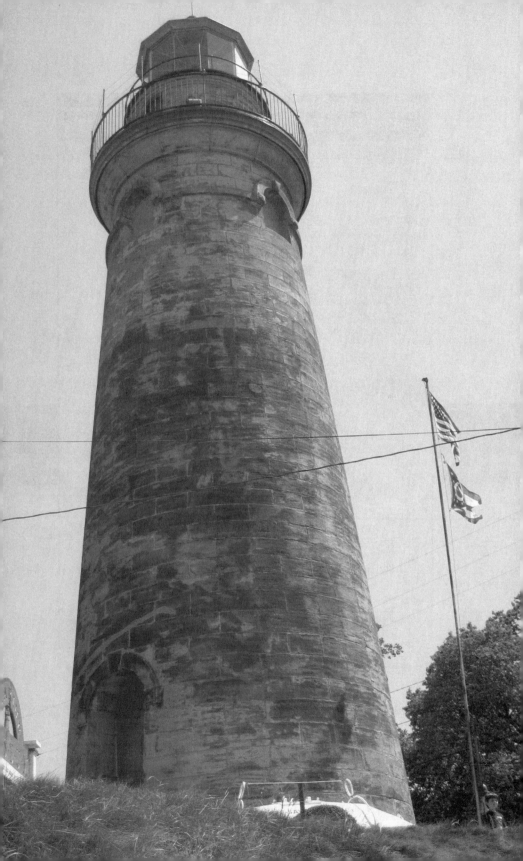

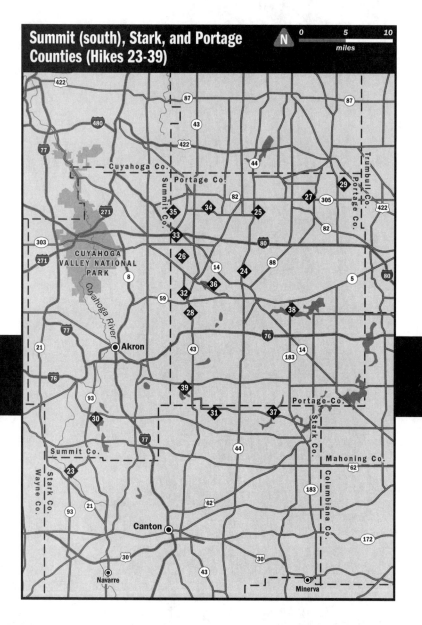

Summit (south), Stark, and Portage Counties (Hikes 23-39)

N

| 0 | 5 | 10 |

miles

422
87
87
480
43
77
422
44
Cuyahoga Co.
Portage Co.
29
271
Summit Co.
35 34 82 25 27 305
Trumbull Co.
Portage Co.
422
33
82
303
80
271
CUYAHOGA 26 88 5 80
VALLEY NATIONAL
PARK 14 24
8 36
Cuyahoga River 59 32
28 38
77
21 76
Akron 43 14 183
76
39
93
Portage Co.
30 31 37
Stark Co.
77
Summit Co. Mahoning Co.
23 62
Stark Co. 183
Wayne Co. 93 21 Columbiana Co.
62
Canton 172
30
30
Navarre 43
Minerva

SUMMIT (SOUTH), STARK, AND PORTAGE COUNTIES

23 CANAL FULTON, TOWPATH, AND OLDE MUSKINGUM TRAIL

 KEY AT-A-GLANCE INFORMATION

LENGTH: 5.5–11 miles

CONFIGURATION: Loop (or end-to-end with shuttle)

DIFFICULTY: Moderate

SCENERY: Historical town Canal Fulton; Tuscarawas Riverbed, with wildflowers and working canal lock

EXPOSURE: Mostly shaded; very exposed when leaves have fallen

TRAFFIC: Busy, especially on warm weekend afternoons

TRAIL SURFACE: Towpath, crushed limestone; Olde Muskingum, grass and gravel

HIKING TIME: 4.5–5 hours

DRIVING DISTANCE: 41 miles from I-77/I-480 exchange

ACCESS: Daily, sunrise–sunset

WHEELCHAIR TRAVERSABLE: Parts of Towpath rough but manageable

MAPS: USGS Canal Fulton; also at visitor center and starkparks.com

FACILITIES: Restrooms in visitor center and along Towpath

CONTACT INFORMATION: For *St. Helena* and Towpath, see discovercanalfulton.com or call (330) 854-5530. For Olde Muskingum, see starkparks.com or call (330) 477-3552.

IN BRIEF

Settled in the early 1800s, Canal Fulton has maintained and celebrated its rich canal history. Following the Towpath Trail on the eastern side of the river and the Olde Muskingum Trail on the west, hikers and bikers can enjoy historical landmarks and scenic views on both sides of the Tuscarawas River.

DESCRIPTION

As you step up onto Towpath Trail in Canal Fulton, you may plod alongside a couple of draft horses pulling the *St. Helena*, a restored canalboat. About 1 mile south of your starting point, you'll lose the horses and find a canal lock that still works. If you're lucky, you might catch a live lock demonstration, thanks to the Canal Fulton Heritage Society. Even if you don't see the demo, stop at Lock 4 and read the interpretive sign.

Continue south, enjoying the view as you stroll along about 10 feet above both the canal bed on your left and the river on your right. In many places from this point south, the canal bed is overgrown with cattails and duckweed, providing a haven for birds, butterflies, and ducks. Pick a quiet evening for your trip and you're almost certain to see warblers, finches, robins, jays, and cardinals.

GPS Trailhead
Coordinates
Latitude   40° 53.266983'
Longitude 81° 35.819099'

Directions ───────────────▶

Follow I-77 South toward Akron and take Exit 136/OH 21 south to Massillon. Turn left onto Arcadia Street NW, which becomes Cherry Street West. Follow Cherry to Tuscarawas Street Northwest. Turn left into the parking area for Canalway Visitor Center and the *St. Helena* boarding area.

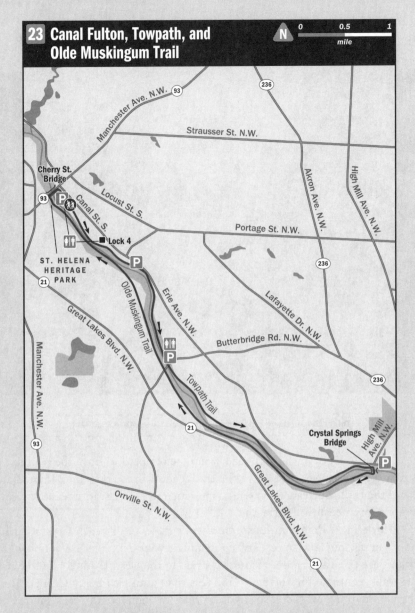

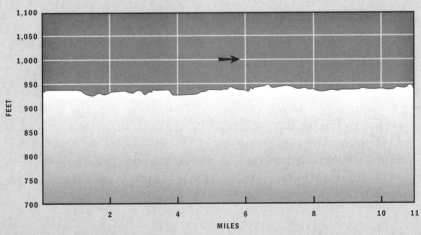

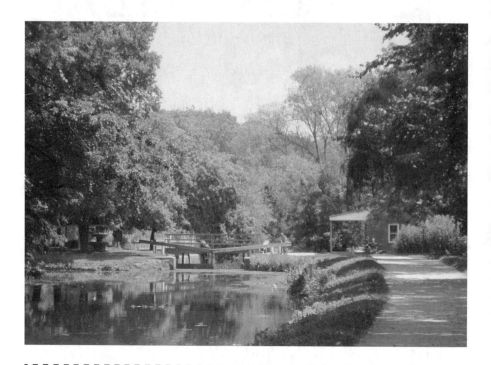

This section of the trail was created as a canal towpath in 1825–1827.

One mile south of the trailhead, you'll be tempted to leave the trail for the shops at Butterbridge, just east of the trailhead of the same name. Immediately west of the trail, a private farm with a majestic red barn paints a scene typical of Stark County's beautiful farmland.

A little more than 5 miles south of your start, you'll reach Crystal Springs Bridge, an obvious spot to rest and contemplate your next move. A couple of restaurants are open to visitors across the street to the west. If you'd like to extend your walk, continue on Towpath Trail less than a mile to Forty Corners Road. (There's a parking lot there, so if you'd prefer to complete this as a shuttle, you can.) Before going anywhere else, however, you'll probably want to learn more about the bridge.

Built in 1914, the iron bridge replaced one damaged in a flood. The slightly newer iron grid floor has an almost lacy appearance. In 1996 the bridge was saved from demolition and the area around it was designated Crystal Springs Bridge Park. This small park—no facilities are here other than a convenient spot for the canoe livery to collect tired paddlers—closes the gap between the Olde Muskingum Trail on the west and the Towpath Trail on the east bank of the river, creating an obvious loop for hikers who want to get two different perspectives on Canal Fulton's history. The route described here follows this loop, so turn right, crossing Crystal Springs Bridge to the north, and then turn right again to travel north on the rail-trail.

(*Note:* Here you cross paths with the southern portion of the Akron Little Loop of the Buckeye Trail, so you may notice blue paint on nearby trees.)

If you've timed your hike correctly, you'll be able to watch the sun sink slowly in the sky as you head back to Canal Fulton. Stretches of farmland reach out to the west; the panorama is quite pretty. Toads, rabbits, and deer will join you, bumping along this old railroad right-of-way. You may also share the road with horses, as equestrian traffic is allowed all along the Olde Muskingum Trail, which is managed by Stark County Parks.

After crossing to the north side of Butterbridge Road, the trail winds back by Community Park, bending slightly to the right before depositing you onto Cherry Street. Turn right and cross over the bridge, heading east. Pause to look upstream, and perhaps to wave at a canoe as it drifts under the bridge that has carried traffic through town for nearly 100 years.

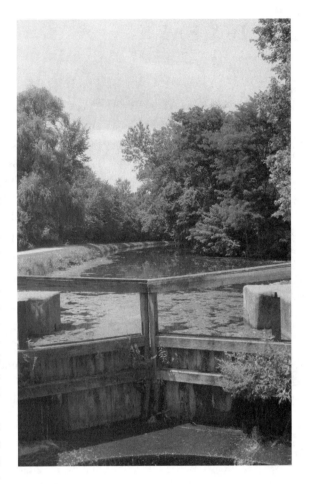

The view from inside a still-working canal lock

NEARBY ACTIVITIES

Canal Fulton was incorporated in 1814, and visitors can relish a sort of time-warp feeling here, walking along brick streets lined with historical street lamps. From May through September, the *St. Helena* offers an authentic canalboat ride experience; call (330) 854-3808 for a schedule and rates. Those who prefer to paddle down the river can rent canoes from a livery just north of Community Park.

Budding botanists may want to visit Jackson Bog, just 2 miles east of Crystal Springs Bridge. The bog is managed as a state nature preserve; more than 20 endangered plants can be viewed from its 1.3-mile boardwalk trail.

24 DIX PARK

KEY AT-A-GLANCE INFORMATION

LENGTH: 2.2 miles

CONFIGURATION: Out-and-back connecting a loop

DIFFICULTY: Easy

SCENERY: Working farm, plus a variety of trees and spring wildflowers

EXPOSURE: Mostly shaded

TRAFFIC: Moderate

TRAIL SURFACE: Trillium Trail and Fox Loop, dirt; Farm Lane, gravel

HIKING TIME: 45–50 minutes

DRIVING DISTANCE: 35 miles from I-77/I-480 exchange

ACCESS: Daily, sunrise–sunset; no bikes or horses permitted, and farm fields not open for public use. On occasion, agricultural activity may temporarily close the Farm Lane and subsequently the other trails.

WHEELCHAIR TRAVERSABLE: No

MAPS: USGS Ravenna; also posted at trailhead and portagepark district.org

FACILITIES: Picnic tables in parking lot; portable restroom

CONTACT INFORMATION: To check on farming activity before you go, call the Portage Park District at (330) 297-7728. Other information can be found at portageparkdistrict.org.

- -

GPS Trailhead Coordinates

Latitude   41° 11.399217'

Longitude   81° 14.690580'

IN BRIEF

This small, unique Portage Park District property offers a short woodlands trail set amid lovely farm fields. Depending on the time of year, you may get to watch planting, harvesting, or other farmwork. Go in the early spring to enjoy the best wildflower display.

DESCRIPTION

In 2000, the Dix family donated the property and funds to create a new county park in memory of Robert Dix. There was one request, however: that the neighboring dairy located on a 25-acre portion of the land be allowed to continue operations. The park district agreed, and Dix Park came into being. While the farm operations are not part of any formal programming, visitors can gain a little understanding of what a working farm looks like while making their way to rich woodland trails.

A trail system loops through approximately 60 of the park's 103 acres. Bluebird nesting boxes sit near the parking lot; the rest of the property has been left for cultivation.

From the parking lot, follow Farm Lane east. This lane is in use by the farm, and hikers will occasionally meet farm equipment here. This is the most exposed portion of the hike, and good birding opportunities exist along the hedgerow that parallels the gravel lane. The farm is on your left; maple and cherry trees line the fields of corn, soybeans, and hay.

About 0.6 miles east of the parking lot, a trail sign invites you to turn left onto Trillium

- -

Directions ────────────────→

Take I-77 South to I-80 East. Take turnpike Exit 193 to OH 44 south. The park entrance is about 4 miles south of the turnpike exit.

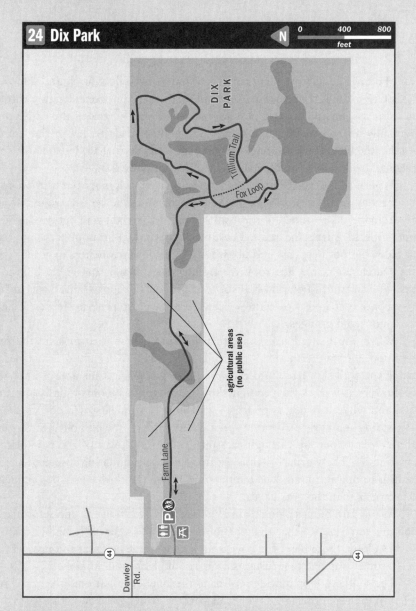

N

0   400   800
feet

DIX PARK

Trillium Trail

Fox Loop

agricultural areas
(no public use)

Farm Lane

P

44

Dawley Rd.

44

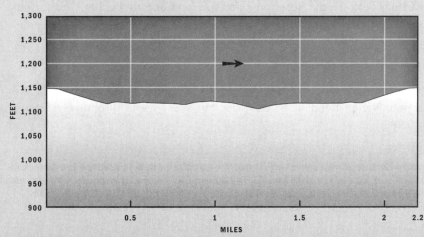

1,300
1,250
1,200
1,150
1,100
1,050
1,000
950
900

FEET

0.5   1   1.5   2   2.2

MILES

Trail. Follow the narrow dirt trail as it wanders by yellow birch and a few sassafras trees. You'll tramp across footbridges to save you from slogging through the wettest spots in the trail. What looks like a small creek in the early spring is actually an ephemeral (or seasonal) water flow. Usually dry in the summer months, the temporary drainage provides a perfect setting for buttonbush and a breeding ground for a number of winged insects as well.

Typical of Portage County, the woods here are rich in glacial history. You'll notice many small erratics strewn about as you skirt the higher ground around the drainage depression. As the trail bends to the right and returns to Farm Lane, look for sugar and red maples, black cherries, tulip poplars, white oaks, red oaks, bigtooth aspens, and dogwoods. Wildflower watchers may spot trilliums, Dutchman's breeches, toothworts, anemones, marsh marigolds, blue cohoshes, violets, trout lilies, and bellworts. See if you can spot a spicebush. Its light brown bark is coated with white speckles, and when you rub the leaves, it smells like lemons and oranges.

When you reach Farm Lane, turn left and follow it to pick up the short Fox Loop, the southernmost of the trails here. You'll turn right off the lane, following the trail sign back into the woods. In the spring, this area is alive with wildflowers as well as the peculiar skunk cabbage. Its blooms usually appear in May, and while it is not as pretty as wildflowers, it has its own odd charm. In early spring—as early as February in a warm winter—the bulbous heads of new cabbage plants pop up through the soil. Inside the flower of the new plant, it warms itself. The warmth is thought to appeal to pollinating insects that need the heat to move around. The temperature inside the flower may be as much as 10° warmer than the outside air.

As the path bumps along through the woods, wildflowers, and self-warming cabbage, you'll notice that this portion of the trail is generally higher than the northern loop. From here, you have a good view of the landscape in progress and the seasonal drainage that sustains a variety of plants and animals.

The southern loop quickly returns to the lane. Turn left onto the gravel road to return to the parking lot. As you walk past the farm fields again, it's easy to draw comparisons between the water flow and the farm operations. Both are seasonal and supply the land—and the park—with a measure of diversity and richness.

NEARBY ACTIVITIES

To explore more woodland trails, visit nearby Towner's Woods (see page 171) or go north to Nelson-Kennedy Ledges State Park (see page 139) for a very different hiking experience.

Thanks to Portage Park District (PPD) staffer Brad Stemen, who created the trail, for a special tour of Dix Park and for identifying many of its natural attractions. Thanks also to PPD executive director Christine Craycroft for reviewing this hike description.

HEADWATERS TRAIL 25

IN BRIEF

This rail-trail in Portage County makes for peaceful, easy walking (as well as jogging and biking). Running east and west between Mantua and Garrettsville, it abuts the Mantua Bog and Marsh Wetlands state nature preserves, making it a great trail for bird-watching.

DESCRIPTION

Step onto the crushed limestone trail, walk up a short slope to meet the old rail bed, and turn left to head east. The trail more or less follows Eagle Creek, a tributary of the Mahoning River, but you won't see much of it.

Starting 0.5 miles east of the trailhead, you'll reach the northwestern edge of the 152-acre Marsh Wetlands State Nature Preserve. On the west side of Peck, you'll walk alongside a different wetland—Mantua Bog (actually an alkaline fen). It was designated as a National Natural Landmark in 1976 and as a state nature preserve in 1990. Both the wetlands and the bog are protected by the Ohio Department of Natural Resources and are open by permit only. So, while you can't see the beavers in the marsh or the cranberries in the bog, you can enjoy the migrating waterfowl as you stroll by the edge of these protected areas. You might also find a generously

KEY AT-A-GLANCE INFORMATION

LENGTH: 7 miles with options to extend

CONFIGURATION: End-to-end; out-and-back approximately 16 miles

DIFFICULTY: Easy

SCENERY: Beech forests, creek ravine, lots of waterfowl; Western Reserve architecture in Mantua and Garrettsville is worth a look too

EXPOSURE: About half exposed

TRAFFIC: Moderate

TRAIL SURFACE: Crushed limestone

HIKING TIME: 3 hours

DRIVING DISTANCE: 32 miles from I-77/I-480 exchange

ACCESS: Daily, sunrise–sunset; pets must be leashed; horses and bikes frequent the trail.

WHEELCHAIR TRAVERSABLE: No

MAPS: USGS Garrettsville and Hiram; also available at portageparkdistrict.org

FACILITIES: Restrooms and water available at trailheads at Buchert Park in Mantua and Garrettsville Village Park

CONTACT INFORMATION: For more information, see portagepark district.org or call (330) 297-7728.

Directions ⟶

From I-77 head east on I-480 to Exit 26/US 422 East (follow signs toward Warren). Take OH 44 south toward Ravenna approximately 7 miles, and then turn left onto East High Street in Mantua, where trailhead parking is available on the south side of the road. Additional parking is available behind the McDonald's Restaurant on OH 44, south of Mennonite Road.

GPS Trailhead Coordinates

Latitude 41° 17.013237'

Longitude 81° 12.985382'

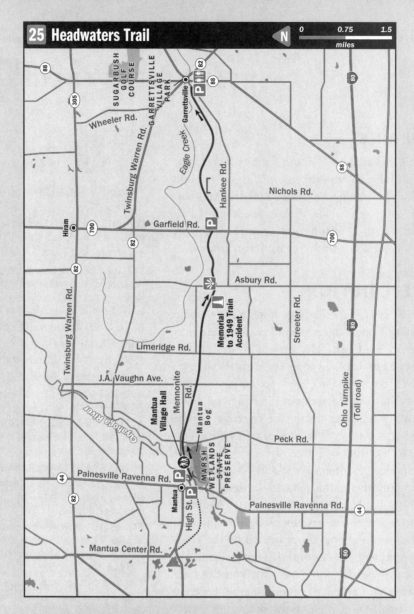

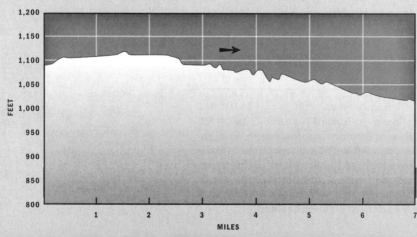

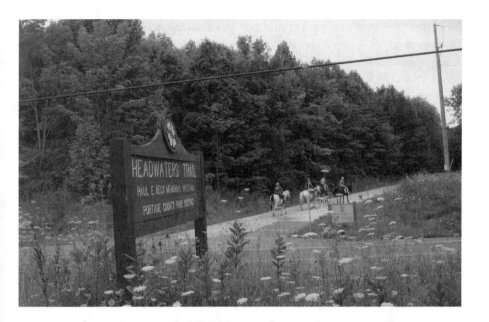

Share the trail with equestrians.

sized garter snake, or even a skunk that has wandered away from its protected habitat to gawk at the funny two-legged creatures plodding along the trail.

Along this stretch you'll probably notice some sights indicative of 21st-century trailways, such as a horse grazing on one side of the road and a mini-storage facility or a convenience store on the other. Keep going, and be happy that the trail managed to cut a swath through this interesting place and time.

About a mile into the hike, the trail offers some gradual changes of scenery: shallow but pretty ravines, cornfields, and a mix of both old and new homesites.

As you pass Vaughn Avenue heading east, you'll soon cross the Lake Erie–Ohio River Divide. While it hardly marks a cosmic shift, trivia fans should note that water east of here flows into the Ohio River, while waters west of here make their way to Lake Erie. Most hikers will notice instead—depending on the season—cattails, thistles, and other delicious butterfly food growing on either side of the trail.

This portion of the trail east of Limeridge Road is nestled in between banks of tall trees, which may make your trek feel extra dark and quiet. It's easy to forget that this trail came about largely thanks to the railroad that came through here long ago. A reminder is coming up: on the south side of the trail you'll soon see a large rock with a plaque describing a deadly train accident in 1949. After reading the somber story, you'll head up an ever-so-gentle slope to reach a clearing and greet Asbury Road. Stop and look north to enjoy a lovely vista.

Continuing east, you'll notice that the landscape changes on both sides of the trail rather quickly. Now instead of being flanked by banks of trees, you can look into a ravine on either side of the trail. (It's steep in places, a good reminder to stay on the trail.) For less than a mile, the trail follows along a wide access road for several private driveways—it sees very light traffic, but hikers should be aware and especially alert on this stretch.

Less than a mile farther down the trail, you'll reach OH 700, where additional parking is available. (This is a good place to park a shuttle vehicle if you're not sure that your hiking group is up for the full 7 miles.) At this intersection you'll also notice signs marking a spot where the Buckeye Trail joins Headwaters Trail for a time. It's a pretty spot to end your hike, and there's no need to feel like a quitter because you've logged more than 4 miles since leaving Mantua at OH 44. If you continue on, you'll reach the official end of the trail about 3 miles east, behind Garrettsville Village Park, another spot you can park a shuttle vehicle. In the late summer, you'll find big milkweed pods at the end of the trail (more butterfly food!) and quite possibly get to watch a ball game in progress.

Whether you walk, ride, or drive back to Mantua, you'll have great sunset views for company in the late afternoon or evening. Upon your return to Mantua, you can continue east on the path about 0.5 miles toward town to find a pretty footbridge. When you cross it and follow the path to the right, you'll see a wooden deck on the north side of the river that's perfect for fishing, reading, conversation, and contemplation.

You can also choose to continue on Headwaters Trail east another mile, at least—the trail is young and still growing! Enjoy.

NEARBY ACTIVITIES

Interested in Western Reserve history? Have a look around Garrettsville, which, like Hiram and Mantua, was settled before Ohio became a state in 1803. All three towns conjure up visions of New England—including central village squares with imposing churches surrounded by large frame-style houses.

Garrettsville came into being when John Garrett of Christian Hundred, Delaware, purchased 300 acres of land in Nelson, obtaining Silver Creek waterpower rights so he could build a gristmill. Unfortunately, Garrett soon died of pneumonia, but Mrs. Garrett managed the mill, and it and the town thrived. A clock from the gristmill-era still chimes at the corner of Main and Center streets. And before you leave Garrettsville, you might want to pick up a pack of Lifesavers. Clarence Crane invented the candy here in 1912.

More hiking can be found at Eagle Creek State Nature Preserve, heading east from the village by way of Center Street to Hopkins Road. The preserve is open sunrise–sunset year-round; call (330) 527-5118 or see **ohiodnr.com** for more information. (Note that no pets are allowed in the nature preserve.) Also nearby: the not-so-flat Nelson-Kennedy Ledges State Park (see page 139).

Special thanks to Christine Craycroft, executive director of the Portage Park District, for reviewing this section.

HERRICK STATE NATURE PRESERVE 26

IN BRIEF

Who knew carnivorous plants could be so cute? Who knew beavers could cause such trouble? As pretty and peaceful as this place is, you may not notice the battles raging all around you. This fen harbors the tiny insect-eating sundew plants, endangered bayberries, and rare sedges. While only careful observers will spot many of the rare and endangered species here, the tamarack trees are easier to spot. Tamaracks, Ohio's only native deciduous conifer, are not evergreen. They have needles that turn bright yellow in autumn and then fall off. Visit in autumn to see the tamaracks' remarkable display; visit anytime to watch for birds and stay, perhaps, for a sunset.

DESCRIPTION

If you know the difference between a fen and a bog, you probably paid very close attention in biology class. (Unfortunately, I didn't.) While bogs, swamps, fens, and other wetlands have some commonalities, they're not the same.

So what is the difference between a bog and a fen? An overly simplified explanation: A fen is alkaline and a bog is acidic. Both areas are ecologically important, too scarce these days, and generally damp. Bogs receive their water from aboveground sources (mostly

KEY AT-A-GLANCE INFORMATION

LENGTH: 1.5 miles

CONFIGURATION: Out-and-back, with a small turnaround loop

DIFFICULTY: Easy

SCENERY: Rare plants, herons, beavers, muskrats; good bird-watching

EXPOSURE: Mostly shaded

TRAFFIC: Moderate

TRAIL SURFACE: Wooden boardwalks and dirt trail

HIKING TIME: 45 minutes

DRIVING DISTANCE: 28 miles from I-77/I-480 exchange

ACCESS: Daily, sunrise–sunset; pets, bicycles, and motorized vehicles prohibited

WHEELCHAIR TRAVERSABLE: The northernmost portion allows handicapped-equipped vans to access the boardwalk, but the gate to the road is locked. To arrange access, contact the Nature Conservancy through nature.org. ADA-compliant boardwalk has turnaround points.

MAPS: USGS Kent

FACILITIES: None

CONTACT INFORMATION: Owned by Kent State University and managed by the Nature Conservancy. Visit nature.org or call (614) 717-2770.

Directions

Follow I-480 East to OH 14 in Streetsboro. Turn right onto OH 43, following it 0.2 miles to Seasons Road. Turn right. Approximately 2 miles west of OH 43, Seasons Road curves sharply to the left and crosses a railroad track. Turn left into the preserve access driveway on the eastern side of Seasons. Follow the drive past a stream crossing to the small parking lot on the right.

GPS Trailhead Coordinates

Latitude 41° 12.839098'

Longitude 81° 22.267921'

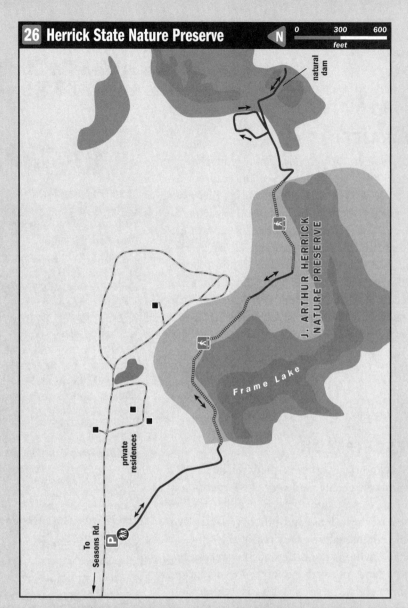

N

0   300   600
feet

natural dam

J. ARTHUR HERRICK NATURE PRESERVE

Frame Lake

private residences

To Seasons Rd.

P

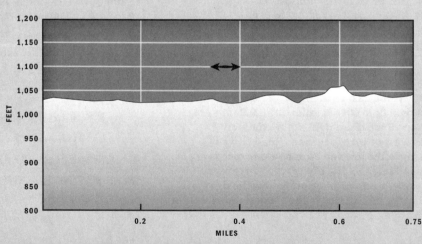

1,200
1,150
1,100
1,050
1,000
950
900
850
800

FEET

0.2   0.4   0.6   0.75
MILES

rain and snow), and they may have a surface outflow. Groundwater seeps and springs, usually coming out of permeable glacial deposits, feed fens. True bogs are isolated from groundwater—sometimes from impermeable soil conditions but often also from an impermeable layer of compressed, humified peat. Peat is what really sets bogs and fens apart from other wetlands. Peat, combined with the continual wetness, causes and perpetuates extreme soil conditions. You don't have to be a science whiz to realize that different types of plants live in alkaline and acidic soils. But shades of gray exist in nature, and in the relative acidity of bogs and fens. Because bogs and fens are both generally wet with nutrient-poor soil, some plants exist in both, and some of those species cannot exist anywhere else. This concludes the science lesson; now it's time for a field trip. Well, make that fen trip.

While the fen isn't well marked from the road, the drive can be found just east of a (privately owned) red barn. The barn sits on a small hill on the eastern end of the preserve and trailhead. Follow the wide gravel path past tall marsh grass and seasonal wildflowers. When the goldenrods explode under a sunny fall sky, the scene is as colorful and glossy as a still-wet painting. But behind the pretty picture, there is turmoil. Battles rage, quietly but constantly, among the fen's inhabitants.

About 0.2 miles from the trailhead, you'll come to a large stone recognizing the work of the Nature Conservancy and the Akron Garden Club in preserving this land. Step onto the boardwalk, where you'll have a chance to stop at three inviting benches. These are good seats for watching the herons and marsh wrens that commonly appear here. Believe it or not, these seats are in the middle of the battlefield.

A few cattails appear here and there, almost like sentries on guard along the boardwalk. But are they here to protect or invade? The answer depends on whom you ask. Cattails provide high-energy food for migratory birds and butterflies; so birds and butterflies, and people who watch them, may root for the cattails. But the answer also depends on the type of cattails. Some are native and nonaggressive, content to enjoy their view of the fen without overtaking it. Other cattail species are invasive and quite aggressive, threatening some of the fen's indigenous plants. What needs protection here? Bayberries, for one, are on the state's list of endangered plants. This fen is one of just three spots in Ohio where it grows. Unfortunately, the cattails and bayberries aren't the only species at odds in this preserve. The invasive cattails and reed canarygrass threaten the open fen as a whole, driving out the sedge meadow and shrubby cinquefoils. Glossy buckthorns, small trees or large shrubs (distinguished by their shiny oval leaves and speckled bark), threaten the tamarack population as well as the bayberries. The skirmishes among the plants and animals here started long ago, and along the way, people have stepped in—for better or for worse.

The lakes and dams on this property—although on portions not open to the public—date back to the 1940s and 1950s, when the Frame family raised

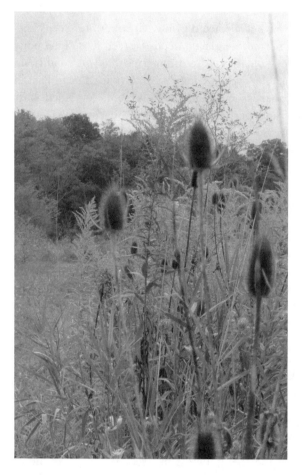

Native and alien species vie for space at Herrick Fen.

mink and muskrats here. J. Arthur Herrick bought the initial tract of land that would form the preserve in 1969; for some time after that the area was known as Frame Lake Bog. The muskrats (who didn't care what the place was called) stayed, and beavers joined them. But beavers, like cattails, can be troublemakers. Beaver dams cause the water levels to rise, threatening the tamarack population. The tamaracks in this fen comprise one of the few reproducing populations of this tree in the country.

What can—and what should—be done to tip the balance in favor of the bayberries and the tamaracks? Again, the answers vary depending on whom you ask, and a resolution is not expected in the near future. The good news is that the fen has been preserved, so the battles may continue. The Nature Conservancy sends aid in the form of volunteers. They diligently thin the ranks of invaders in hopes that the natives can continue to fight for themselves. While some of the natives are under duress, the volunteers who visit typically report finding the battlegrounds overwhelmingly beautiful. So march on . . .

As you continue south on the boardwalk, tamarack trees line the trail; you're likely to see or hear a catbird at this point. It's easy to spot the mayapples and skunk cabbages growing along the boardwalk. Skunk cabbage is probably most noticeable in the spring, thanks to its white flower that resembles a lily. In the fall, however, its fruit is worth a look. Waxy and dark brown, with a hint of purple, its shape might be described as oblong, somewhat reminiscent of a hand grenade (in keeping with the battlefield imagery).

Notice, too, the fen-loving shrubby cinquefoils, whose bright yellow flowers bloom from spring through mid-summer. You'll have to look hard for the less common sundews, small but mighty carnivorous plants resembling a sunburst. When an insect lands on the plant's hairy, sticky leaves, it triggers an enzyme reaction that makes a leaf grow very quickly—so quickly that it wraps up the insect like a burrito before absorbing the bug's nutrients. Another unusual plant to look for is turtlehead. It has dark, waxy, green stems and white flowers. Each bloom is about a half-inch long. When viewed from the side, with just a bit of imagination, the bloom indeed forms the outline of a turtle's head. Also look for poison sumac, cousin to the more common sumacs that only occur in fens. (Admire, but don't touch it if you are remotely sensitive to poison ivy!)

Just 0.4 miles into the trail, the boardwalk ends, and you'll step down onto a narrow, rooty dirt trail that winds between the base of a wooded hill and the shrub swamp. Soon, the boardwalk begins again, curves to the left, and then redeposits you on the dirt trail.

The hard-packed dirt path bends left, leading you up a small hill into a beech-maple wood that offers color-charged spring wildflower displays. Circling back down the hill you'll find two shallow lakes separated by a narrow dam. The water levels are dropping here, by design. Releasing the dams that created the man-made lakes allows more native wet meadow plants to return.

The trail loop rejoins the original path at this point; you will retrace your steps back to the boardwalk and return home from here. You probably won't have any war stories to tell when you return, but you should bring home some lovely pictures.

NEARBY ACTIVITIES

This nature preserve sits about 5 miles north of Towner's Woods (see page 171) and about 5 miles south of Tinker's Creek State Nature Preserve in Aurora/Streetsboro (see page 167).

Special thanks to Nature Conservancy volunteer Mark Purdy for plant identification and insight into the ongoing battles at Herrick Fen. Interested in volunteering to protect Ohio's natives? Contact the Nature Conservancy at nature.org.

27 HIRAM FIELD STATION

KEY AT-A-GLANCE INFORMATION

LENGTH: 4.5 miles

CONFIGURATION: Loop

DIFFICULTY: Moderate

SCENERY: Wide variety of trees, ferns, wildflowers, wildlife

EXPOSURE: Mostly shaded

TRAFFIC: Light

TRAIL SURFACE: Dirt and leaves

HIKING TIME: 1.5 hours

DRIVING DISTANCE: 36 miles from I-77/I-480 exchange

ACCESS: Daily, sunrise–sunset; dogs on leash are permitted, but bikes, horses, and motorized vehicles are not.

WHEELCHAIR TRAVERSABLE: No

MAPS: USGS Mantua; also posted at the trailhead and available inside Frohring Laboratory Building

FACILITIES: Public restrooms in the lab building/interpretive center near entrance to the trail; emergency phones available on the Hiram College campus

CONTACT INFORMATION: As part of Hiram's outreach program, the field station offers educational visits for preschool through high school students. For information, call (330) 569-6003.

IN BRIEF

Wandering through these woods, you can breathe easy. One of the largest beech-maple forests in Ohio, the Hiram College Field Station is quiet, beautiful, and teeming with diverse plant and animal life. Watch for barred owls and pileated woodpeckers in the trees.

DESCRIPTION

If urban sprawl is getting to you, this is the place to come. The woods are thick and quiet, and the trail is not well worn. Established in 1967 by Hiram College, the James H. Barrow Field Station is one of the largest forests of its kind in Ohio and the fourth largest in the United States. The 260 acres of woods are essentially an oxygen factory situated between Cleveland and Youngstown's industrial development, where you can get a lungful of scents, including pine, sassafras, and other truly organic smells.

Start your hike in the small gravel parking lot by the green museum building known as Frohring Lab. Inside, you'll learn about some of the animals you're likely to find on the trail, such as the American toad and the painted turtle.

From the museum, take the gravel road west to the Observation Building. There, on the edge of a pond, you can enjoy watching

GPS Trailhead Coordinates

Latitude   41° 18.389761'

Longitude   81° 6.715379'

Directions

Take I-480 East to Exit 26/US 422. Follow US 422 east (toward Solon) to OH 44, heading south toward Ravenna. At OH 82, turn left to head east and veer left to continue onto OH 305 (Wakefield Road). Turn right onto Wheeler Road. The entrance to the James H. Barrow Field Station will be on your right.

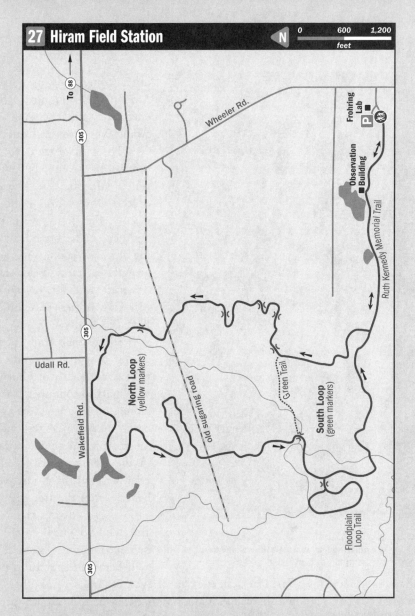

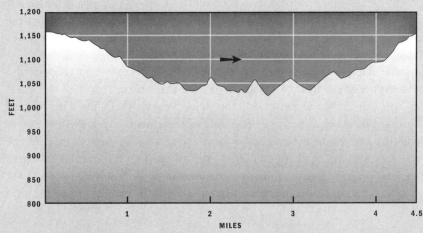

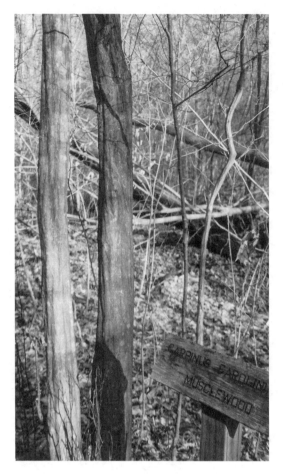

Take a quiet, educational walk through the forest.

birds from inside or outside. Among the wild birds you'll encounter, a pair of trumpeter swans lives here year-round.

The official trail sign for the Ruth E. Kennedy Memorial Trail stands to the left of the Observation Building. Follow the signs west past another smaller pond. Walking through young but dense growth, a farm field slants down to your left, revealing a nice view of the gentle hills of Portage County.

Soon the trail begins to roll downhill as well. The path is not well worn but it is well marked. Numbered signs along the South Loop (with green markers) correspond to an interpretive guide available in the lab/interpretive center. Even without the guide, you'll benefit from the tree identification signs listing the common and botanical names for some common species. They will help you spot tulip poplars, white pines, sassafras, black cherries, musclewoods, and several others. As the trail begins to go up a slight hill, a junction occurs where the South (green) and North (yellow) loops split. Here, at about the 1-mile point, you can turn left to follow the shorter green trail (about a 2-mile loop), but this hike follows the longer (4-mile) yellow trail by veering right. Follow the longer trail as it heads east, then wiggles north, from here.

As you wiggle with the trail, five little platform bridges help you through the softer spots of the trail. You're on your own at a stream crossing—but don't worry. You can cross the shallow, 3-foot-wide expanse with the aid of a few large rocks. Like a beacon on the other side of the stream, a yellow tree marker tells you that you're going the right way. Soon after crossing the stream, you'll be able to hear cars passing along OH 305 to the north. That's about the only time that civilization will re-enter your thoughts on this trail.

You'll soon cross a long narrow clearing (a right-of-way for communication utilities). The trail continues north toward OH 305 and crosses an old sugaring road; continue west. A map posted by this dirt road crossing indicates that you've gone about 2 miles. The trail parallels OH 305 for a few more steps before bending left (south), taking you into a dense wood.

Pines, pin oaks, and Christmas ferns keep you company as you head, generally, south. But to go south, you must zigzag along each wiggle of the tributaries here on the forest floor.

While you're generally heading south, several sharp turns in the trail may shake your sense of direction; just wiggle on down the path to cross another footbridge where the path seems to narrow.

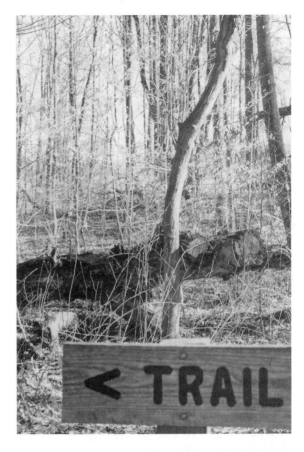

Wear boots here; you'll need them to splash through the creek.

The trees that grow along here are young and skinny, so although they don't impose on you with their size, they do give the unmistakable impression that you are outnumbered.

As you proceed, this thick forest of slender trees changes to the more mature forest of fewer, more widely spaced trees similar to those you encountered at the start of the trail. You'll head up a slight hill and then go down a fun, sharp incline to cross another small stream. No bridge; no problem. The rocks make for another easy crossing. Across the stream, a map indicates that 1.7 kilometers (about 1 mile) remains ahead of you. The trail goes right, then up a few steps, to reach a bench overlooking a floodplain and stream.

After descending a steeper set of stairs, the yellow and green trails meet again, sharing a single path heading south by southwest. You're heading downstream, at this point, along the shallow but friendly creek. Its babble provides a bit of conversation here in the middle of the woods.

Soon you'll reach a large wooden bridge marking the intersection of the short (0.3-mile) Floodplain Loop Trail. Turn right and follow the loop around and return to the bridge and main trail. Just beyond the Floodplain Loop Trail, you'll traverse a boardwalk over a wetland of cinnamon ferns. The trail curves right from here as it follows Silver Creek. Another small footbridge across a tributary leads to a crooked bench, which has shifted due to erosion from high flows in the creek. (Sit down and it's almost guaranteed to alter your perspective!) Moving on, you'll cross the creek again and bound over a pair of bouncy wooden bridges, bearing left and uphill a bit to reach another observation bench. Walking on acorns, you'll pass shagbark hickory trees as the path twists right, then left, then right again before leveling out to find a bitternut hickory tree. You'll travel about 0.3 miles up a gradual slope to reach the second-highest point of the field station.

There, you'll see grapevines that create a natural arch—you may need to duck to walk under it. Soon after you'll come to a grove of white pines and the sign marking the point where the yellow and green trails originally split. They join again by a dogwood tree. At this point, you've logged about 4.3 miles. From here, you'll follow the trail back to the smaller pond, then east past the observation pond, reaching the Observation Building. Follow the driveway east back to the green lab building and to the parking area where you began your exploration.

NEARBY ACTIVITIES

Before leaving Hiram, you may want to tour the college and the town, both of which reflect their Western Reserve heritage. You may also want to visit the Headwaters Trail (see page 121), about a five-minute drive from the field station. To get there, follow Wheeler Road south to Twinsburg-Warren Road (OH 82). Turn right, heading west to OH 700. Turn left and follow OH 700 south about 1 mile to the bike/hike trail parking lot.

Special thanks to James H. Barrow Field Station associate director Laura Collins for supplying additional information on the station and for reviewing this hike description.

KENT BOG (COOPERRIDER) STATE NATURE PRESERVE 28

IN BRIEF

Kent Bog is one of only three places in Ohio where small cranberries make a stand. It is also home to what may be the largest stand of tamarack trees in Ohio and is possibly the southernmost grouping of the trees in all of the United States. Ancient history and modern technology are both on display here: visitors can see what's left of this 12,000-year-old bog from a boardwalk made of recycled plastic.

DESCRIPTION

Long, long ago, a retreating glacier left behind a giant ice cube. It was buried with silt, clay, and gravel. Eventually, the ice melted, forming a glacial kettle lake. Over the next 10,000 years or so, the lake was covered by boreal plants and then completely filled in with peat. Today, in what is left of that ice cube, a tiny bog hosts rare plants, including sphagnum moss, Virginia chain ferns, small cranberries, and tamarack trees. It is the best stand of tamaracks in Ohio and probably the southernmost stand of tamaracks in the continental United States. It is a bog full of history, firsts, and rarities.

In 1985 Kent Bog (Cooperrider) State Nature Preserve was the first state nature preserve purchased with money donated by Ohioans through the state income tax refund

KEY AT-A-GLANCE INFORMATION

LENGTH: 0.5 miles

CONFIGURATION: Loop

DIFFICULTY: Easy

SCENERY: Rare bog plants and the birds and animals that relish them

EXPOSURE: About half shaded

TRAFFIC: Moderate

TRAIL SURFACE: Flat boardwalk trail

HIKING TIME: 30 minutes

DRIVING DISTANCE: 33 miles from I-77/I-480 exchange

ACCESS: The bog is open sunrise–sunset, but sometimes the gate is locked; when the lot is closed during open hours, you may park on the grassy shoulder of Meloy Road. Pets, bikes, and skates are prohibited here.

WHEELCHAIR TRAVERSABLE: Yes, the entire boardwalk is ADA compliant

MAPS: USGS Kent; also available at trailhead kiosk and at dnr.state.oh.us

FACILITIES: None

CONTACT INFORMATION: More information is available at dnr.state.oh.us or (330) 527-5118.

Directions

From Cleveland, take I-480 East to OH 14 in Streetsboro. Turn right, heading south on OH 43, through Twin Lakes and into Kent. (Follow signs, taking a hard left to stay on OH 43 at OH 59.) About 0.5 miles south of OH 261, turn right (west) onto Meloy Road. The bog's entrance is about 0.5 miles west of OH 43 in Kent.

GPS Trailhead Coordinates

Latitude 41° 7.759981'

Longitude 81° 21.224699'

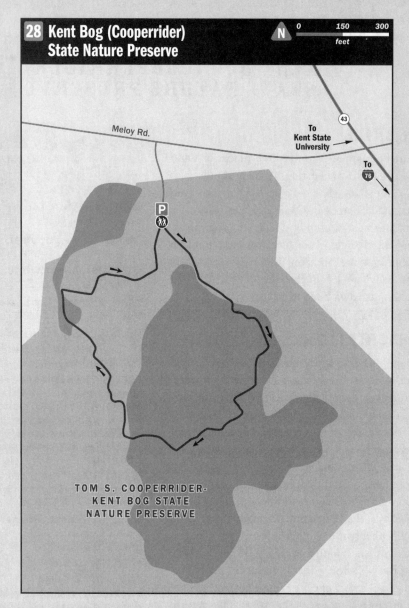

0   150   300
feet

Meloy Rd.

To
Kent State
University

To
76

P

TOM S. COOPERRIDER-
KENT BOG STATE
NATURE PRESERVE

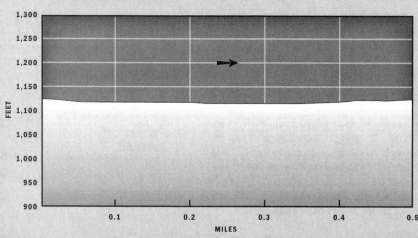

1,300
1,250
1,200
1,150
1,100
1,050
1,000
950
900

FEET

0.1   0.2   0.3   0.4   0.5

MILES

Checkoff program. The boardwalk was added in 1993, which also was a first. Paid for in part by a grant from the Division of Litter Prevention and Recycling, the walkway is made of recycled plastic shopping bags, stretch wrap, and bottles. (See? What you recycle at home today, you may find underfoot tomorrow!)

A bog is a harsh environment; its climatic conditions are called limiting factors. Extremes in temperature, wetness, nutrient levels, and acidity significantly limit the plants that can survive in a bog. During summer, root level temperatures in the peat can be as much as 40° cooler than the surface temperature. Bogs favor plants that can thrive in an acidic, mineral-poor environment because nutrients

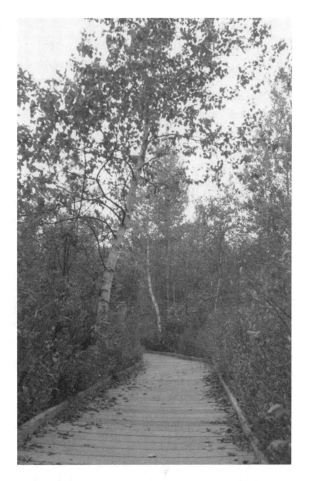

The boardwalk is made of recycled plastic.

from dead plants are tied up in peat and therefore not available to nourish the plants. That's one reason carnivorous plants tend to show up in bogs. Many other unusual species thrive here as well.

Sphagnum moss is one. A rootless moss, it continually grows from the top while dying at the bottom. Sphagnum moss can hold up to 27 times its own dry weight in water, is more than twice as absorbent as cotton, and has antiseptic properties. Where it grows, it lowers root temperatures and oxygen levels. Its peculiar properties have earned it at least two footnotes in history: Native Americans used sphagnum to diaper their babies, and during the Civil War and World War I, doctors used the moss as emergency field dressings.

Small cranberries also grow here—one of the very few spots in Ohio they call home. Most people are surprised to see that cranberries are not so much trees as viny, woody shrubs that creep over the ground. Poison sumac is here too. Like its mean, nasty cousin poison ivy, poison sumac has white berries. (Several other sumac species, which sport red berries, are harmless.)

If you visit the bog in the fall—October is your best bet—you'll notice that the needles on the tamarack trees have changed from green to yellow, and they may be falling off. They're not dying! Tamaracks are deciduous conifers, so they shed needles like other trees shed leaves. Tamarack trees love the cold; they grow as far north as trees can grow in Canada. This far south, however, they are rare. Walk through the bog in the winter, when the tamaracks are nearly bare, and you'll be able to spot catberry, a bog holly identified by its bright red berries.

To see all these and many other bog oddities, step onto the boardwalk trail from the south end of the parking lot. Turn left, following the loop clockwise. The walkway circles a sedge meadow and runs northeast through a marsh and wooded stretch of land. As you stroll through, you can stop along the way to read many educational plaques describing some of the bog's unusual conditions and inhabitants.

Six park benches placed along the boardwalk provide good places to observe wildlife. Birders will watch for Rufous-sided towhees and berry-loving wax-wings. The bog is also home to deer, foxes, and cottontail rabbits. Rare spotted turtles also live here, but it's unlikely that you'll see one. The spotted turtle is palm-sized, with brilliant yellow spots on its shell. To protect these slow bog residents, turtle tunnels were built into the boardwalk's underside. They allow the turtles to move freely about the bog, out of sight of most visitors as they walk over the boardwalk.

As you are leaving the bog, you'll cross a dry moatlike depression that surrounds it. This trough around the bog brings excessive shade and leaf litter from the adjacent upland trees. That and the well-oxygenated runoff that enters here allow other species to creep into the bog. The main peat mass, with its limiting factors that control bog ecology, is reduced and threatened by the invaders. Eventually, the bog will naturally go the way of the glacier, and its long history will be, finally, just history. Visit now, so you can say you were here when.

NEARBY ACTIVITIES

Head north from Kent on OH 43 to visit the bog's nearest relative, an alkaline fen. Herrick Fen (see page 125) in Streetsboro is about a 15-minute drive from here.

This state nature preserve was named to honor Tom S. Cooperrider, PhD, a nationally recognized botanist who played an instrumental role in discovering and protecting this unusual and important area.

NELSON-KENNEDY LEDGES STATE PARK

IN BRIEF

Nelson-Kennedy Ledges offers what may be the wildest 2-mile walk in the eastern United States. Don't let the short distance fool you; you could easily spend several hours here. Dramatic ledges and tight crevasses team up with a waterfall and several small caves, creating striking beauty. Bring a flashlight to peer into some of the narrower passages in this small, surprising state park. Beginners longing for a rocky hike should start with Gorge Trail (see page 222) or Whipp's Ledges (see page 270) and work their way up to this one.

DESCRIPTION

With formation names such as Devil's Hole and Fat Man's Peril, these trails sound a little scary. Dire warnings posted on park bulletin boards don't offer any warm fuzzies either. The park service strongly (and effectively) discourages horseplay here by posting recent accident information at the trailhead. Unfortunately, life-flight rescue has been called to the park several times for serious injuries. In short, the rock formations that give this park its amazing beauty also make it dangerous. By heeding the posted warnings and proceeding with respect and caution, you will certainly enjoy the cliffs, caves, and crooked trails here

KEY AT-A-GLANCE INFORMATION

LENGTH: 2 miles

CONFIGURATION: Two connecting loops and an out-and-back

DIFFICULTY: Difficult

SCENERY: 60-foot cliffs, creek, caves, crevasses, and a tall, skinny waterfall

EXPOSURE: Mostly shaded

TRAFFIC: Moderately heavy

TRAIL SURFACE: Rock surfaces, dirt, and peat

HIKING TIME: 2 hours

DRIVING DISTANCE: 37 miles from I-77/I-480 exchange

ACCESS: Daily, half hour before sunrise–half hour after sunset; cars in the lot 30 minutes after sunset are subject to towing. Do not attempt hiking here when icy conditions exist. Pets are allowed on leashes; however, I don't recommend bringing them or young children here.

WHEELCHAIR TRAVERSABLE: No

MAPS: USGS Garrettsville; also available at dnr.state.oh.us

FACILITIES: Restrooms at parking lot; picnic tables on both sides of OH 282

CONTACT INFORMATION: Visit dnr .state.oh.us or call (440) 564-2279.

Directions

From Cleveland, take I-480 East to Exit 26/US 422. Follow US 422 east (toward Solon) to OH 700. Turn right on OH 700 and continue south for about 5 miles into Hiram. Turn left onto OH 305 and go east about 3 miles to OH 282 (Nelson Ledge Road). Turn left. The park entrance is about 1 mile north of OH 305. Parking is on the eastern side of the road; the trails are on the western side of OH 282.

GPS Trailhead Coordinates

Latitude 41° 19.706283'

Longitude 81° 2.337778'

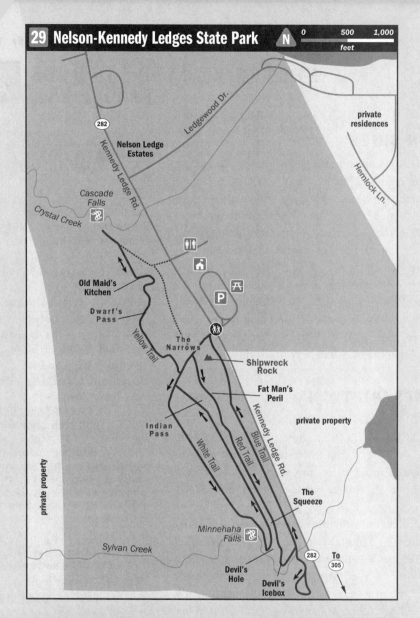

N

0   500   1,000

feet

Ledgewood Dr.

private
residences

Hemlock Ln.

282

**Nelson Ledge
Estates**

Kennedy Ledge Rd.

*Cascade
Falls*

Crystal Creek

**Old Maid's
Kitchen**

**Dwarf's
Pass**

Yellow Trail

**The
Narrows**

P

Shipwreck
Rock

**Fat Man's
Peril**

**Indian
Pass**

White Trail

Red Trail

Blue Trail

Kennedy Ledge Rd.

private property

**The
Squeeze**

private property

*Minnehaha
Falls*

Sylvan Creek

282

**To
305**

**Devil's
Hole**

**Devil's
Icebox**

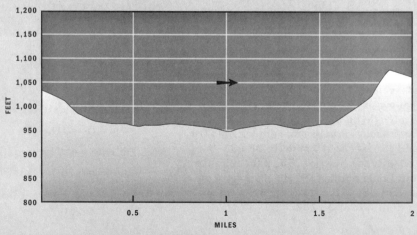

1,200				
1,150				
1,100				
1,050				
1,000				
950				
900				
850				
800				

FEET

0.5   1   1.5   2

MILES

on this little plot of land in Portage County.

Four trails run through the park; their combined length is about 2 miles. While the park's direction is HIKE ONLY ON THE MARKED TRAILS, you may be hard-pressed to do so. The trails dart in and out of huge rock formations, and it's easy to lose the trail. Study the map and take care in your exploration. With warnings duly noted, start with the easy, relatively speaking, White Trail.

Head west a few strides from the trailhead sign, passing the Blue, the Red, and then the Yellow Trail, before turning left (south) onto the White Trail. Even though the White Trail is rated the easiest to walk, part of it follows along the top

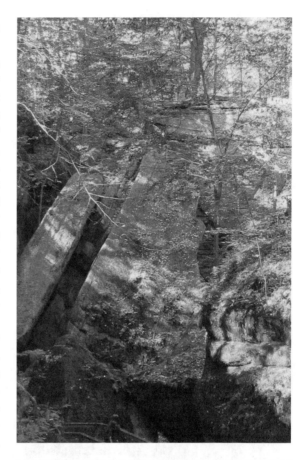

Stunning ledges beg to be explored, but heed the warnings.

ridge of 65-foot cliffs—highlighting the need to use caution on all of the trails, regardless of their individual ratings.

The White Trail gives you a good overview of the south end of the park and a glimpse of what to expect on the trails below. About 0.4 miles south, the path loops to the left (east), where you'll see the trickle of Minnehaha Falls tumbling into Sylvan Creek below. A chain-link fence here marks the southern boundary of the park. Follow the trail as it loops back to its beginnings, and turn right, going downhill a few steps to find the Red Trail.

You'll enter the Red Trail through a "tunnel" of 20- to 25-foot-tall boulders. The Red Trail is rated difficult. No kidding. It leads through a 20-foot-long corridor that will not accommodate much larger than a size 44 belt. If you make it through there, two more tricky maneuvers await: The Squeeze and Devil's Icebox.

Once through Devil's Icebox (where you and an assortment of moss and ferns emerge by Sylvan Creek), you'll find a short set of steps leading down to

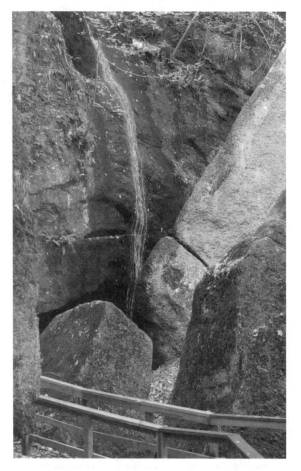

Cascade Falls

the Blue Trail. At the bottom of the steps, turn right, heading south among some relatively small rocks (still taller than you) and loop around to head north, back to the trailhead. While the Blue Trail is rated moderate, it has much in common with the Red Trail: both give you a squeeze, challenge your knees, and cause you to wonder at the trees, with their roots hanging onto the rocks for dear life. The blue line on the park map is a straight line, but don't be fooled. The actual trail wiggles through the woods and rolls over lots of small rocky bumps—all the way, however, it is well marked.

When the Blue Trail returns you to the trailhead sign, turn left and head uphill again. This time you'll pass the Red Trail. Beyond it, turn right to follow the Yellow Trail (also rated moderate). Yellow metal signs point you north; you'll also find yellow markers painted on rocks and trees. Even with these clues, you'll find that it's easy to lose the trail.

Like the White Trail, Yellow leads you along the top edge of the cliffs. From there it takes you downhill fast—first on a dirt path and then along makeshift stone steps. It bottoms out, cools off, and lurches to the right. The Yellow Trail heads into a closet of sorts, created by two massive boulders. Moving north from there, you'll jog left then right again to pad along a sturdy wooden bridge into Old Maid's Kitchen. The "kitchen" is about as big as a New York City loft apartment. When you exit the dark and drafty "room," it's nice to see the sky again! You can also see the parking lot across the road—but don't leave yet. Follow the trail abruptly west, turning left and heading along a wooden boardwalk to the bottom of Cascade Falls. The small stream that tumbles over a 40-foot drop eventually makes its way to the St. Lawrence River. (For trivia buffs: This park

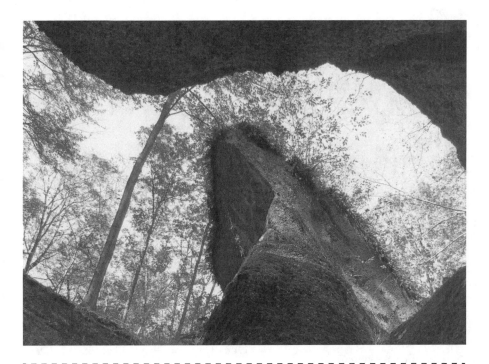

Looking up at Shipwreck Rock

sits on a watershed divide. This stream, and water north of here, runs into the St. Lawrence River; Sylvan Creek, on the park's south side, runs to the Mississippi.)

At the bottom of the falls, you can peer into Gold Hunter's Cave. Although the cave is not open to explorers, you can see inside from the wooden platform at the bottom of the falls. Retrace your steps back to the trailhead, or just cross OH 282 to the east to return to the parking lot.

NEARBY ACTIVITIES

You probably passed through Hiram to get here. Why not visit the field station (see page 130) on your way back?

Thanks to naturalists Laurie Wilson and Megan Acord for reviewing this description.

30 PORTAGE LAKES STATE PARK

KEY AT-A-GLANCE INFORMATION

LENGTH: 2.5 miles

CONFIGURATION: Loop and out-and-back

DIFFICULTY: Flat and easy

SCENERY: Thick deciduous forest, pines, wetlands, sandy lakefront

EXPOSURE: Mostly shaded

TRAFFIC: Light

SURFACE: Dirt with some gravel; beachfront is sand

HIKING TIME: Allow about 45 minutes per trail

DRIVING DISTANCE: 35 miles from I-77/I-480 exchange

ACCESS: Daily, sunrise–sunset

WHEELCHAIR TRAVERSABLE: No

MAPS: USGS Akron West; also available online at ohiostateparks.org and at camp office, 5031 Manchester Road

FACILITIES: 900-foot sand beach swim area, boat launch ramps, restrooms, playgrounds, and picnic shelters throughout the park; campsites available.

CONTACT INFORMATION: Visit ohiostateparks.org or call (330) 644-2220.

IN BRIEF

Portage Lakes State Park extends from Akron's southwest side well into the heart of Summit County. These two short hikes showcase just two of the park's many assets: its popular swim beach and little-known observatory.

DESCRIPTION

The Portage Lakes area south of Akron boasts eight or more lakes (depending on how you classify reservoirs), and none are named Portage. Most are kettle lakes formed by glacial activity long ago, which created the habitats that allow unique plant communities to thrive here.

One of the species you'll see here is *Larix laricina*, commonly known as tamarack trees, which are rarely found this far south. Not just pine trees, tamaracks are deciduous conifers. Every autumn their needles turn yellow and then fall off, to be replaced in the spring.

Interspersed among the lakes are dams and canals created by people to serve their own needs—first industrial, then recreational. Today, Portage Lakes State Park encompasses more than 400 acres of land and 2,000 acres of water, ensuring that the habitat for wetland-loving birds and animals remains more or less undeveloped and creating a popular destination for outdoors enthusiasts.

GPS Trailhead Coordinates

Latitude   40° 58.078737'

Longitude   81° 32.744279'

Directions ⟶

Take I-77 South to Exit 129, following I-76 West toward I-277/Canton. Exit at Exit 2/Waterloo Road/OH 93 and turn left onto Waterloo, and then right onto OH 93 South/Manchester Road. Follow signs to the entrance to Turkeyfoot Beach and Picnic Area, on the right.

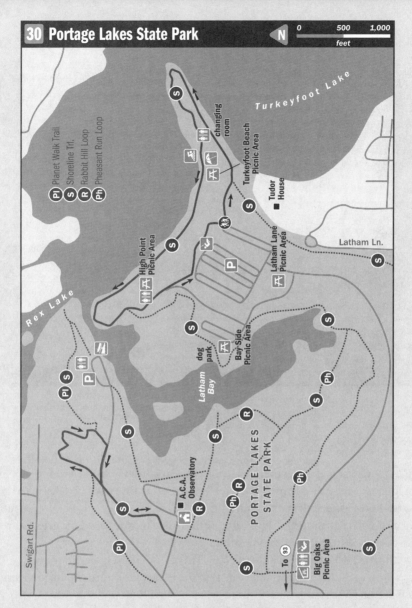

30 Portage Lakes State Park

N

0   500   1,000
feet

Turkeyfoot Lake

Pl Planet Walk Trail
S Shoreline Trl.
R Rabbit Hill Loop
Ph Pheasant Run Loop

changing room

Turkeyfoot Beach Picnic Area

Tudor House

Latham Ln.

High Point Picnic Area

Latham Lane Picnic Area

Rex Lake

P

dog park

Bay-Side Picnic Area

Latham Bay

A.C.A. Observatory

PORTAGE LAKES STATE PARK

Swigart Rd.

To 93

Big Oaks Picnic Area

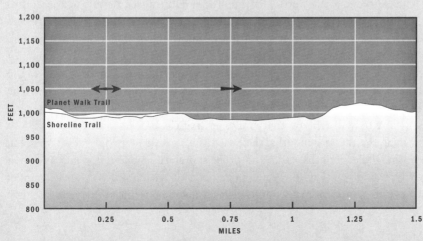

FEET

1,200
1,150
1,100
1,050
1,000
950
900
850
800

Planet Walk Trail

Shoreline Trail

0.25   0.5   0.75   1   1.25   1.5

MILES

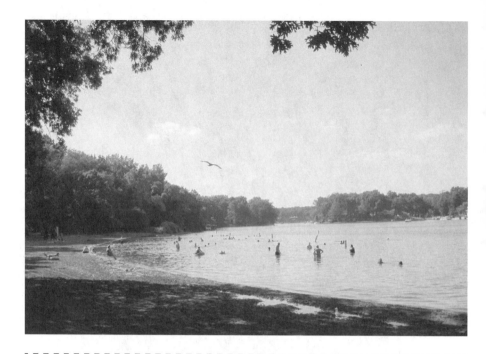

Swimmers can enjoy watching small boats on Turkeyfoot Lake.

The southern end of Portage Lakes State Park sees more fishing and camp-
ing activity than the northern side of the park, which attracts more picnickers, hikers, sunbathers, and stargazers. The two trails described here are good
starter hikes, and either one could be easily included in a family swim outing.
Because both trails are fairly level and flat, they're also good choices for those
just starting a hiking or fitness routine.

Starting from the eastern end of Turkeyfoot Beach parking area, follow
signs to the Tudor House and join the Shoreline Trail already in progress, as
they say in TV land.

After surveying the outside of the Tudor House (see details at the end of
this section), turn left and follow the shady dirt trail northeast as it rambles
toward the beach. The narrow path isn't all shoreline as its name suggests. Poison ivy, mayapples, and Virginia creeper all crowd the path, but there's room for
you too. You'll likely enjoy solitude along this stretch of trail and all the way to
the end of Turkeyfoot Lake, where the path bends sharply to head for the swim
beach. And although trees will obscure your view of the swim beach for several
yards, your ears will tell you that you're getting close.

During the warmer months, the beach is well used by people of all ages, but
even in the cooler months, gulls and other shorebirds make the scene, and their
cries will remind you that you're not alone here. Up a slight hill to your left, under
the shade of magnificent maples and other hardwoods, picnic tables, grills, a small

changing/restroom area, volleyball court, and a children's playground dot the landscape. Once your feet hit the sandy beach, to your right you may see windsurfers and other small crafts out on Turkeyfoot Lake.

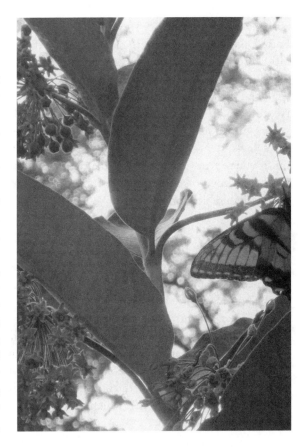

Take off your shoes or boots if you like to feel the sand beneath your feet and walk across the beach and then past a restroom and assorted picnic tables, leaving the swimming area as you amble toward the edge of Turkeyfoot Lake under the shade of big trees once again. No swimming is allowed at this point of land, but you won't stay long as the trail bends sharply and heads away from the water, leading you to High Point Picnic Area and the small playground. Now back to the parking

Explore the solar system on Planet Walk Trail.

lot, you've had a taste of what this park has to offer. Ready for more? Head for the "otherworldly" experience of the Planet Walk Trail.

From the swimming beach parking area to the Astronomy Club of Akron's Planet Walk Trail, the distance is just about 1.3 miles along lightly traveled park roads, an easy walk or drive. If you choose to walk it, you'd be smart to reapply sunscreen, as it's entirely exposed.

To reach the trailhead, follow the park road on which you entered, turning left before you reach Manchester Road. (A sign indicates that the road leads to the ACA's observatory and park offices.)

The trailhead sits behind the ACA building, marked by a sign that describes Mercury's hot spot in the solar system, located *only* 36 million miles from the sun. Not far behind you'll find Venus, 67.2 million miles from the sun and 900°F on the surface. You'll veer left and into the woods to find Earth a much more inviting place, at 93 million miles from the sun and with a surface made mostly of water.

Continuing along the narrow path, you'll encounter Mars and its moons as well as an asteroid belt. The trail is a little bumpy and the woods can be buggy, but we all know that space travel has yet to be perfected. There's good news for Earth hikers, though. The thick young growth creates terrific birding opportunities along Planet Walk Trail, and many different butterflies enjoy this wetland woods. Have a camera at the ready; they don't sit still very long.

The path rolls downhill to visit Jupiter and eventually bumps along to find Neptune (2.79 *billion* miles from the sun) and the end of this odyssey. When you've landed here, it's time to turn around and retrace your steps back through the solar system—or cheat a little, and walk back along the edge of the road. Or, if you're ready for a longer hike, you can continue past Neptune to join the northwest edge of Shoreline Trail and finish out its 5-mile loop, here in our watery, habitable world.

NEARBY ACTIVITIES

If it's a longer hike you want, stay here and take the whole Shoreline Trail, which covers 5 miles of the park, including attractions such as the dog park and Big Oaks Kids Zone, a gated, paved playground that appeals to kids and their parents alike. If you've got a special event coming up, you might want to revisit the historical, 20-room Tudor House and its lavish grounds (accessible from the Turkeyfoot Beach parking area), which can be rented for parties, reunions, and other events. For information, contact the city of New Franklin at **newfranklin.org** or (330) 644-1728. Also worth considering: more hiking at nearby Quail Hollow State Park (see the next page), which also features a beautiful manor house, open to the public year-round.

QUAIL HOLLOW STATE PARK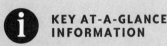

IN BRIEF

From an herb garden with a sundial to rough-and-tumble mountain bike trails, Quail Hollow State Park will satisfy a wide range of interests—even if you want to stay indoors. A unique, glass-enclosed nature viewing area in the lodge allows you to watch birds and small critters up close.

DESCRIPTION

From the manor house parking lot, head south through stone gates to the herb garden. Established in 1986 by the Quail Hollow Herbal Society, the garden includes a rose arbor and features a traditional sundial. The beds are divided in wagon-wheel style, with plantings of irises, lamb's ears, and Oriental poppies that bloom from late May through early June. Thankfully, almost all of the plantings are labeled, so you don't have to wonder what's blooming. You'll have to identify the buzzing on your own; the butterflies and other insects that frequent the garden in late summer are so colorful that they compete with the flowers. Several benches in the herb garden provide rest in the shade of tall trees and offer a view of the manor house.

Wander just a few hundred feet north of the herb and flower garden to a waiting picnic

KEY AT-A-GLANCE INFORMATION

LENGTH: 1.3 miles
CONFIGURATION: Loop
DIFFICULTY: Easy
SCENERY: Marsh and prairie, pine and deciduous forest, herb and rose garden, evidence of beavers
EXPOSURE: Woodland trail is shaded; herb garden and marsh are exposed.
TRAFFIC: Moderate
TRAIL SURFACE: Dirt and grass
HIKING TIME: 1 hour
DRIVING DISTANCE: 46 miles from I-77/I-480 exchange
ACCESS: Daily, 6 a.m.–11 p.m.
WHEELCHAIR TRAVERSABLE: No
MAPS: USGS Hartville; also available inside visitor center and at ohiostateparks.org
FACILITIES: Restrooms, water, phone, and drink vending machine by manor house/visitor center parking lot; picnic tables and grills scattered throughout park
CONTACT INFORMATION: Visit ohiostateparks.org or quailhollowpark.org or call (330) 644-2220.

Directions

From Cleveland, follow I-77 South through Akron, past I-76 and US 224, taking Exit 120 onto Arlington Road, heading south. Turn left on OH 619, following it east into Hartville past OH 43 to Congress Lake Road. Turn left and then right into the park entrance at 13480 Congress Lake Avenue. Follow the long park driveway approximately 1 mile, following signs to the manor house on the park's eastern side.

GPS Trailhead Coordinates

Latitude 40° 58.786261'
Longitude 81° 18.274384'

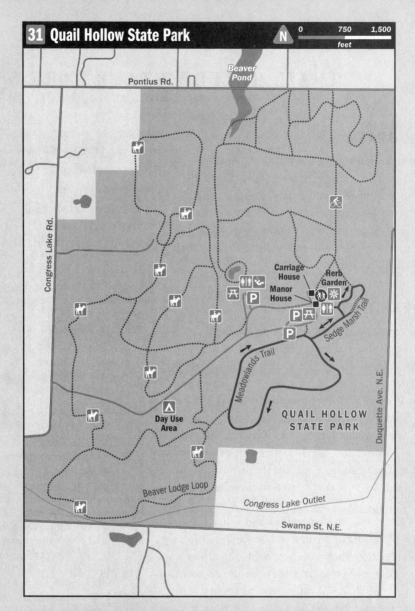

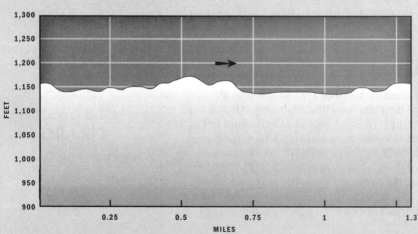

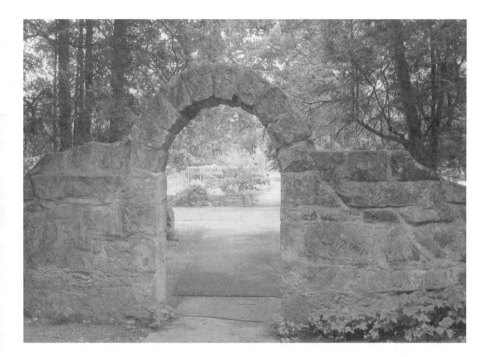

Enter to find Quail Hollow's extensive gardens.

table and quiet fountain for a picturesque stop. Returning to the herb garden, have another look at the manor house from below, and then turn left (east) and step onto the short Tall-Grass Prairie Trail. As you might expect, it follows a mown grass trail amid taller prairie grasses. Soon you'll turn right, stepping onto Sedge Marsh, a half-mile trail that bends south and then west. Along the trail you'll find sweet flag and cattails and perhaps see some of the many frogs (spring peepers, chorus frogs, and American toads are common here) or birds that frequent this marsh. In the summer, watch and listen for yellow warblers.

A small quiet creek runs along the eastern side of Sedge Marsh Trail. On wet spring days, Sedge Marsh can be impassable unless you're wearing high, dry boots. That's OK because the natives can still get around—the marsh teems with animal life, although much of it is microscopic. Squishy marshes, not surprisingly, are important foundations in food webs. As you move south on a long stretch of boardwalk, you approach a meadow where larger links in the food chain live.

At the southern end of the marsh, you'll connect with the 1.5-mile Meadowlands Trail loop and turn left to follow the trail clockwise. About 0.3 miles from the marsh, the wide grassy trail turns into a sea of pine needles. You'll rise and fall over several 10- and 20-foot hills as the trail turns along a pine stand. Now you're heading west, and deciduous trees 30 and 40 feet tall line the trail. Among them are crabapples, beautiful in bloom in the late spring.

It's important to note that the thick grass here camouflages some deep

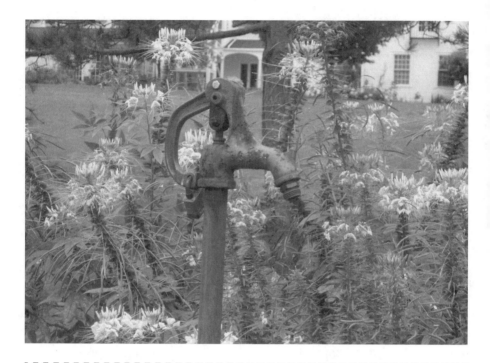

Tours of the Manor House (in the background) are offered throughout the year.

holes in the trail; folks with weak ankles should watch their steps through here. If you stop and look into the woods, you may see a red fox, white-tailed deer, or a wild turkey on this trail. If you miss them, don't despair. Look carefully and you'll surely see some smaller life-forms. Signs along the Sedge Marsh and Meadowlands trails encourage you to get down on your hands and knees to look for caterpillars and other small insects and unusual plants. (Unfortunately, the signs don't tell you how to explain yourself to other hikers when they stumble upon you, crawling about.)

As the path bends and rolls along, you'll pass a sign pointing the way to mountain bike trails and to the Beaver Lodge Loop. Stay on the Meadowlands Trail and, as you turn right, you'll come to a clearing where you'll have a view of the entire meadow. It's one of those wide-open spaces where—just for an instant—you'll wish that this were your own backyard. The view is fantastic.

Looping eastward, the Meadowlands Trail leads you back to the manor house; it sits north and to the left of the end of the trail. From here you can go up a dozen wide stone steps into the manor house. The house started life as a humble farmhouse back in 1838. Harry Bartlett Stewart, chief executive officer of the Akron, Canton, and Youngstown Railroad, began acquiring adjacent land in the early 1900s, and he passed it down to his son, Harry Jr. The Stewart family lived here and enlarged the home several times until 1975, when they offered the property to the state for half its appraised value.

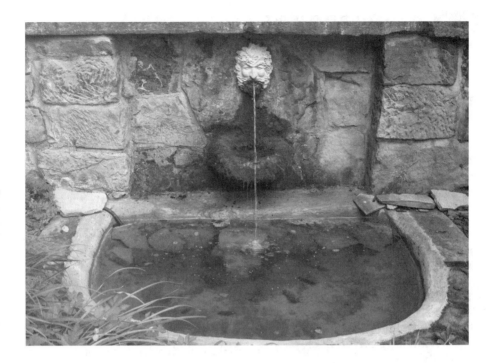

The gardens boast many unique features.

Today, the 40-room manor house is used as a natural history study center, hosting a variety of nature-oriented educational programs and workshops throughout the year.

Part of the home's lower level serves as a visitor center and is open weekends 1–5 p.m. A glass-enclosed room looks out onto a stone landscape featuring a small fountain and bird feeders. Inside, visitors enjoy watching chipmunks, squirrels, bright cardinals, and jays year-round, from the warmth of an old farmhouse.

NEARBY ACTIVITIES

Tours of the manor house are offered throughout the year—call (330) 877-6652 for available dates. Educational programs are also offered regularly, both inside the visitor center and on the trail. Quail Hollow's 698 acres include mountain bike and bridle trails, ice-skating, and cross-country skiing (equipment rentals are even available from the park). Once you've worked up an appetite here, you won't have to go far to satisfy it. Several restaurants in Hartville, near the junction of OH 43 and OH 619, serve hearty meals in the Mennonite tradition. Two wineries in or near Hartville are also popular stops—if you don't have a designated driver, though, buy a bottle to open at home.

32 RIVEREDGE TRAIL AND CITY OF KENT

KEY AT-A-GLANCE INFORMATION

LENGTH: 2.5 miles

CONFIGURATION: Figure eight

DIFFICULTY: Easy

SCENERY: Great variety—from river fowl and ravine views to a rail station from the 1870s

EXPOSURE: Mostly shaded, with a few short exposed stretches

TRAFFIC: Moderate

TRAIL SURFACE: From dirt and wooden boardwalks along the river to sidewalks along city streets

HIKING TIME: 50 minutes

DRIVING DISTANCE: 31 miles from I-77/I-480 exchange

ACCESS: Daily, sunrise–sunset

WHEELCHAIR TRAVERSABLE: No

MAPS: USGS Kent; also available inside the Kent Parks and Recreation Department office in Fred Fuller Park

FACILITIES: Restrooms at east end of Fred Fuller Park and at the Kramer ball fields; a drinking fountain is also located in the parking lot by the ball field.

CONTACT INFORMATION: Visit kentparksandrec.com or call (330) 673-8897.

IN BRIEF

This stroll along the Cuyahoga River and through the city of Kent highlights the town's history since the 1800s. It will lead you through a pioneer cemetery, by Ohio's oldest masonry dam, and by some of Kent's historical buildings, many of which are still in use. You'll also visit a large city park, filled with tall shade trees and fun playground areas.

DESCRIPTION

Legend has it that Captain Samuel Brady leapt across the Cuyahoga River to escape from Native Americans in 1780. The river is narrow as it runs through Kent; still, it must have been a mighty leap. We'll never know just how far he jumped or how much credence to give the story. Nevertheless, Riveredge Trail in Kent is the setting for this and many other interesting tales in American history.

Start your hike at John Brown Tannery Park, where a paved path leads from the parking lot down a slight slope toward the river. A seasonal canoe livery operates here in the warmer months, and in addition to paddlers you're likely to see ducks and Canada geese at this spot. The pavement ends and you'll follow a limestone path south (to the right) along the river. As with any river path, you

GPS Trailhead Coordinates

Latitude   41° 9.033o1'

Longitude   81° 21.795480'

Directions

Take I-480/OH 14 into Streetsboro. Turn right onto OH 43, heading south into Kent. Turn left onto Main Street and then right onto Water Street. Follow Water Street about 1 mile south to Summit Street and turn right. Tannery Park is about 0.3 miles east on your left.

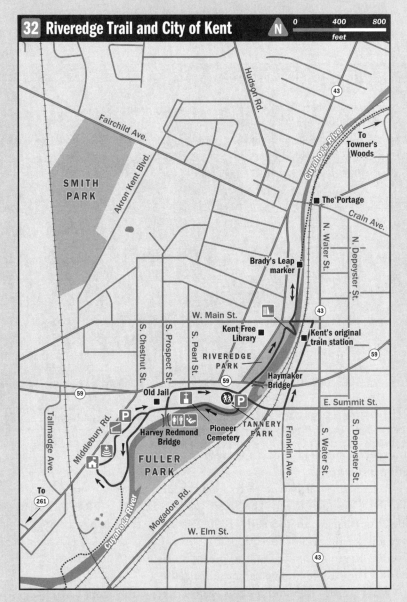

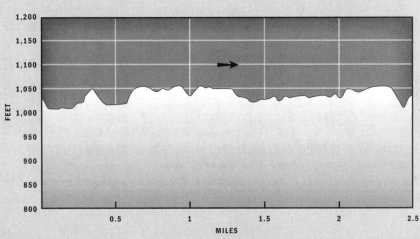

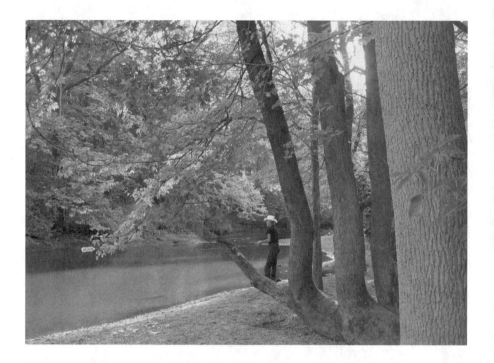

Fishing here can be interrupted by the occasional canoe or kayak launch.

can expect some mud here. (Improvement plans in the works will address this section of the trail.)

Riveredge Trail is true to its name; it doesn't stray more than a few feet from the Cuyahoga River. The river was the primary reason that Kent was a popular settlement in the early 1800s. At first, the town was simply named Franklin, for the son of the original landowner. In 1805 the Haymaker family moved to Kent and built a dam to power a gristmill. As other mills popped up, the town came to be known as Franklin Mills.

What was then Franklin Mills is now a busy university town, full of folks with flexible schedules, so the trail sees a fair share of traffic all week long.

As you continue south, the trail is a mix of mostly dirt and roots, although gravel has been laid in the wettest spots and plans call for paving, eventually, to allow bicycles to roll alongside the river. You'll cross two wooden bridges as the path follows the river south (downstream) and then west. On your left, a steep hill blocks the afternoon sun, making the trail cool and shady, even on summer afternoons.

About 0.3 miles into the trail, you'll pass the Harvey Redmond Bridge. It leads to the Kramer ball fields, on your left. A small fenced-in playground and portable restrooms are situated near the ball fields.

Cross the street and continue on the trail. To your right, a set of wooden stairs climbs up a steep hill to one of the park's many swing sets and picnic

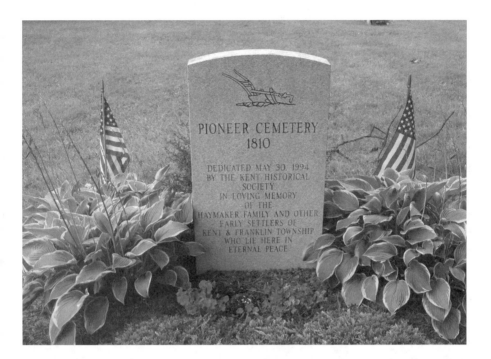

Originally established as Stow Street Cemetery, on land deeded to the city by the Haymaker family

areas, but you'll want to stay on the trail going straight to enjoy the thick of the woods along the river.

The path forks again about 0.2 miles later. The rocky path to the right leads to Fred Fuller Park's main shelter and picnic area. Veer left instead, following the narrow path that winds along the riverbed. You're likely to see deer here in any season; herons also frequent this quieter portion of the river.

Continue another 0.3 miles or so to the edge of the park property. (You'll know you're there when shade trees are replaced with a view of the city's water treatment plant.) From here, you can look downstream to see an old bridge truss and remnants of the canal bed. If you choose to, you can follow the trail south another 1.5 miles. The wide wooden boardwalk turns into a paved path and ends, for the time being, at Middlebury Road. Eventually the paved portion in Kent will meet up with the Summit County Metroparks Bike & Hike Trail and continue into Tallmadge and Akron. For now, though, turn right and take a walk in the park.

A gravel trail leads you up a steep, shady hill, and you'll emerge at the southern end of Fred Fuller, Kent's largest city park. Restrooms and a playground are located here to the left; you'll spot a small amphitheater to the right.

Follow the dirt road to the right. Cars are permitted here, but traffic is light. Walk 0.2 miles past the shelter house and park office to the historical Old Jail.

The jail was built in 1869 by the order of Mayor John Thompson, though

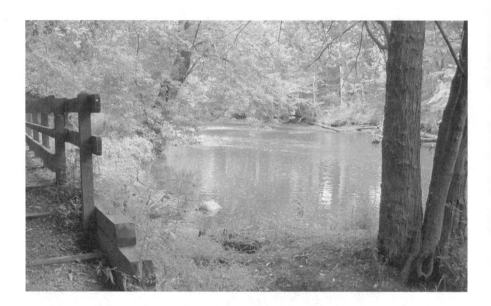

Many wildflowers and waterfowl can be found along this portion of the Cuyahoga River.

it might easily have not existed, as Mayor Thompson won the office by just two votes. (Votes for Thompson totaled 145; runner-up Luther Parmelee had 143.) The jail was moved to the park in 1999 and completely renovated, and while it's now used for meetings and other events, elements of the original building remain.

From the jail, you'll head north down a steep, grassy hill. Swings, grills, and another picnic shelter sit at the bottom of the hill. Cross Stow Street, now heading west, and follow the sidewalk to the left to find Kent's Pioneer Cemetery, dating to 1810. Headstones here represent the families who figured prominently in Kent's history, including Haymaker, DePeyster, and Franklin. The cemetery gate is open sunrise–sunset.

Back on Stow Street, follow the sidewalk down to the Tannery parking lot. Cross Stow to the north to continue along the river trail. A sign here marks the entrance to Franklin Mills Riveredge Park. Head down about 20 wooden steps, under the Haymaker Bridge. At the bottom of the stairs, the path bends left; shallow river rapids gurgle to your right.

From wooden stairways and elevated boardwalks, you'll see some of Kent's historical industrial buildings on the left; the old downtown is on your right. From the top of a set of stairs, you'll get a good look at the Kent Dam, the oldest masonry dam in the state of Ohio. This area, including the Kent Dam (constructed around 1836) and Canal Basin from the Main Street Bridge to the Stow Street Bridge, comprises the old industrial district that is listed on the National Register of Historic Places. The dam was modified in the first few years of the 21st century to allow the river to flow freely again. Spared demolition because of its historical significance, the structure was retrofitted to become the centerpiece of a small park. Climb the steps to the top of the dam and enjoy a unique view of the town. To the west, at the corner of Mantua (OH 43) and Main streets, is Kent Free Library. At first glance, it doesn't hint at its age. In fact, the library has been there for well over 100 years. The original building, built with Andrew Carnegie's money on land donated by Marvin Kent, was incorporated into a much larger building that opened in 2005.

Looking east, you'll see the iconic two-story redbrick structure that was the city's original train station, built in 1875. The railroad's arrival here meant that the town would continue to grow, even as canal transportation declined. The man most responsible for bringing the new Atlantic and Great Western line to town was Marvin Kent. In 1864 the grateful citizens of Franklin Mills changed the town's name to honor him; since then, the name has stuck.

After descending from your observation point atop the old dam, continue north on Riveredge Trail, crossing under the bridge, where the path becomes relatively new brick walkway. Follow it about 0.3 miles, and you'll find a large rock and plaque marking the spot of Captain Brady's famous leap and describing how he managed to outsmart his would-be captors. (Believe it or not.)

From here, you can simply turn around and retrace your steps on Riveredge Trail, returning to Tannery Park along the river. If you'd like to keep going, the trail will take you east (following The Portage) to Towner's Woods (see page 171) and beyond. Or, you can take one of several exits from Riveredge Trail to explore the city of Kent. Now that you know its history, its modern style might surprise you. Main Street is a center of activity, lined with several art galleries, unique shops, and restaurants for every taste. If you decide to explore the city, you can return to Tannery Park along Franklin Avenue, turning right where Summit Street intersects Franklin.

NEARBY ACTIVITIES

While children probably won't want to leave Fred Fuller Park's playground equipment, Kent's downtown and the university offer much more to see and do. Local merchants host numerous festivals and activities all year long. (For a schedule, see **mainstreetkent.org**.) An adventure outfitter managed by the university offers daily pedal-and-paddle trips along the Cuyahoga throughout the spring and summer. (See **kent.edu/recservices/crookedriver**.)

Kent State University is located 1 mile east of the Tannery Park parking lot. There, you can visit the May 4 Memorial—a somber spot recalling the day in 1970 when four students were killed during an anti-war protest. Or visit the nationally known fashion museum (call [330] 672-3450 for hours and visitor information).

Thanks to John Idone, director of Kent's Parks and Recreation Department, for reviewing this description and offering a glimpse into the future of Kent's trails.

33 SENECA PONDS

KEY AT-A-GLANCE INFORMATION

LENGTH: 1 mile

CONFIGURATION: Loop

DIFFICULTY: Easy

SCENERY: Deciduous forest, wetlands, three ponds, swans, beavers, wildflowers

EXPOSURE: Shaded in spring and summer, when trees are full

TRAFFIC: Moderately heavy on weekends, evenings, and weekday lunchtimes

TRAIL SURFACE: Dirt, mulch, grass, and gravel

HIKING TIME: 35 minutes

DRIVING DISTANCE: 23 miles from I-77/I-480 exchange

ACCESS: Daily, sunrise–sunset

WHEELCHAIR TRAVERSABLE: No

MAPS: USGS Kent; also posted at trailhead

FACILITIES: None

CONTACT INFORMATION: Visit Portage Park District online, portageparkdistrict.org, or call (330) 297-7728.

IN BRIEF

Surrounded by corporate offices and light industry, a small parcel of land protects wetlands, breeding pairs of swans, and possibly our sanity.

DESCRIPTION

As has happened in countless outlying suburbs, Streetsboro's commercial district developed quickly. The urban sprawl steamroller of big-box retailers, manufacturers, and other employers threatened to engulf the entire city. Fortunately, Western Reserve Land Conservancy and Portage Park District were able to create a small preserve in the middle of an office park. The trail loops around two of the three ponds on this rustic 48-acre preserve.

While visitors can see neighboring businesses from at least two spots on the trail and will never completely escape the droning sounds of traffic coming from the Ohio Turnpike, the unassuming little path through wetlands and forest is a welcome addition to the neighborhood, drawing walkers from nearby employers at lunchtime and evenings throughout the workweek. Seneca Ponds is also a popular fishing destination; bass and sunfish can be hooked here. (See tips for successful catch-and-release techniques at **dnr.state.oh.us.**)

GPS Trailhead Coordinates

Latitude   41° 15.017402'

Longitude   81° 23.064902'

Directions

From the I-480/I-77 exchange, follow I-480 East into Streetsboro, where I-480 becomes OH 14. Turn right onto Mondial Parkway, following it to the park entrance on the north side of Mondial.

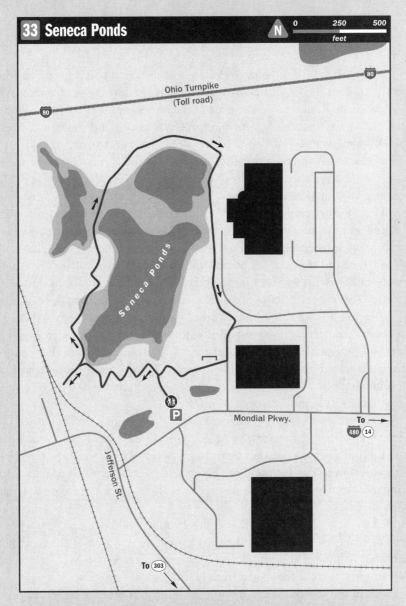

N

0   250   500
feet

Ohio Turnpike
(Toll road)

80

80

Seneca Ponds

Mondial Pkwy.

To →
480 14

P

Jefferson St.

To 303

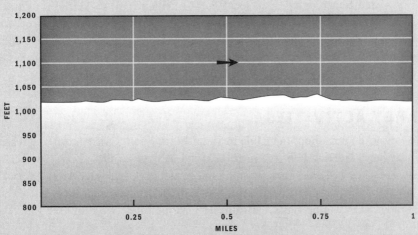

1,200
1,150
1,100
1,050
1,000
950
900
850
800

FEET

0.25   0.5   0.75   1

MILES

Enter the trail from the northern edge of the small parking lot, heading up a gentle slope to the first of many trail markers. Follow the trail as it curves to the left and you'll soon be on the edge of the largest of the three ponds. A bench is perched on the water's edge. Be quiet and look closely and you may see beavers at work—and even if you don't, you're almost certain to see anglers at work. Proceed clockwise and note the different types of rocks you find along the trail. These erratics, typical of the area, were deposited by glacial activity 10,000 years ago, give or take a few years. As you cross over a couple of footbridges to avoid some very squishy sections of the trail, Beaver Trail meanders slightly west, and you can peer through the trees at a still-active railroad track. (Trains chug through infrequently, however.)

Much of the trail and its boardwalks were built by local Boy Scouts from the Seneca District; the park's name is a nod of appreciation to their hard work that made this property more accessible without damaging its natural assets.

Soon you'll leave the woods to cross over a narrow strip of earth between two ponds, then return to the shaded path where another wooden park bench greets you. A sign alerts you to another trail, marked by a swan. It's essentially a shortcut through the middle of the property. Ignore it and continue venturing left, following Beaver Trail, where you'll also have a chance to see the swan family that makes its home at Seneca Ponds.

Curving east around the northern edge of the large pond, you'll walk over a variety of different surfaces, including gravel, grass, and mulch, each doing a good job of keeping the trail dry in this wetland habitat. Numerous marsh-loving wildflowers can be found on this short stretch of exposed trail. Naturally, during most of the spring and summer, this is also a good spot to spy dragonflies and damselflies.

Before the path returns to the shade of young oaks, you might see a bear—a statue of one, that is—gracing the picnic/patio area of one of the neighboring businesses. (Although it's not marked as such, the statue stands on private property and visitors are discouraged from getting too close.)

Back in the woods, heading south, you'll find another park bench, this one ideally situated for enjoying a sunset. (Insect repellant will make the watching that much more enjoyable, as the mosquito population comes out in force on summer evenings.) The path rolls up a slight incline before veering east and returning you to your starting point, a stark reminder that you just might have to go to work tomorrow.

NEARBY ACTIVITIES

Don't get sucked into shopping while in Streetsboro; instead, visit another natural area near here. Herrick Fen (see page 125) is less than 2 miles away, Towner's Woods (see page 171) less than 3, and Sunny Lake Park (see page 163)—a park with a completely different personality—is just about 5 miles north of here. A highly rated KOA campground is also nearby, about 1 mile west on OH 303.

SUNNY LAKE PARK 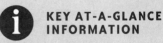 34

IN BRIEF

Sunny Lake serves many different interests. Want to soak up lazy lake views or watch great blue herons come in for long-legged landings? There are plenty of birds (and benches) to keep bird-watchers happy. Green thumbs will admire the Memorial Tree Garden on the park's south side. And active visitors of all ages can enjoy bocce and volleyball courts, boat rentals, an exercise circuit, and two playgrounds.

DESCRIPTION

From the shelter/office, follow the paved path east across a short wooden bridge; then begin your tour of the Memorial Tree Garden. It features a wide variety of trees, including flowering crabs, ivory silk lilacs, dawn redwoods, Kentucky coffees, red buckeyes, and several varieties of oaks and ash. In 1999 the Aurora Garden Club planted a garden celebrating Aurora's 200th birthday. Day lilies, 'Overdam' reed grass, autumn joy sedum, and flame grass grow there amid other decorative trees and bushes.

The paved trail curves to the left, hugging the lake's eastern shore. In places, cattails grow so thick and tall that they obscure views of the lake. Sunny Lake is indeed sunny;

KEY AT-A-GLANCE INFORMATION

LENGTH: 2.3 miles

CONFIGURATION: Loop

DIFFICULTY: Easy

SCENERY: Arboretum, natural forest, birds, lake

EXPOSURE: Mostly exposed

TRAFFIC: Moderate–heavy during warm weather

TRAIL SURFACE: Mostly paved; stretches of dirt, wood-chip trails

HIKING TIME: 50 minutes

DRIVING DISTANCE: 19 miles from I-77/I-480 exchange

ACCESS: Daily, sunrise–sunset; if gate at main parking is closed, park at Memorial Tree Garden, east of main entrance, off Mennonite Road

WHEELCHAIR TRAVERSABLE: Yes; lake loop is paved, but nature trails are not.

MAPS: USGS Aurora; also available from City of Aurora Parks & Recreation Department, (330) 562-4333

FACILITIES: Restrooms and water by main parking lot; picnic tables, shelters, and grills throughout park

CONTACT INFORMATION: More information about the park and events held there is available from the parks department at parks .auroraoh.com or (330) 562-4333.

Directions

From the I-77/I-480 exchange, follow I-480 East and take Exit 41 at Frost Road. Follow Frost Road east to OH 43; turn left. Turn right onto Mennonite Road. Follow Mennonite about 1.5 miles east to the park's main entrance on the left at 885 East Mennonite Road.

GPS Trailhead Coordinates

Latitude 41° 17.472839'

Longitude 81° 19.096076'

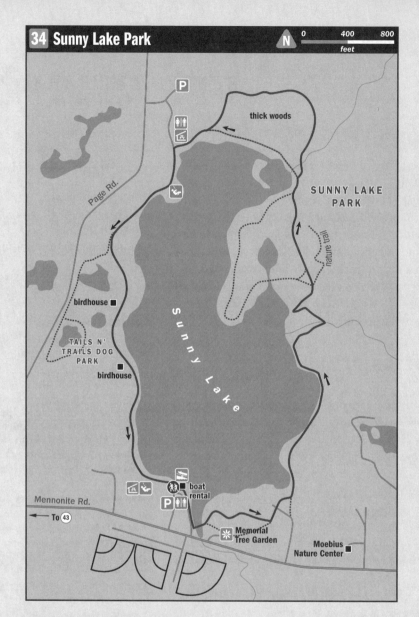

N

0   400   800
feet

thick woods

SUNNY LAKE PARK

Page Rd.

nature trail

birdhouse

TAILS N' TRAILS DOG PARK

birdhouse

S u n n y   L a k e

boat rental

Mennonite Rd.

To 43

Memorial Tree Garden

Moebius Nature Center

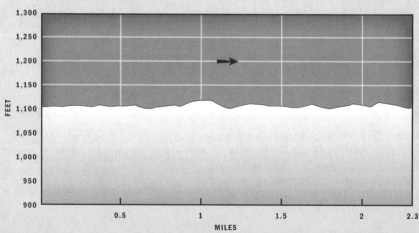

1,300
1,250
1,200
1,150
1,100
1,050
1,000
950
900

FEET

0.5   1   1.5   2   2.3

MILES

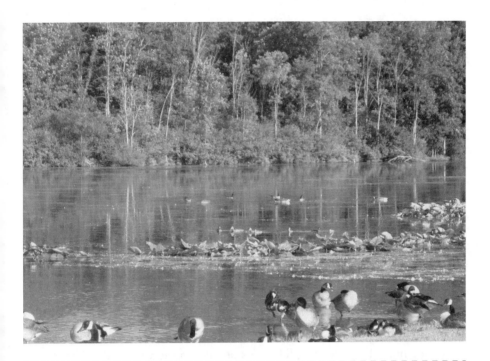

The city of Aurora operates a seasonal boat rental concession here.

most of the trail around it is exposed. That's not unusual for a lake trail.

At 0.5 miles into the trail, you can't see the lake for the trees. A couple of well-traveled but unmarked dirt trails on the left head through the woods toward the lake. (They're very short and loop back to the main trail quickly, so follow them if you want.) As the woods thin out, you'll be able to see most of the lake again from its mid-point. There's a lot to see.

Great blue heron sightings are almost guaranteed here. There's a rookery at Tinker's Creek State Nature Preserve, about 2 miles from here as the crow—or heron—flies, and the birds often travel between the parks. Gulls and goldfinches gather here as well. At 0.8 miles into the trail, you'll come to a small clearing and several birdhouses. A mown but unmarked utility path leads east, to your right. The paved path veers left, curling down to the lakeshore. Pass both and head straight for the woods on the northern edge of the park. A hard-packed dirt trail winds through the oak and maple trees, over a couple of small hills, before leaving the woods via a short limestone path facing the Page Road parking lot. The path curves left and meets the paved trail near a small picnic shelter. As you head south from here, you can see the whole lake. Lily pads cover the water in places; this is an ideal spot to listen as frogs, birds, and bugs sing to you. The woods are thick again as you round the lake's western edge; several park benches are placed to take advantage of the resulting shade and birding opportunities.

Other than the trail shoulder being mown, and the obvious care put into the Memorial Tree Garden, Sunny Lake's trees and vegetation have been left to their own devices. The snarled brush shelters a large population of rabbits, black and gray squirrels, fat robins, noisy jays, singing spring peepers, and a few harmless garter snakes.

Returning to the main parking lot, you've logged about 2.3 miles. (Keeping to the paved path around the lake and avoiding the extension through the woods makes it a total of about 2 miles.) The two short nature trails—both of which can be quite muddy—add another 0.5 miles or so to the trip. In that time, you've probably met up with a number of dog walkers, stroller pushers, and maybe a bike or two. Sunny Lake's loop is also a popular spot at lunchtime, as workers escape the nearby industrial parks, if only for an hour.

As you complete your trip around the lake, you'll come to a bench swing just north of the main shelter. Sit and swing a spell; if you took advantage of only some of the park's amenities, you've earned a rest.

NEARBY ACTIVITIES

Sunny Lake Park's 463 acres offer plenty of activities. On the western side of the main parking lot, there are swings, volleyball and bocce courts, and four horseshoe pits, plus a sledding hill that's popular in the winter. Pedal boats and rowboats can be rented at the park office. Aurora residents can launch their own nonmotorized crafts here for free; nonresidents pay a nominal fee for the privilege. Details are available at the website, **parks.auroraoh.com/parks-sunnylake.html,** or by calling (330) 562-1204. About 1 mile from here, Moebius Nature Center hosts a variety of educational programs for folks of all ages. See the events schedule at the website, **moebiusnaturecenter.org,** or call (330) 562-2592. For more hiking options, visit Tinker's Creek State Nature Preserve (see page 167), just about 2 miles southwest of Sunny Lake.

TINKER'S CREEK STATE NATURE PRESERVE   **35**

IN BRIEF

This 786-acre nature preserve offers great waterfowl and other wildlife viewing opportunities, as well as a peaceful, quiet marshland in which to be still and enjoy a bit of solitude.

DESCRIPTION

Although the parking area is on the north side of Old Mill Road, the main entrance to the preserve is across the street. But before you head south, make your way to the northeast end of the parking lot and follow the short Eagle Point Trail through the woods. The dirt trail through young deciduous trees may not impress you at first, but once you reach the raised observation platform, you'll be glad you made the trip. The vista that greets you—a wide expanse of marshy wetlands—is outlined by tall trees that eagles like to call home.

State naturalists found a nest that had fallen out of a tree here (it happens; the nests are quite heavy!) and rehabbed the fallen home, so visitors could appreciate it. It sits on the wet ground just out of reach, but close enough to get a good look at the amazing construction techniques of our national bird. Once you've had plenty of time to admire the marvel of avian engineering, retrace your steps back to the parking lot to begin the real hike.

KEY AT-A-GLANCE INFORMATION

LENGTH: 2 miles

CONFIGURATION: Out-and-back plus two loops and a short spur

DIFFICULTY: Easy

SCENERY: Seven ponds, marshlands, herons, nesting Canada geese and wood ducks, beavers, raccoons, deer, snapping turtles

EXPOSURE: Mostly shaded

TRAFFIC: Light

TRAIL SURFACE: Dirt trail with some boardwalk

HIKING TIME: 1 hour for three trails and observation time at the overlook

DRIVING DISTANCE: 22 miles from I-77/I-480 exchange

ACCESS: Daily, half hour before sunrise–half hour after sunset; pets not allowed

WHEELCHAIR TRAVERSABLE: No

MAPS: USGS Twinsburg; also available at the trailhead and online at dnr.state.oh.us

FACILITIES: None

CONTACT INFORMATION: Call (330) 527-5118 or visit dnr.state.oh.us.

Directions ————————————➤

From Cleveland, take I-480 East to Exit 37/ OH 91. Turn right (south) on OH 91/Darrow Road. Turn left at Old Mill Road and head east 2.6 miles to the small parking lot on the left (north) side of the road.

GPS Trailhead Coordinates

Latitude 41° 17.088783'

Longitude 81° 23.498397'

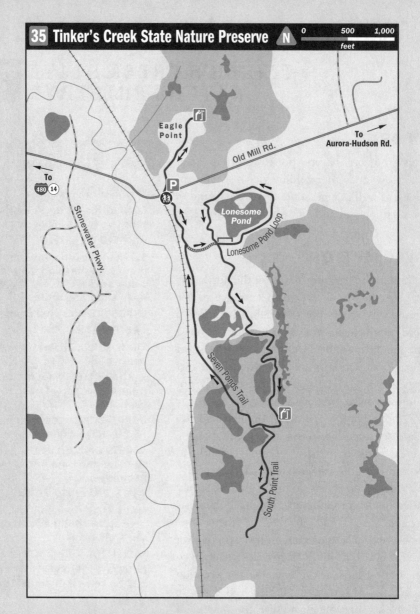

N

0   500   1,000
feet

To 480 14

Eagle
Point

Old Mill Rd.

To
Aurora-Hudson Rd.

P

Lonesome
Pond

Lonesome Pond Loop

Stonewater Pkwy.

Seven Ponds Trail

South Point Trail

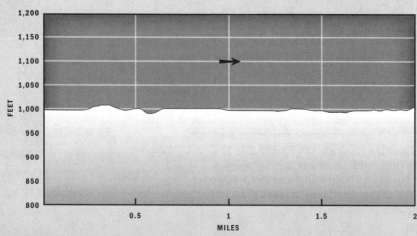

FEET			
1,200			
1,150			
1,100			
1,050			
1,000			
950			
900			
850			
800			

0.5   1   1.5   2
MILES

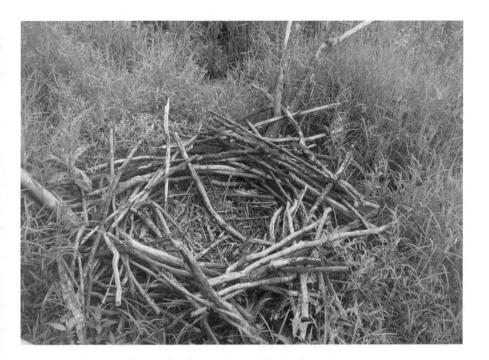

Eagle nests are so heavy that they sometimes fall to the ground, like this one did.

When you cross Old Mill, you'll enter the preserve on a path that runs parallel to and just a few hundred feet from active railroad tracks, but they don't detract from what you're about to see.

About 0.3 miles south of the trailhead sign, turn left onto Lonesome Pond Loop. The path can be quite muddy (this is a wetland, after all), and if your insect repellent fails here, you'll be sorry. Continue across the trail intersection and circle around the pond. Old-growth pines and younger deciduous trees almost completely shade the trail. In the spring and summer, an abundance of ferns and wild purple violets line the trail. The path narrows as it heads south. Not long after it narrows, the path forks—turn left (east). You'll soon step up on a wooden boardwalk. About half of this 0.5-mile loop is boardwalk, necessary because it travels over marsh. Ohio's early pioneers liked to hunt here, but they were also wary of the squishy ground. Some referred to it as a "perilous" place, full of sinkholes and quicksand. Although the thick peat is messy, deerflies and mosquitoes are really all hikers in this area have to fear today. You're likely to come upon deer or hear the slap of a beaver's tail as you near the pond. The boardwalk ends just about the time the pond comes into sight. The marsh, full of cattails, is on your right; the pond is on your left. Lonesome Pond Loop is mostly shaded by young oak trees. Water in the pond itself is clean enough to watch crappie and turtles swimming around below the surface.

Several types of ferns dot the trail; in spring, a thick covering of mayapples appear. Their umbrella-like leaves shade the pretty white flowers. On the north side of Lonesome Pond, grass and roots have overtaken much of the trail, making for less sloppy footing, even on wet days. After circling the pond, leave it lonesome once more and head south. A bench at the intersection of Lonesome Pond Loop and Seven Ponds Trail is a good place to contemplate what you've seen and consider your next steps.

Seven Ponds Trail heads south from here. Follow it as it weaves around the small ponds (that total seven, as advertised) and leads to a wooden observation deck. The deck faces east, and from here you can see almost all of the marsh. Herons like to fly between Tinker's Creek and nearby Sunny Lake (see page 163). It's a rare visit to either park that doesn't include a heron sighting. While this trail (and the whole preserve) sees little traffic, you may meet an avid birder or photographer here on the deck; it's popular with both.

When you can tear yourself away from the view, follow the path around a gentle bend to the right. Soon after, the path splits. Follow the left fork south to the tip of the "peninsula" surrounded by the open marsh. Shaded by beeches, oaks, and maples, this spur is especially pretty in the fall. When you return to the loop and head west, you'll make your way by and between the remaining ponds.

As you head north, the trail straightens out and, for the most part, it dries out as well. The railroad tracks are on your left, and the trail returns you to the intersection of Lonesome Pond Trail. With footsteps cushioned by the pine needles, you'll exit as quietly as you came in, slipping past the trailhead sign and crossing Old Mill Road.

NEARBY ACTIVITIES

If watching the waterfowl dive and splash made you want to drop a line in the water, go around the corner to "sister" Tinker's Creek State Park. There, just off Aurora-Hudson Road, you'll find plenty of fish-friendly spots and a completely different set of trails. Serious bird-watchers will want to visit Aurora Sanctuary State Nature Preserve, a 164-acre property owned by the Audubon Society. Access is available through the Aurora City Hall parking lot, 130 South Chillicothe Road. For more information, contact the local Audubon Society at (440) 285-2721.

TOWNER'S WOODS 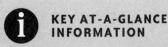 36

IN BRIEF

The 175-acre Towner's Woods is home to an ancient Native American mound, as well as to a number of creatures that require a variety of habitats: woodpeckers, owls, and deer claim the forest, while eagles like to perch high above Lake Pippen, which is closed to recreation. The grassy fields along the southern perimeter of Towner's Woods provide the perfect spot for the rare American woodcocks, or timberdoodles, who perform their unusual mating dance on early spring evenings.

DESCRIPTION

Tucked away, unassuming Towner's Woods park, established in the mid-1970s, has evolved in its first four decades. Visitors enjoy its riches in many different ways. When the trails are snow-covered, sledding and cross-country skiing make the park a popular destination. During the summer months, it's a cool and shady spot to hike (or bike along the rail-trail), and fall draws folks who admire the forest's flurry of color, as well as many young runners who use the cross-country ski trails to train.

In spite of all those visitors, the park somehow maintains its peaceful demeanor, inviting those who just want to enjoy a bit of nature's refreshing tranquility.

KEY AT-A-GLANCE INFORMATION

LENGTH: 5.5 miles

CONFIGURATION: Interconnecting loops; out-and-back rail-trail

DIFFICULTY: Easy, with a few hills

SCENERY: Fields, forests, wetlands, remnant prairie, lake views, a Hopewell Native American mound

EXPOSURE: Mostly shaded

TRAFFIC: Light–moderate

TRAIL SURFACE: Dirt and grass

HIKING TIME: 1.5 hours

DRIVING DISTANCE: 31 miles from I-77/I-480 exchange

ACCESS: Daily, sunrise–sunset. Lake Pippen, part of the city of Akron's watershed, abuts the park. The lake is off-limits to all but City of Akron Water Department workers.

WHEELCHAIR TRAVERSABLE: No

MAPS: USGS Kent; also available at portageparkdistrict.org

FACILITIES: Restrooms and water in parking lot near trailhead; sledding hill, picnic tables, shelters, gazebo, benches. A portion of The Portage Hike & Bike Trail runs through Towner's Woods, extending west to Kent and east into Ravenna.

CONTACT INFORMATION: To reach Portage Park District, call (330) 297-7728 or visit portageparkdistrict.org.

Directions ————————————→

Take I-480 East to OH 14 East in Streetsboro. Turn right onto OH 43, heading south about 3 miles to pass through Twin Lakes. Turn left onto Ravenna Road, following it about 2.5 miles to the well-marked park entrance.

GPS Trailhead Coordinates

Latitude 41° 10.329423'

Longitude 81° 18.702843'

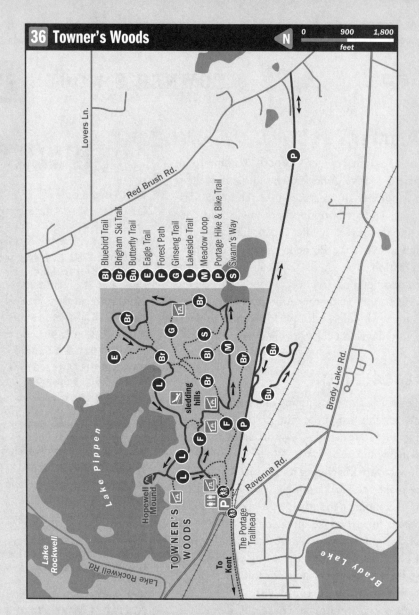

N

0   900   1,800
feet

Bluebird Trail — Bl
Brigham Ski Trail — Br
Butterfly Trail — Bu
Eagle Trail — E
Forest Path — F
Ginseng Trail — G
Lakeside Trail — L
Meadow Loop — M
Portage Hike & Bike Trail — P
Swann's Way — S

Red Brush Rd.

Lovers Ln.

Lake Pippen

Lake Rockwell

Lake Rockwell Rd.

Hopewell Mound

TOWNER'S WOODS

sledding hills

To Kent

The Portage Trailhead

Ravenna Rd.

Brady Lake Rd.

Brady Lake

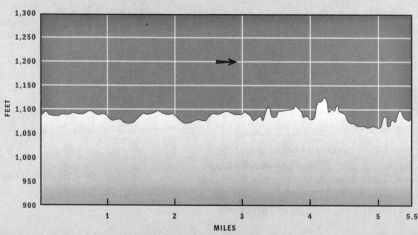

FEET

1,300
1,250
1,200
1,150
1,100
1,050
1,000
950
900

1   2   3   4   5   5.5

MILES

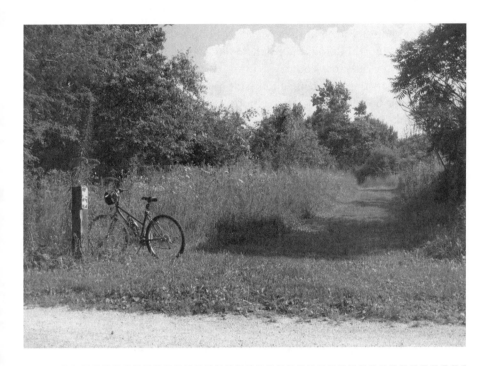

The cross-country ski trails at Towner's Woods are well-used in the winter months.

This hike explores two distinct areas: the rail-trail known as The Portage Hike & Bike Trail and Towner's Woods park. Trailheads for both sit on the eastern side of the parking lot. The park's wooded, hilly trails lead off to the left, but this hike begins to the right of a large park bulletin board, where you'll see a sign for The Portage. Tall oak and hickory trees stand on your left; a railroad track lies to the right. Follow the rail-trail about 100 yards into the trail where it forks. Turn right and follow the Butterfly Trail into the former farmland, strolling along a gentle, grassy hill. Birds and flying insects abound here, and it's a good spot to let your eyes glaze over and imagine how wide expanses of Portage County looked before trains and people rolled through in ever-increasing numbers. The Butterfly Trail is only about a half-mile long, so you'll soon return to the harder, flatter trail.

From there you can continue east on The Portage, which is mostly shaded, at least until it crosses Red Brush Road at the edge of the park property. From there, it continues east into the city of Ravenna and beyond. It's a great trail for cyclists and pedestrians too, but if you're here to hike through the woods, you'll want to return to the Towner's Woods Trailhead. From here, turn left onto the rail-trail, returning to the parking lot and the main trailhead.

Most of the trails through Towner's Woods wind through thick forests of oaks, maples, and pines to find shady and strikingly beautiful views of Lake Pippen on the west. More than 4 miles of interconnected trails are located throughout the park; all are well marked. My favorite route goes like this.

Follow Forest Path and then Meadow Loop to the east, past the sledding hill. Turn left (north) to join the Brigham Ski Trail. Follow it north, over lots of hills. Soon after the cross-country ski trail turns left, heading west toward the lake, it intersects the aptly named Lakeside Trail. Tall oaks and pines run alongside, reaching heights of 50 feet or more. Lakeside Trail is skinny and rather sharply banked in some places. It drops down several railroad-tie steps to the lowest point in the park, just a couple of feet above the water level. Soon after, Lakeside leads you north onto a small peninsula, where you'll find the Hopewell Native American mound.

The Hopewell people (and the mound) date to between 300 BC and AD 600. The mound was excavated in 1932, and 11 burials were found inside. The Hopewell culture is thought to have included worship of the dead, although admittedly, we're not quite sure what it involved.

Unfortunately, the excavations weren't conducted as carefully as most are today, and some artifacts were undoubtedly lost in the process.

Whatever its prehistoric significance, the mound sits rather artfully on the top of a sandy knoll overlooking the lake. It's probably safe to say, at least, that long ago, the Hopewell found this spot as beautiful as we do today. Once you're done exploring the mound, head south to return to the trailhead.

NEARBY ACTIVITIES

In the middle of Towner's Woods, you'll find a sizeable sledding hill and two large picnic areas with grills. Beckwith Orchards (**beckwithorchards.com**) is just around the corner from Towner's Woods. The orchard is open seasonally, and the Beckwith family is usually happy to allow visitors to wander through its gardens—a nice extra hike in itself.

Officials from the park system, the cities of Ravenna and Kent, and Kent State University (**kent.edu**) have worked together to connect Towner's Woods with other recreational venues via The Portage. The path is paved as it goes west from Lake Rockwell about 2.5 miles into the city of Kent; heading east, the grass-and-gravel trail extends from Red Brush Road to Peck Road in Ravenna.

Each September, a hot-air balloon festival is held in Ravenna, just beyond the western edge of the park. Depending on the wind, you'll see the balloons for a few minutes or the better part of an hour after their evening launch. Call the Balloon-A-Fair committee at (330) 297-2247 or see **ravennaballoonafair.com** for details about the annual event.

Special thanks to Christine Craycroft, executive director of Portage Park District, for reviewing this section.

WALBORN RESERVOIR 37

IN BRIEF

Wander through lush, fertile landscape typical of Stark County farmland in this park. The reservoir offers excellent opportunities for bird-watching. When the water is low, you may find the bleached-white skeletons of tiny crayfish dotting the shore.

DESCRIPTION

In northern Stark County, near Alliance, Stark County Park employees are busy. Not only do they host many activities and classes at Walborn Reservoir, but they're also eagerly awaiting the opening of a new trail that will connect this park to nearby Deer Creek Reservoir. But there's already plenty to explore at Walborn.

From the northeast end of the parking lot, follow along the edge of the farm field, drinking in the fresh honest smells that only good growing soil can provide. As you wind right (south), you'll eventually head into the woods, quite possibly meeting up with some horses out hiking (with their riders). You'll soon join up with the Loop Trail, which takes you west to reach the shore, where you'll be able to see the dam to your left. Follow the trail as it continues to crank clockwise, and listen. Few things are as peaceful and calming as water lapping gently on a shore. The

KEY AT-A-GLANCE INFORMATION

LENGTH: 2.5 miles

CONFIGURATION: Figure eight with parking in the middle (do either side as separate loop if you choose) and short out-and-back

DIFFICULTY: Easy

SCENERY: Bluebirds, wildflowers, ospreys, eagles, loons, possibly signs of beavers

EXPOSURE: Mostly shaded

TRAFFIC: Marina is busy; trails lightly used

TRAIL SURFACE: Dirt and grass

HIKING TIME: 1 hour

DRIVING DISTANCE: 53 miles from I-77/I/480 exchange

ACCESS: Park: Daily, sunrise–half hour before sunset; marina open April–September

WHEELCHAIR TRAVERSABLE: No

MAPS: USGS Limaville; also at park kiosk and at starkparks.com

FACILITIES: Restrooms, water, concession, and pay phone at marina

CONTACT INFORMATION: Visit starkparks.com or call (330) 409-8096.

Directions

Follow I-77 South to Exit 129 for I-76 West toward I-277/Canton/US 224. Take Exit 18 to I-277 East/US 224 East toward Canton. Follow US 224 East about 13 miles to OH 44 South/Ravenna Louisville Road and turn right. At Pontius Street NE, turn left and then veer right onto Price Street NE. Trailhead parking is on the east side of the reservoir.

GPS Trailhead Coordinates

Latitude   40° 58.661699'

Longitude   81° 10.804617'

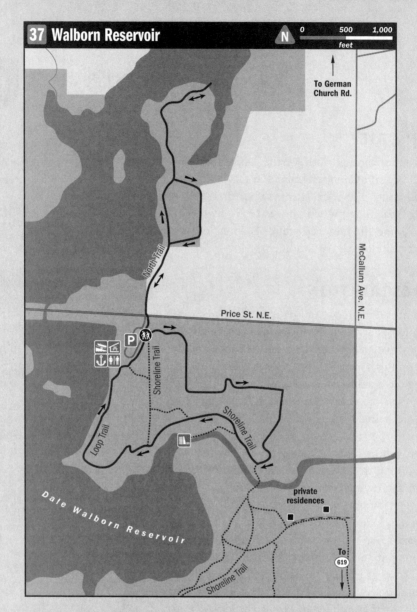

N

| 0 | 500 | 1,000 |

feet

To German
Church Rd.

McCallum Ave. N.E.

North Trail

Price St. N.E.

P

Shoreline Trail

Loop Trail

Shoreline Trail

Dale Walborn Reservoir

private
residences

To
619

Shoreline Trail

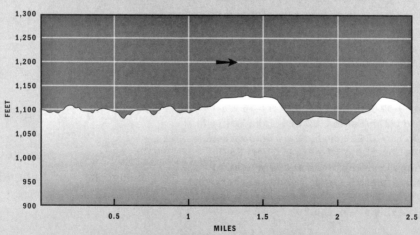

1,300				
1,250				
1,200				
1,150				
1,100				
1,050				
1,000				
950				
900				

FEET

0.5   1   1.5   2   2.5

MILES

going is relatively easy, as long as you don't mind a bit of slogging through the sandy soil.

While visiting here in the summer, you'll probably see bright-yellow cloudless sulphur butterflies along this stretch. From spring through fall, keep an eye out for herons, a pair of bald eagles, and the occasional ospreys, especially in August and September when the low water beckons waterfowl with tasty surprises. The Ohio Department of Natural Resources' (ODNR) work to repopulate this area with ospreys has paid off, and you may see one circling overhead. They resemble gulls, but if what you think is a gull dives feet-first into the water, then you've spotted an osprey.

As you make your way along the shore, you'll find

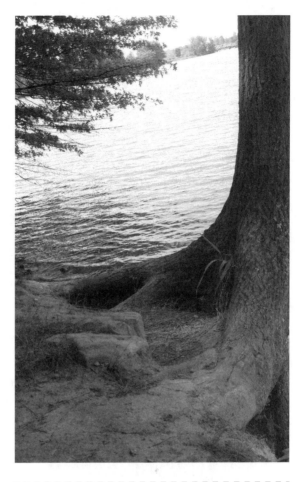

Fishing is popular at Walbourn Reservoir.

yourself crawling over fallen tree branches and creeping over the carcasses of expired crayfish. Ohio has about 20 species of crayfish. Many varieties burrow in the mud and are active only at night. That's fine with the owls, which like to eat the little crustaceans. Live crayfish also make good bait, but when you fish here (or anywhere!), it's important to use only native species. The bait that swims away can establish itself in the new habitat, and some nonnative species, such as the rusty crayfish, are so aggressive that they can wipe out native varieties and wreak havoc on a delicate ecosystem.

As you skirt the shore, you'll have to be nimble to stay dry, clambering over trees and tree roots that hug the bank. With roots half in water, half in soil, some of the roots appear to have grown into thin air when the water is low. Also, when the water is low, especially along the western shore, you'll appreciate displays of driftwood and rock art. Over the years, water and wind mold unique shapes and etch unusual patterns in both media. The pieces are displayed against a background of variegated dirt and clay. Take a flat rock and skip it into the lapping water before you return to the marina, at about 0.7 miles. Follow the boardwalk around the dock, and then cut across the parking lot (northeast) to return to your starting point.

This time, cross Price Street and head north to visit the typically quieter side of Walborn. You'll go up a slight hill and find yourself amid tall maple, chestnut, hickory, and pine trees. The soft dirt path wiggles through the woods, turning slightly away from the water before bending left to offer you another look at Walborn's wet playground. Fish and frogs keep the insect population hopping; ducks, herons, and other birds let their voices be heard. As you near the water's edge (and the northern edge of the short North Trail), you might see some evidence that beavers are working here; park employees are working just as diligently to keep them from creating their own dam here. Time will tell who will win. Flip a coin, place your bets, and turn around to follow your path back to Price Street and the parking lot.

NEARBY ACTIVITIES

There's a six-horsepower limit on the reservoir, making Walborn a good place to bring small sailboats or canoes. The marina also rents kayaks by the hour. Fishing is good here year-round; bass is a common catch.

For more hiking and boating nearby, follow Price Street east about 3 miles to Deer Creek Reservoir, another Stark County Park. For information about interpretive programs or about the status of connecting trails, go to **starkparks .com** or call (330) 477-3552.

WEST BRANCH STATE PARK 38

IN BRIEF

Like a lazy roller coaster, this hike follows gentle ups and downs on the south side of Michael J. Kirwan Lake. Pretty woodlands and lake views combine to make this a pleasant trek.

DESCRIPTION

The trails on the south side of the Michael J. Kirwan Lake's boat launch area were designed for snowmobiles and mountain bikes, and they also make delightful hiking paths. While the boat launch ramp is crowded (especially on warm weekends), the trails see little traffic during the week. However, hikers are warned to be on the lookout for mountain bikers, who can build up speed and round a blind corner quickly.

(*Note:* All bike/snowmobile trails lie within an Ohio Department of Natural Resources (ODNR) public hunting area. Small game is in season mid-August–mid-April. Wear bright colors when on the trails.)

Start your hike at the south side of the parking lot, entering the trails behind the bulletin board where park notices and a map are posted. You'll head up a short hill and turn left to follow the main Cable Line Trail east toward the reservoir.

KEY AT-A-GLANCE INFORMATION

LENGTH: 4 miles

CONFIGURATION: Out-and-back

DIFFICULTY: Moderate

SCENERY: Heavily wooded beech-maple forest, a few stands of pine, lake views, overlook

EXPOSURE: Mostly shaded

TRAFFIC: Moderate weekdays; heavy on weekends

TRAIL SURFACE: Partially paved

HIKING TIME: 1 hour

DRIVING DISTANCE: 35 miles from I-77/I-480 exchange

ACCESS: Daily, 6 a.m.–11 p.m.

WHEELCHAIR TRAVERSABLE: No

MAPS: USGS Ravenna; also posted at the trailhead and available at the park office, 5708 Esworthy Road

FACILITIES: Restrooms, pay phone, picnic shelter, and grills by boat ramp

CONTACT INFORMATION: For more information about hunting and fishing opportunities, see wildohio.com. To reach the park office, call (330) 296-3239 or visit westbranchstatepark.com.

Directions

From I-271/I-480 East, take OH 14 south to OH 5. Follow OH 5 about 5 miles east of Ravenna to Rock Spring Road. Turn right on Rock Spring Road and go about 2 miles to Cable Line Road. Turn left, following signs to the boat ramp parking lot.

GPS Trailhead Coordinates

Latitude   41° 7.923417'

Longitude   81° 8.536863'

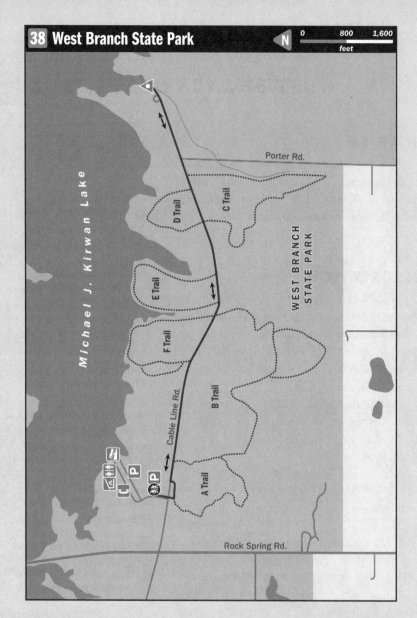

N

| 0 | 800 | 1,600 |

feet

Michael J. Kirwan Lake

Porter Rd.

D Trail

C Trail

WEST BRANCH STATE PARK

E Trail

F Trail

Cable Line Rd.

B Trail

P

P

A Trail

Rock Spring Rd.

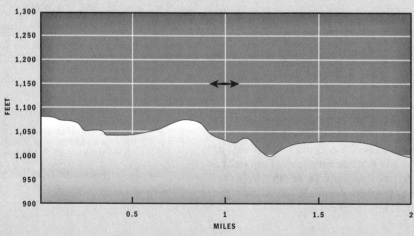

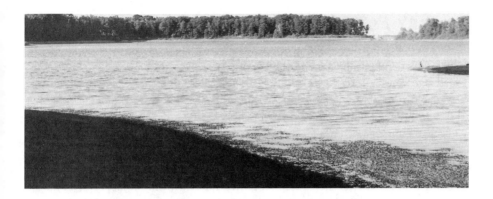

The sprawling reservoir features many quiet inlets like this one.

This partially paved road rolls along under the remainder of a beech-maple forest that once stretched from Mansfield, Ohio, to Pennsylvania. As the path rolls upward, the pavement holds its own, but by the bottom of the hill, it has lost ground to the encroaching grass. And so it goes. The battle between grass and asphalt continues all along the path, over five distinct hills, each offering at least a 20-foot climb. The grass has taken most of the low areas; the pavement still holds the tops of the hills. In between battles, on both sides of the path, small streams snake their way through the woods on their way to the reservoir.

The path rolls up to Porter Road, which you'll recognize by a circular turn-around, where there's room for several cars to park. This area, too, is zoned as a public hunting area; however, most folks here are armed with fishing poles. Cross Porter Road and continue east. You can see the reservoir from here, and a culvert wall on your left serves as a make-do bench. (On early spring evenings, this is a good seat from which to listen to the chorus of spring peepers.) About 0.3 miles east of here, the trail dead-ends into a lovely overlook and a popular fishing spot on the water's edge. After admiring the view, turn back and head west.

From this point, you can return directly to the trailhead. However, if you plan to follow the mountain bike/snowmobile trails on the way back, you have a lot to look forward to. The park map labels them alphabetically, but the trails themselves lack signs. The four short loops on the north side of Cable Line Trail wind through shady beech-maple and small stands of pine. Each loop bumps along to reach the water's edge and then turns south again, looping back to the main trail. Short wooden bridges carry you across the many twisting tributaries winding their way to the reservoir. On the south side of Cable Line, two longer loops (A and B, about 1 mile each, and F, about 0.9 miles) are more exposed than the northern paths, and just as hilly. If you follow the main trail and all the loops here, you'll have covered just over 7 miles.

NEARBY ACTIVITIES

West Branch State Park—named for the west branch of the Mahoning River, which was dammed in 1965—offers a variety of wet and dry activities for folks of all ages and interests. In addition to the snowmobile/bike trails, an 8-mile segment of the Buckeye Trail loops through the park's eastern end. Add to that about 20 miles of nature and bridle trails, including a paved path across the dam causeway, and there's enough day hiking here to keep you and your boots busy for a month.

The park's campground is extremely popular and hosts a variety of family-friendly events, such as the Grassman Festival in May, Christmas in July, and the Annual Halloween Campout in October. Call the park office at (330) 296-3239 for more information.

A 700-foot swimming beach, complete with restrooms and a vending area, is located on the southeastern side of the reservoir. Admission is free. The marina rents boats ranging from canoes and rowboats to ski boats and WaveRunners. The marina also offers a 90-minute pontoon boat cruise for groups. To arrange a tour, call the marina at (330) 296-9209 or visit **westbranchmarina.com.**

Special thanks to John Wilder, regional park manager, for reviewing this hike description.

WINGFOOT LAKE STATE PARK 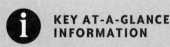 39

IN BRIEF

This property was operated as a recreation area for employees of the Goodyear Tire & Rubber Co. for several decades. When word spread that it would open in 2010 as Ohio's 74th state park, interest in its history was revived; once it opened, the park began building a new generation of fans. (*Note:* The park had recently opened as this book went to press, and more trails may be added in the future. The best way to see what Wingfoot Lake offers is to visit!)

DESCRIPTION

It's a safe bet that most visitors to Wingfoot Lake State Park don't go just to hike the 80-plus-acre property. Land-based attractions here include a miniature golf course, tennis courts, a dog park, and several large and well-appointed picnic shelters; in addition, the 444-acre lake offers fishing and boating opportunities. And while hikers almost certainly won't find solitude here, they will find a wide and gently rolling paved path circling the park. From that path, visitors can enjoy plenty of people-watching opportunities as well as gain an interesting perspective on the Goodyear Airdock and its place in history.

From the northeast side of the main

KEY AT-A-GLANCE INFORMATION

LENGTH: 1.5 miles

CONFIGURATION: Loop

DIFFICULTY: Easy

SCENERY: Lake and cultivated woodlands, unique view of the Goodyear Airdock

EXPOSURE: Mostly shaded

TRAFFIC: Moderate–heavy

TRAIL SURFACE: Paved

HIKING TIME: 35 minutes

DRIVING DISTANCE: 41 miles from I-77/I-480 exchange

ACCESS: Daily, 6 a.m.–11 p.m.

WHEELCHAIR TRAVERSABLE: Yes

MAPS: USGS Suffield; also posted at kiosk

FACILITIES: Boat rental, disc golf, miniature golf, playgrounds, sledding hill, tennis and volleyball courts, several enclosed shelters, grills and picnic tables, dog park

CONTACT INFORMATION: For shelter reservations, events information, maps, and more, visit ohiodnr.com. Shelter reservations can also be made by phone at (866) 644-6727. For information about fishing and hunting on the adjacent Ohio Division of Wildlife property, visit wildohio.com.

Directions

Follow I-77 South toward Akron, taking Exit 129 to I-76 West, then Exit 18 to I-277/US 224 East toward Canton. From US 224, turn right onto Martin Road and then left on Waterloo Road. Follow Waterloo about 1 mile east to the park entrance at Goodyear Park Boulevard.

GPS Trailhead Coordinates

Latitude   41° 1.085343'

Longitude   81° 21.7o7160'

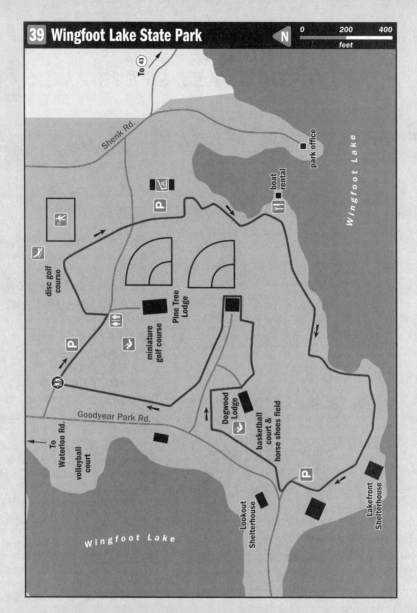

0   200   400
feet

N

To 43

Shenk Rd.

park office

boat
rental

Wingfoot Lake

disc golf
course

P

Pine Tree
Lodge

miniature
golf course

P

Goodyear Park Rd.

To
Waterloo Rd.

volleyball
court

Dogwood
Lodge

basketball
court &
horse shoes field

P

Lookout
Shelterhouse

Lakefront
Shelterhouse

Wingfoot Lake

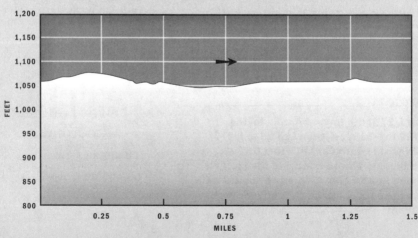

1,200						
1,150						
1,100						
1,050						
1,000						
950						
900						
850						
800						

FEET

0.25   0.5   0.75   1   1.25   1.5

MILES

parking lot, you'll probably see some disc golf or sledding enthusiasts—depending on the season—before you reach the paved trail, near one of the large enclosed picnic shelters. The path heads slightly downhill under the shade of mature oaks, maples, and other deciduous trees. You'll soon come to the park's boat concession area, where visitors can rent pedal boats and small pontoon boats in the warmer months.

As you continue along the gently rolling path on the edge of Wingfoot Lake, you're likely to encounter a few anglers hoping to hook bass, bluegills, crappie, brown bullheads, walleyes, or yellow perch. But while the landscaped grounds and lake views are sure to please visitors, for most, those sights will take a backseat to the supersized structure on the northwestern edge of the lake: the Goodyear Airdock.

The massive blue-and-silver building where more than 239 airships have been erected is a rather obvious reminder that The Goodyear Tire & Rubber Co. makes more than tires. In fact, Wingfoot Lake Airship Base is the oldest airship base in the United States; Goodyear built and operated the first U.S. commercially licensed blimp in 1925 and has sold several different airship models to the U.S. Navy. On clear days from late spring through early fall, visitors will often see (and hear!) the company's blimps take off and land across the lake.

Regardless of the activity in the air, there's plenty to see and do on the ground on the north side of the lake. Follow the path as it curves along the shore and then inland, and you'll see multiple structures enjoying new life in this new park, from the canteen where Goodyear employees and their families once purchased candy and other items (now used primarily for office space) to three large enclosed picnic shelters, one with a built-in sound system. Approximately in the center of the park, you can stop to enjoy a game of miniature golf or watch younger visitors frolic on two large playgrounds.

As the paved path continues to loop around the park's perimeter and back to the main parking lot, you'll pass volleyball and bocce courts before reaching a dog park on the northwestern side of the property.

Returning to the main parking lot, you'll know just where you are: the historical stone sign featuring Goodyear's distinctive winged-foot logo marks the spot.

NEARBY ACTIVITIES

This new park is situated near other well-used Ohio state parks, including Quail Hollow to the south (see page 149). Mogadore Reservoir to the north is owned by the city of Akron (call [330] 678-0077) and is managed by the Ohio Division of Wildlife (call 800-945-3533 or visit **dnr.state.oh.us**).

Special thanks to Todd Metz, assistant park manager, for sharing his knowledge about this property and his vision for its future as a much-loved Ohio state park.

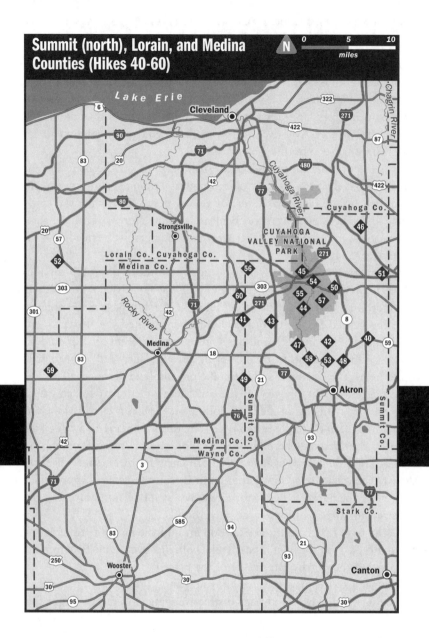

Summit (north), Lorain, and Medina Counties (Hikes 40–60)

N

0   5   10
miles

Lake Erie

Cleveland

322

271

422

87

6

90

83

20

71

480

Cuyahoga River

Chagrin River

42

77

422

80

Strongsville

CUYAHOGA VALLEY NATIONAL PARK

Cuyahoga Co.

46

20

57

52

Lorain Co. Cuyahoga Co.
Medina Co.

56

271

45

54

50

51

303

303

55

57

301

Rocky River

60

44

8

42

71

41

43

47

42

40

59

Medina

18

58

53

48

83

59

49

21

77

Akron

76

Summit Co.

Summit Co.

93

Medina Co.
Wayne Co.

3

42

71

585

94

77

Stark Co.

250

83

21

93

Wooster

30

30

Canton

95

30

SUMMIT (NORTH), LORAIN, AND MEDINA COUNTIES

40 ADELL DURBIN PARK AND ARBORETUM

 KEY AT-A-GLANCE INFORMATION

LENGTH: 1.1 miles

CONFIGURATION: Three intersecting loops

DIFFICULTY: Easy

SCENERY: More than 80 identi-fied species of trees and shrubs; ravine overlook and creek-crossing opportunity

EXPOSURE: Mostly shaded when trees have leaves

TRAFFIC: Moderately busy, especially on weekends

TRAIL SURFACE: Dirt and grass

DRIVING DISTANCE: 27 miles from I-77/I-480 exchange

ACCESS: Daily, sunrise–sunset; dogs and other pets are not allowed.

WHEELCHAIR TRAVERSABLE: No

MAPS: USGS Hudson; self-guided tour brochures available at the trailhead bulletin board

FACILITIES: Restrooms, water, vending machines, and pay phone in main parking lot

CONTACT INFORMATION: Reach the city of Stow's parks office at (330) 689-5100 or visit stow.oh.us.

IN BRIEF

This beautifully maintained arboretum and trail system sits on a surprisingly rugged 34 acres in the heart of Stow. Many drivers passing by every day might be surprised to discover the natural beauty that lies beyond the tennis courts and kiddie playground visible from OH 91. You'll have to pull off the road and put on your hiking boots to find out.

DESCRIPTION

This hike follows the park's three trails: The Hiker's Trail (marked in red), Cliff Trail (blue), and Tree and Shrub Trail (yellow). If you're short on time, take the 0.6-mile Cliff Trail. Regardless of which trail you choose, be sure to take along the self-guided brochure that identifies dozens of trees and shrubs in the park. The trees are marked with round numbered tags; their names are listed numeri-cally on the brochure.

Before your hike begins, you'll surely notice that you're being watched—the statue of a Native American chief presides over the parking lot. Perhaps he's daring you to ven-ture into the relative wildness just behind him. Rattlesnakes, wolves, and mountain lions roamed here not so long ago. So be brave and step onto the Yellow Trail (also called the

GPS Trailhead Coordinates

Latitude   41° 9.278641'

Longitude   81° 26.445000'

Directions

From I-77 take I-480 East (toward Youngstown) to I-271; then take the OH 8 South exit, turning right. Take the Graham Road exit (toward Silver Lake/Stow). Turn left onto Graham, then right onto Darrow Road (OH 91). After you cross OH 59 (Kent Road), the park is about 0.3 miles south, on the right (west) side of OH 91.

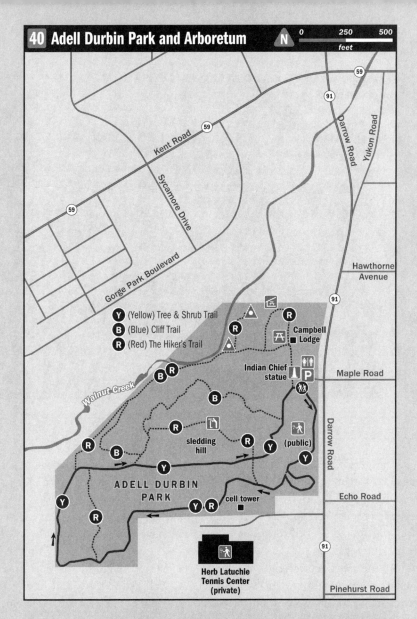

N

0   250   500
feet

Y (Yellow) Tree & Shrub Trail
B (Blue) Cliff Trail
R (Red) The Hiker's Trail

Kent Road
Sycamore Drive
Gorge Park Boulevard
59
59
59
91
Darrow Road
Yukon Road
Hawthorne Avenue
91
Maple Road
Darrow Road
Echo Road
91
Pinehurst Road

Campbell Lodge
Indian Chief statue
(public)
sledding hill
ADELL DURBIN PARK
cell tower
Herb Latuchie Tennis Center (private)

Walnut Creek

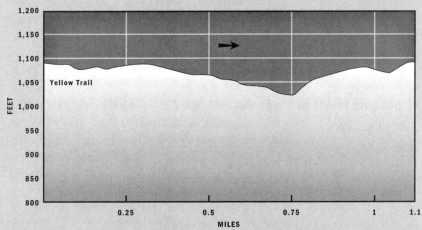

1,200					
1,150					
1,100					
1,050	Yellow Trail				
1,000					
950					
900					
850					
800					

FEET

0.25   0.5   0.75   1   1.1

MILES

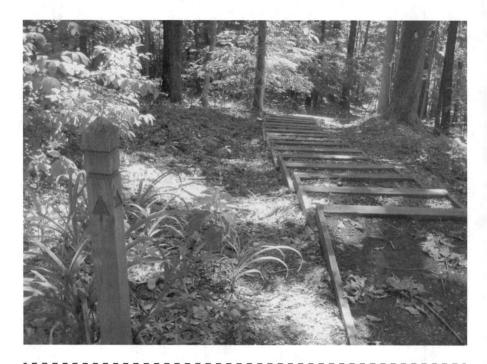

Step on the Cliff Trail, and into the ravine.

Tree and Shrub Trail) at the southern end of the parking lot. Take the concrete steps down from Campbell Lodge and follow the mulched path in a clockwise direction. You will briefly walk parallel to OH 91, and when you reach the end of the tennis courts, you'll notice quarter-size silver tags on some of the trees. After you've logged a third of a mile, you may have spotted as many as 25 tree-identifying tags.

As the path veers right, you'll skirt the western edge of the park to find a wide variety of grasses and wildflowers, as well as the birds and insects that are attracted to them. Look north to enjoy a lovely panorama: a diverse ring of deciduous trees. In the fall, of course, the panorama is at its boldest, brightest best; even the poison ivy vines that wrap around the tree trunks turn bright orange-red, like ribbons tying up the season. In the spring, the beauty is subtler but worth contemplation. As the various trees awake in slow progression, each buds in its own time, providing evidence (especially welcome in Northeast Ohio) that while winter slows us all down, life goes on.

Continuing west, you'll pass a sign for the Red, or Hiker's, Trail. The sign marks one of several spots where the park's trails intermingle. This can cause some confusion if you attempt to follow the trails without a map. There's little danger of getting lost (the park is relatively small at 34 acres), but you could miss a significant, and pretty, section of the trail and the park. So swallow your pride, grab a map, and refer to it as needed.

Where the Red Trail crosses your path, turn left (south) following the Yellow Trail through the thick forest. A number of tall, old pines grow along here, and the forest floor is strewn with pine needles and rotting logs of all sizes. In various states of decay, they provide both food and shelter for a host of animals, birds, and insects.

As you walk near the park's southern border, you'll pass the short and pretty balsam fir (its tag is number 95) and a few hardy strands of goldenrods poking up though the forest floor looking for the sun. The path veers right, heading north and a bit east as you pass near some apartment buildings. Here you'll see English ivy that has escaped domesticity

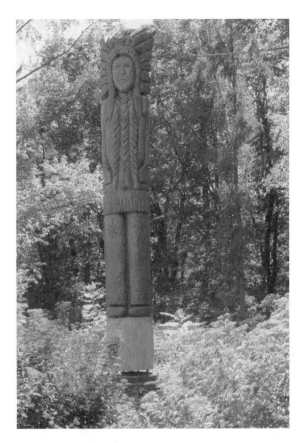

You're never quite alone at Adell Durbin.

for the relative wilds of this little park—score one for houseplants! Red-bellied woodpeckers like to dart about here, 10–20 feet above, tapping on dead branches to scare out a snack. (*Note to novice birders:* The name *red-bellied* is a bit misleading, as its head is dark red, but its belly is actually rather light—a pinkish white. Don't let this discourage you from developing a bird-watching habit; it's a hobby that develops keen observation skills and, if you're lucky, patience too.)

A sign at about 0.6 miles confirms that you have been following the yellow and red paths. A few steps later, on your right, you'll see tree number 87. Old number 87 is the rigid hornbeam; its gray, taut bark gives it a face as distinguished as its name. Its pretty bark is almost too smooth, as if it had a facelift that pulled too tight. Not surprisingly, it is also commonly referred to as musclewood.

Before you cross the Red Trail again, you'll go up a small hill, past a small wooden observation deck, and pass beneath a row of chestnut trees to reach a persimmon tree. In the late summer and early fall, the fruits reach the size of cherry tomatoes. In the fall, this section of the trail might be considered a falling nut zone, as it is full of shedding oak, beechnut, and chestnut trees. When the winds

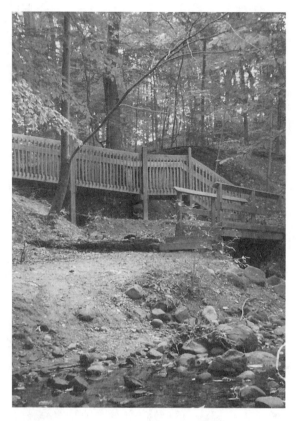

Walnut Creek is clear and shallow.

or squirrels are very active, nuts literally rain down from the trees along here. You'll hit the bottom of a short hill at about 0.9 miles, trek uphill a few steps to pass the nature center, and then return to the parking lot. Long before you reach this point, you'll probably realize that you've followed the Yellow Trail backwards— at least according to the "Tree and Shrub Guide" provided by the park. Your reward for following the path south to north is that when you reach the end (or the beginning?), you come to the heart of the park, the deep gorge that cradles Walnut Creek.

In the parking lot, look for the Blue Trailhead and follow the 100-plus steps down into the ravine. The 0.6-mile Blue Trail is also known as the Cliff Trail, and you'll see why about halfway down the steps. A large wooden deck there overlooks the creek, which is clean, shallow, and, in most places, about 7 feet wide. If you follow the Blue Trail, you'll cross the creek and have a choice of veering left to join up with the Red Trail or turning sharply back to the north and then venturing east again, through the thick of the forest. However, you don't have to follow the Blue Trail to enjoy the creek and ravine.

NEARBY ACTIVITIES

Adell Durbin Park features a small fenced-in play area, perfect for toddlers, as well as volleyball and tennis courts and a sledding hill. Just south on OH 91, you can access Brust Park ([330] 867-5511; **summitmetroparks.org**) on the Summit County Bike & Hike Trail for miles.

Special thanks to Nick Wren, of the Stow Parks and Recreation Department, for reviewing this description.

ALLARDALE LOOPS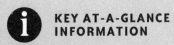

IN BRIEF

When Stan and Ester Allard donated 336 acres of their farm to the Medina County Park District in 1992, they guaranteed that at least some of the rolling landscape would remain beautifully undeveloped. What they did with the land before they gave it away is as impressive as their generosity.

DESCRIPTION

The best advice about hiking Allardale is this: walk the outer loop counterclockwise. That way, you're treated to the marvelous overlook view at the end of your hike. It is a deserved reward for your effort; to reach it early on makes the rest of the trip almost anticlimactic. Walking the trail clockwise isn't wrong, exactly; it's sort of like having dessert first.

The 1-mile outer loop of dirt and grass winds through a valley and former farmland. Along the way you'll find many examples of the careful planning and maintenance this land enjoyed under the Allards' ownership. When you reach the dedication overlook, you may be overwhelmed at the generosity that they demonstrated in giving it away.

From the trailhead sign, turn right and head down a paved hill. As the trail curves to the left, the pavement ends and you'll follow

KEY AT-A-GLANCE INFORMATION

LENGTH: 1.5 miles

CONFIGURATION: Two nested loops

DIFFICULTY: Easy

SCENERY: Forest, farmland, wide variety of identified trees, one incredible view

EXPOSURE: About half shaded

TRAFFIC: Moderate

TRAIL SURFACE: Inner loop trail, paved; outer loop, hard-packed gravel and dirt

HIKING TIME: 1 hour

DRIVING DISTANCE: 21 miles from I-77/I-480 exchange

ACCESS: Daily, 8 a.m.–sunset

WHEELCHAIR TRAVERSABLE: Shorter paved loop, yes; longer loop, no

MAPS: USGS Medina; also posted on a signboard at the trailhead

FACILITIES: Water and flush toilets at main parking lot; sheltered picnic area also available

CONTACT INFORMATION: Reach the Medina Park District at (330) 722-9364 or medinacountyparks.com.

Directions

From I-271, take Exit 3 onto OH 94 (Ridge Road) and follow it south 0.5 miles to Remsen Road. Turn left and follow Remsen east approximately 3 miles. Allardale is on the north side of Remsen, less than 1 mile west of Medina Line Road.

GPS Trailhead Coordinates

Latitude   41° 11.398559'

Longitude   81° 41.920137'

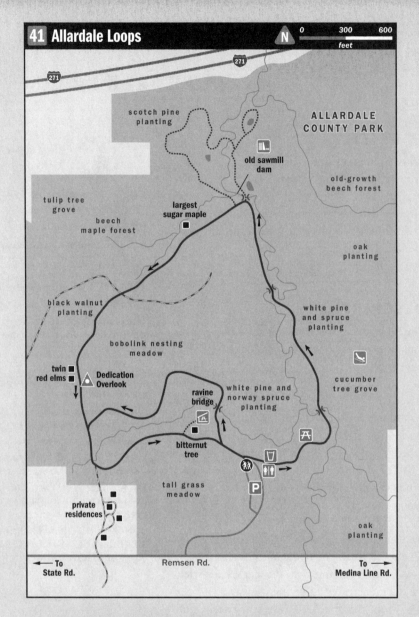

41 Allardale Loops

N

0   300   600
feet

scotch pine
planting

ALLARDALE
COUNTY PARK

old sawmill
dam

old-growth
beech forest

tulip tree
grove

largest
sugar maple

beech
maple forest

oak
planting

black walnut
planting

white pine
and spruce
planting

bobolink nesting
meadow

twin
red elms

Dedication
Overlook

ravine
bridge

white pine and
norway spruce
planting

cucumber
tree grove

bitternut
tree

tall grass
meadow

private
residences

oak
planting

To
State Rd.

Remsen Rd.

To
Medina Line Rd.

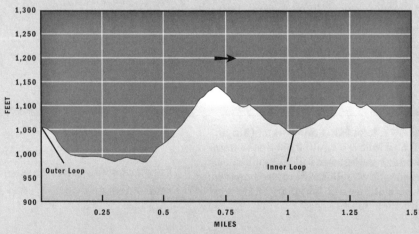

Outer Loop

Inner Loop

FEET

1,300
1,250
1,200
1,150
1,100
1,050
1,000
950
900

0.25   0.5   0.75   1   1.25   1.5

MILES

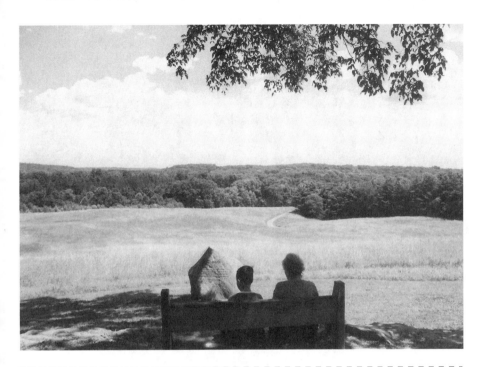

Dedication overlook

a dirt-and-gravel path down a few more feet. Here, the wind rushes across the wide-open trough to meet you head-on. You'll cross a short footbridge into the prairie meadow. Tall pines rise on the west of the hill; young beech trees on the eastern side of the path shade you as you cross over a second footbridge.

At about the half-mile point, you'll pass the remnants of an old sawmill dam marked with a hand-lettered sign. Several other items, such as an old wagon wheel, are also signed; they dot the trail like snapshots decorate a refrigerator. You can imagine them whispering, "Hey, remember this?" Just past the sawmill sign, turn left heading uphill toward the barn. (*Note:* This turn will go against your natural desire to continue west, across an inviting and relatively new footbridge. Don't give in; if you cross the bridge, you'll soon find yourself off the path and on private property.)

Allardale has been recognized, several times, as an outstanding example of forestry and land conservation. In the 1930s, this farm was among the first to practice soil-saving techniques such as contour strip farming and erosion control using pines and spruces planted along steep hillsides. Since then, at least 100,000 trees have been planted—today you'll walk through established collections of black walnuts, red and white oaks, white pines, and a variety of other trees. Allardale has received awards from the Ohio Department of Natural Resources Division of Forestry and is considered one of the finest tree farms in Ohio. Perhaps no one appreciates it more than the myriad moths and butterflies

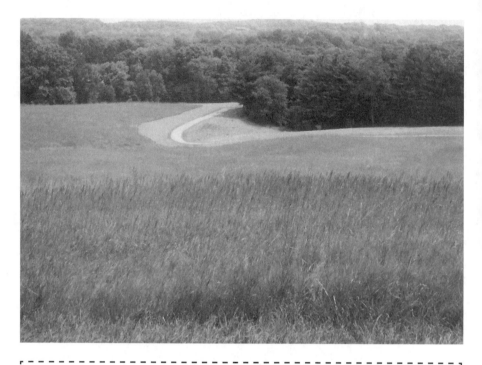

This notable property still speaks to the Allards' stewardship of the land.

that dance happily in the diverse and crowded woods.

You can enjoy their antics as you climb uphill, around a bend, and up another 50 feet or so through the woods, emerging into an open field via a wide, mown path. Look north (to your left) over the tall grass and take in a view that stretches for miles. From this point you'll get a glimpse of the rolling hills, farms, and dales that long ago were all that comprised Medina County.

A few more feet up, at the highest point on the hill, a bench sits under a tree. A large rock directly in front of it doesn't obscure your view; it adds to your overall appreciation. It is inscribed: "Allardale, a gift from Stan and Ester Allard, so others can enjoy the open spaces, the blue sky, the trees, the flowers, the birds, and the hills and valleys that they have loved so much."

If you can tear yourself away from the beautiful vista, take a few more steps east, so you can see the Allards' red barn, standing on the hillside just south of the trails. Until it was given to Medina County, this farm had been in the Allard family since 1877. That being the case, it has a lot of history to relate. A plaque near the shelter explains a bit of the history of the farm and of Medina County.

Just past the plaque, on your left, you'll walk by the western end of the inner loop. Pass by the trail here and enter the shorter loop just east of the shelter, so you can follow it counterclockwise too. The entire half-mile trail is paved. Turn left onto the path and descend a moderately steep hill to a long wooden bridge. As you approach the bridge, your feet will grind over rusty pine needles, releasing a piney fragrance, regardless of the season. You'll have a good look at the ravine from the bridge, which spans about 50 feet. As the loop turns to head west, it leaves the woods and affords another view of the valley, this time from the middle of the hill. When you reach the southwestern end of this short loop, you can turn left to return to the parking lot. More likely, though, you'll turn right—for one more look at the view the Allards left behind.

NEARBY ACTIVITIES

The picnic shelter here, adjacent to the inner loop trail, can be reserved by calling the Medina Park District at (330) 722-9364 or by using the online system at **medinacountyparks.com**. While you're in the area, visit Green Leaf Park (see page 226) just a few miles south on Medina Line Road ([330] 722-9364; **medinacountyparks.com**).

42 BABB RUN BIRD AND WILDLIFE SANCTUARY

KEY AT-A-GLANCE INFORMATION

LENGTH: 3 miles

CONFIGURATION: One loop and one out-and-back

DIFFICULTY: Moderate

SCENERY: The Cuyahoga River and a tributary, sandstone cliffs, a wide variety of ferns, trees, small animals, birds

EXPOSURE: Shady

TRAFFIC: Moderate–heavy in the picnic areas; light on the river's edge

TRAIL SURFACE: Varies from paved to pebbles, dirt, rocks, and roots

HIKING TIME: 1 hour

DRIVING DISTANCE: 29 miles from I-77/I-480 exchange

ACCESS: Daily, sunrise–sunset; pets not permitted. While staying on the trail is difficult (trails are unmarked), use care and common sense— erosion is a constant problem here.

WHEELCHAIR TRAVERSABLE: No

MAPS: USGS Peninsula

FACILITIES: Portable restroom at parking lot

CONTACT INFORMATION: For more information about Babb Run and other park properties owned by the city of Cuyahoga Falls, call (330) 971-8225 or visit cityofcf.com.

IN BRIEF

You'll have to find your own way through here, as Babb Run's sandy paths are unmarked and trodden only by the passing deer and occasional hiker. About 3 miles of trails are fairly easy to find; negotiating them requires a sense of adventure and a good pair of hiking boots. Tread lightly, and your rewards will be close encounters with wildlife and a symphony of sounds—from Babb Run's low babble to the boisterous blare of the river's rapids.

DESCRIPTION

Step onto the paved path from the northwest edge of the small parking lot, marked by a large sign that explains the park's erosion problems. You'll see evidence of those problems as you follow the paved path to the left, heading south down a short, steep hill. The pavement ends at the bottom of the hill where the path splits. For a short detour, you can follow the fork to the right straight to the banks of the Cuyahoga River, where you can look west at the pale cliff rising nearly 40 feet above the river. Sit still for a while and listen as the birds and the water converse. When you're done eavesdropping, retrace your steps to the fork in the path and turn right, heading east.

GPS Trailhead Coordinates

Latitude   41° 7.608483'

Longitude   81° 31.059723'

Directions

Take I-77 South to I-80. Follow the turnpike east to Exit 180/OH 8 south. Exit at Broad Boulevard and turn right. Turn left onto State Road, taking the second right onto Sackett Avenue. Follow Sackett to the park entrance across from Chestnut Memorial Cemetery.

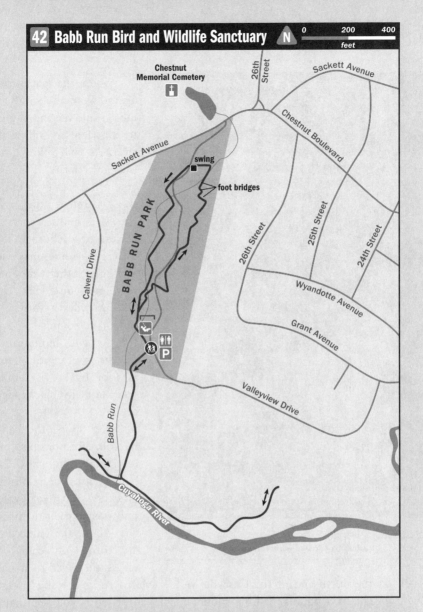

N

0   200   400
feet

Chestnut
Memorial Cemetery

26th Street

Sackett Avenue

Chestnut Boulevard

Sackett Avenue

swing

foot bridges

25th Street

24th Street

BABB RUN PARK

Calvert Drive

26th Street

Wyandotte Avenue

Grant Avenue

Valleyview Drive

Babb Run

Cuyahoga River

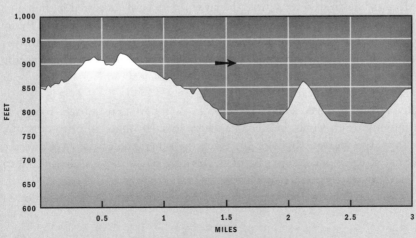

FEET						
1,000						
950						
900						
850						
800						
750						
700						
650						
600						

0.5   1   1.5   2   2.5   3

MILES

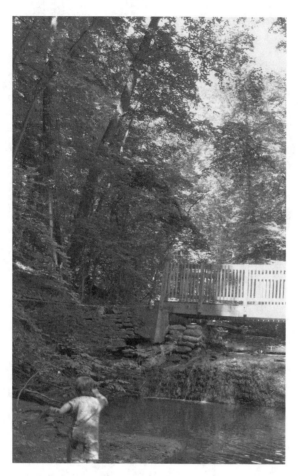

No climbing allowed—but running is OK!

Soon the path forks again. Take the southernmost trail, veering slightly to the right to follow the river. As you follow along the banks of the Cuyahoga, you'll find that even in this short stretch, the river shows its multiple personalities. At each turn it is different—sometimes wide and quiet, other times narrow and noisy. The trail also provides a variety of sights and sounds.

As you bump along on the rooty, sandy soil, 30-foot banks rise up to your left. In places signs declare NO CLIMBING, but in other spots, the banks beckon. Responsible hikers ignore their calls. The banks are deteriorating quickly; your feet would only hasten their demise.

About 0.5 miles into the trail, you can look across the river to a park bench on the north end of the Cascade Valley (Metro Parks Serving Summit County). This is a popular fishing spot; don't be surprised if you see anglers knee-deep in the river here. Where the river is less easily accessed by humans, you're likely to spot a great blue heron fishing for a meal. Kingfishers fly by often too; the nests of both birds are scattered among the tops of the tall trees on the riverbank. A few steps south of the beaten path, you can peer into the shallow, still edges of the river and see minnows lolling about. You may also spot the small white shells of freshwater clams nearby.

Before you've logged a mile on the trail, you'll have to turn back. Your only other options are to climb the steep banks to your left (unwise) or to cross the large, slippery sandstone boulders to reach the other side of the river and the residential street immediately east of it. Turning back, though, doesn't mean you'll have to exactly retrace your steps.

As you head back upstream, you'll soon see that the path you followed along the river splits. Follow the trail to the right. At times it will take you 50 feet or farther north of the path you first followed. In fact, at points along this path you can barely hear—and cannot see—the river at all. Under a canopy of tall oak, maple, and beech trees, you'll encounter a few fallen, decaying limbs and other obstacles across the path. Keep your eyes open (so you don't trip!), and you'll also see a host of ferns, fungi, and mosses taking advantage of the cool ravine climate.

In warm months, you'll enjoy colorful glimpses of the butterflies and moths that flourish here in the cool woods. At least three times, the northern path joins up with its southern sister; then it wanders off again, as siblings often do. The two finally meet up and return, together, to the paved trail.

Now follow the paved path uphill to a small playground area with swings. Just north of the swings you'll follow a dirt path to two footbridges that criss-cross Babb Run. The beauty of the ravine is only marginally interrupted by the drainage pipes inserted here and there. (The drainpipes are necessary to mini-mize erosion in the area. Over time, the tributary will overcome the drainpipes' efforts, so enjoy the walkway while it lasts.) As you continue north along Babb Run, the path veers east and rises up about 20 feet to meet the park's roadway. Alongside the roadway you'll find a 10-foot-long wooden bridge, stuck rather precariously into the steep bank. It is secured by three mature trees, but walking along without the benefit of a railing is slightly unnerving. A few paces farther north, cross the road and continue climbing 15 feet up and to the east.

Turn left at the top of the rise to find three footbridges set close together. At the end of the last bridge, the path bends sharply to the left, twisting down-hill to another bench swing, which faces east. Sit for a spell and wonder what the now-closed path to your left once revealed. The path, blocked by a wooden fence, is overgrown with mayapples, poison ivy, and other vines. Return the way you came, up and down the twisting path, heading south over the bridges. Along the way, you'll notice several patches of English ivy creeping down the hill from the east. Most likely, these vines have escaped from the residential yards high above. One can hardly blame them. Babb Run is indeed a sanctuary from urban life.

NEARBY ACTIVITIES

Chestnut Hills Memorial Park, a small but lovely cemetery, sits across the street from Babb Run. At its entrance, a stone path leads to a bench overlooking a foun-tain. With several bird boxes set in and around the water, it serves to continue the sanctuary for the birds and other wildlife that venture north. Babb Run is situated within a couple of miles of Cascade Valley Metropark ([330] 867-5511; **summitmetroparks.org**) and Gorge Metro Park (see page 222).

43   BATH NATURE PRESERVE

KEY AT-A-GLANCE INFORMATION

LENGTH: 4.5 miles

CONFIGURATION: Four loops

DIFFICULTY: Moderate

SCENERY: Deer and hawks in the oak-maple-hickory forest, frogs and other aquatic life in the ponds, bog-loving tamaracks, broad prairie hillsides

EXPOSURE: Mostly exposed

TRAFFIC: Moderate

TRAIL SURFACE: North Fork is crushed limestone; nature trails are dirt paths

HIKING TIME: 1.5–2 hours

DRIVING DISTANCE: 21 miles from I-77/I-480 exchange

ACCESS: Daily, sunrise–sunset

WHEELCHAIR TRAVERSABLE: No— though a long stretch of trail is paved, most of it is very steep.

MAPS: USGS West Richfield; also available at the trail kiosk at Bath Community Activity Center off North Cleveland-Massillon Road

FACILITIES: Restrooms and water fountain at trail kiosk and at picnic shelters found at either end of this trail

CONTACT INFORMATION: Visit bathtownship.org or call (330) 666-4007.

IN BRIEF

This Summit County nature preserve looms just up the hill from an unassuming community park. Take a tour of the smaller park, and then sneak into the vast preserve through a tunnel.

DESCRIPTION

When you pull into the parking lot off busy North Cleveland-Massillon Road, you may not be expecting much. An oversize wood statue of the Mingo Chief Logan greets you by the trail kiosk, and his imposing figure might distract you for a moment. After you've introduced yourself to the chief, visit the trail kiosk to get a lay of the land, and then head toward the trailhead—just to your right—to wander through a small stand of trees.

The well-shaded path brings you quickly to tennis courts; not far east of there a pretty working water pump stands ready to cool you off. Follow the footpath beyond the tennis courts and you'll soon find two soccer fields and a picnic area.

Traipse by the soccer fields and peer into the woods: you've found King Trail, just a short jaunt through the woods.

The path rolls along under the shade of oak and shagbark hickory trees. Squirrels scurry about picking up their nuts. A picnic

GPS Trailhead Coordinates

Latitude   41° 10.746481'

Longitude   81° 38.163300'

Directions

Follow I-77 South toward Akron and take Exit 143 for OH 176 (toward I-271), getting off the ramp at Wheatley Road. Turn right onto Wheatley, taking a quick left onto Brecksville/Cleveland-Massillon Road. Bath Community Center and trailhead parking are located at 1615 North Cleveland-Massillon Road.

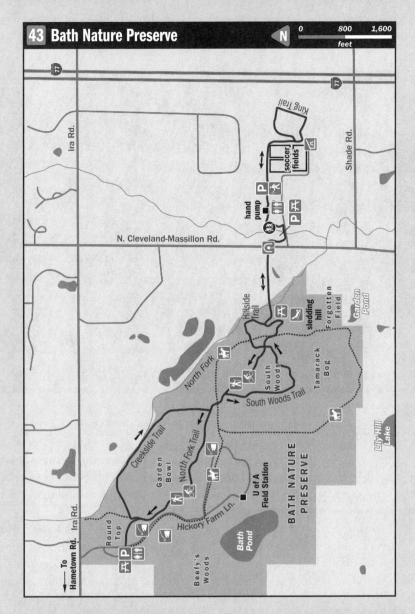

N

0   800   1,600
feet

I-77

Ira Rd.

Shade Rd.

King Trail

soccer fields

hand pump

P

P

N. Cleveland-Massillon Rd.

Hillside Trail

North Fork

North Fork Trail

Creekside Trail

Garden Bowl

South Woods

South Woods Trail

Tamarack Bog

sledding hill

Forgotten Field

Garden Pond

Lily Hill Lake

BATH NATURE PRESERVE

U of A Field Station

Hickory Farm Ln.

Round Top

Beefy's Woods

Bath Pond

Ira Rd.

To Hametown Rd.

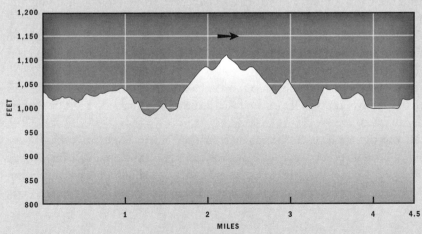

1,200
1,150
1,100
1,050
1,000
950
900
850
800

FEET

1   2   3   4   4.5

MILES

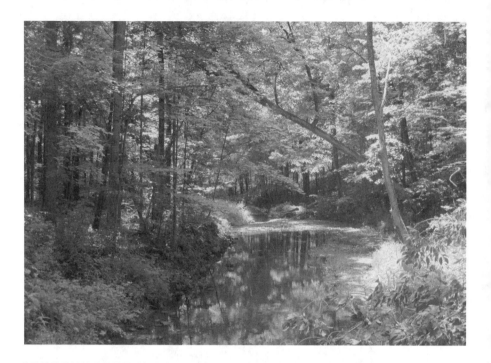

Enjoy the shady spots in this preserve, as the trails are mostly exposed.

might be underway under the covered shelter; if it's a weekend, chances are that you'll catch a ballgame of some sort in progress. Retracing your steps back to where you began, you might shrug and say, "Well, it's just your average community park." But wait, there's more! Much more.

Turn your back to Chief Logan and walk to the north end of the parking lot where a tunnel invites you to slip away. Follow the crushed limestone path through the tunnel and keep going. The trees give way to reveal wide-open sky, and soon you're climbing . . . climbing . . . climbing up to meet it. Just as you're thinking, "Hey, I could use a bench to rest," one appears. When you continue on (and up) the path, it takes a few turns to maneuver around a long sledding hill. At about this point, you have a choice to make: stay on the exposed gravel trail or take a stroll on a shadier path for hikers only. (Bicycle traffic is permitted on the limestone trail, but it's not heavily used.) I suggest staying on the long clear path, named North Fork Trail, until you reach the Round Top, near Ira Road. Along the way, you'll probably see a few trail riders (one trail here is reserved for equestrians only), and you'll also find the entrance to Creekside Trail, for hikers only. Don't go there—yet.

By the time you reach the northern end of North Fork Trail, you'll have passed two small ponds and quite possibly a few folks dropping a line in one or the other. (Catch and release is the only sort of fishing allowed in the preserve.) At the top of the trail, you'll note a few residential developments along

Ira Road. The North Fork Trail has been extended into several of those developments, but once it crosses the road, the trail ventures into private property. From the top of the hill, you can appreciate a sweeping view—and understand why your legs might need a rest.

Once your energy returns, start back down North Fork, but this time, give in to your wanderlust and veer off the wide-open path to enjoy the shadier Creekside Trail that skirts North Fork Creek. Soon after it returns you to the limestone path, follow South Woods Trail to the south for about a 0.4-mile sojourn from North Fork's oh-so-uniform surface. While butterflies love the wide-open prairielike fields along North Fork, you'll hear woodland insects on the two more rugged trails, providing a welcome variety in this relatively new and expansive preserve.

The 410-acre Bath Nature Preserve was once part of the Raymond Firestone Estate. Bath voters approved a bond issue in 1996 that made it possible for the township to purchase the land; it opened for public use in 2001. Students from the University of Akron are permitted to use part of the land for biology and ecology field studies. In 2005 the North Fork Trail was completed and connected to Bath Community Center. And it has been waiting here for you, on the other side of the tunnel, ever since.

Once you've finished exploring the various plant communities—bog, old-growth forest, wetlands, and grasslands—return to Community Park and nod to the Chief. Now you understand why he's looking up the hill.

NEARBY ACTIVITIES

If you forgot your sled, fishing pole, tennis racket, bicycle, and soccer ball and are looking for something else to do, consider taking Cleveland-Massillon Road north to OH 18, and then follow Smith Road to Sand Run Parkway (see page 263) for some more hiking.

44 BEAVER MARSH BOARDWALK

KEY AT-A-GLANCE INFORMATION

LENGTH: 3.5 miles (with optional 2 miles)

CONFIGURATION: Out-and-back

DIFFICULTY: Easy

SCENERY: Beaver marsh and pond, more than 500 types of plants and animals

EXPOSURE: Almost entirely exposed; the southernmost section of this hike is shaded.

TRAFFIC: Moderate–heavy (expect some bikes)

TRAIL SURFACE: Paved Towpath Trail and wooden boardwalk

HIKING TIME: Allow 2.25 hours for walking and watching; allow an additional 30 minutes if you plan to explore Hale Farm too

DRIVING DISTANCE: 17 miles from I-77/I-480 exchange

ACCESS: Daily, 7 a.m.–11 p.m.

WHEELCHAIR TRAVERSABLE: No

MAPS: USGS Peninsula

FACILITIES: Restrooms at Hunt Farm Visitor Center and Ira Road Trailhead

CONTACT INFORMATION: Contact the National Park Service offices by calling (330) 657-2752 or visiting nps.gov/cuva.

IN BRIEF

Once a (real) dump, some enterprising beavers got together and transformed this area into a viable habitat, and not only for themselves. Today the area is home to more than 65 other animal species. Since the National Park Service (NPS) built a wooden boardwalk across the marsh and connected it to the popular Towpath Trail, humans can enjoy its serene beauty too.

DESCRIPTION

Can you say "extreme makeover"? As recently as the early 1980s, this stretch of land was a soggy dumping ground, full of junk from a nearby car repair shop and assorted other trash. Even before the NPS could reclaim the land, a couple of beavers took matters into their own, um, paws. Park volunteers and employees helped the beavers by clearing out the debris, and in 1993 the NPS opened a 530-foot-long boardwalk across the marsh. From a single dam to a community of beavers, muskrats, mink, and many other animals and birds, the marsh and Towpath Trail have grown together, reclaiming the land as habitat for more than 500 types of plants and animals. Pretty impressive, especially for a flat stretch of land less than 2 miles long.

GPS Trailhead
Coordinates

Latitude   41° 12.018363'

Longitude   81° 34.326303'

Directions

Go south on I-77 and take Exit 143/Wheatley Road/Richfield. Go east about 4.5 miles to Riverview Road. Veer left onto Everett Road and then turn right onto Riverview Road, heading north. Turn right onto Bolantz Road. Find trailhead parking on the south side of Bolantz Road.

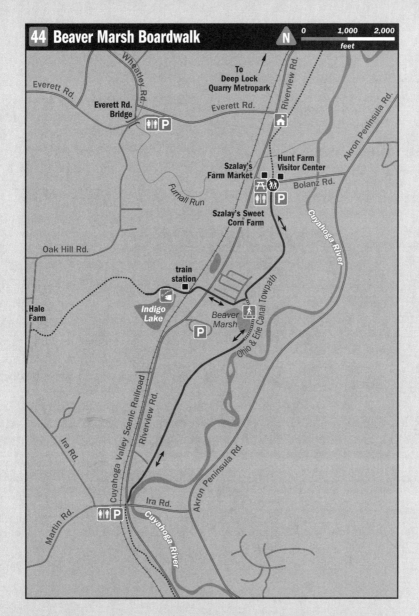

N

0   1,000   2,000
feet

Wheatley Rd.

Everett Rd.

To
Deep Lock
Quarry Metropark

Riverview Rd.

Everett Rd.

Everett Rd.
Bridge

P

Akron Peninsula Rd.

Szalay's
Farm Market

Hunt Farm
Visitor Center

Furnall Run

P

Bolanz Rd.

Szalay's Sweet
Corn Farm

Cuyahoga River

Oak Hill Rd.

train
station

Indigo
Lake

P

Beaver
Marsh

Ohio & Erie Canal Towpath

Hale
Farm

Ira Rd.

Cuyahoga Valley Scenic Railroad

Riverview Rd.

Akron Peninsula Rd.

Ira Rd.

P

Martin Rd.

Cuyahoga River

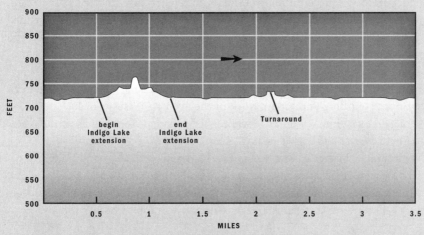

900
850
800
750
700
650
600
550
500

FEET

begin
Indigo Lake
extension

end
Indigo Lake
extension

Turnaround

0.5   1   1.5   2   2.5   3   3.5

MILES

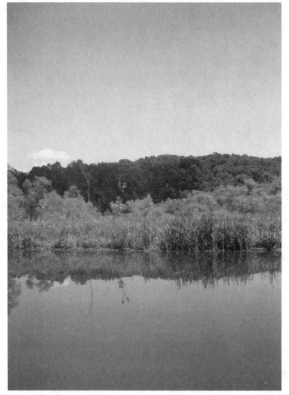

Beavers are sometimes called "park engineers."

The marsh and its adjacent land constitute one of the most diverse spots in the 33,000-acre Cuyahoga Valley National Park. Its diversity and accessibility have earned it a spot on the Ohio Division of Wildlife's list of 80 official Watchable Wildlife sites.

As you follow the Towpath Trail south from Bolanz Road, you'll pass by private farmland, usually sporting cornstalks. During the summer growing season, the loud shots of corn cannons sound periodically in an effort to scare away the crows and other animals that enjoy the corn. (Take home some corn to enjoy without the noise when you purchase it at the nearby farm market.) About 0.3 miles south of your starting point, look to your left and try to imagine the field full of wildflowers as a gravel pit. That's what it was—in the not-so-distant past. Another successful makeover, satisfying thousands of park visitors each year . . . as well as many resident birds, butterflies, and insects.

When you reach Beaver Marsh, you're sure to notice the cattails. They are an important food source for many animals, and when this area was first settled, they were also a staple in the diets of the Native Americans and early settlers, who made meal from their long stems. (Speaking of diets, this might make you grateful for your next salad, hmm?)

Now that you've reached Beaver Marsh, you want to see beavers, right? Here are some basic tips: First, beavers are nocturnal. That means they do most of their home building and repair work in the evening. Visit near dusk and look for them as they swim. Watch for a wake, the V-shaped disturbance in the water created by a beaver's tail as it swims. Keep an eye on the water lilies, and you may see a hungry beaver grab a leaf to eat. He will roll the leaf and hold it in his paw like a green cigar as he nibbles on it. Also look for mink and muskrats that make their homes in and around the water. Muskrats build their homes along the banks of ponds and streams and occasionally on top of beaver lodges.

The boardwalk offers such beautiful scenery, and so much to see, that you may not want to leave at all. But as you head south from the boardwalk, Ira Trailhead (just past Lock 26) makes a natural turnaround point. (Of course, if you don't turn around, you can follow the Towpath Trail into Akron, south into Zoar, and beyond.)

On the way back, you can take a pleasant excursion to Indigo Lake and walk around it, adding about 0.5 miles to your hike distance. Indigo Lake is small but lovely; its name was inspired by its deep-blue hue. As you head north and cross the boardwalk again, it's still hard to imagine that this spot was once a dump. Clearly, this was a successful makeover. The beautiful result: a safe haven for hundreds of animals and plants and a great escape for the humans who make their homes on either side of the valley.

NEARBY ACTIVITIES

If you veer west from the Towpath Trail less than a mile past Indigo Lake, you'll find yourself at Hale Farm and Village and way, way back in time. The working museum is owned and operated by the Western Reserve Historical Society. It offers an accurate representation of life in the Western Reserve, circa 1826. Candle making, glass blowing, and pottery demonstrations are regular fare; special seasonal events, such as the spring sap collection, are even more fun. For an events schedule and admission rates, call (800) 589-9703 or visit **wrhs.org**.

Hunt Farm, just north of the parking lot along Bolanz Road, is a visitor center that doubles as a museum. It highlights the role of the small, family farm as a force in the valley's development. Just a long stone's throw from the visitor center, Szalay's Farm (4563 Riverview Road) sells fresh produce, from spring strawberries and summer sweet corn and apples to fall pumpkins and other squash.

Cuyahoga Valley National Park offers hundreds of educational and recreational events throughout the year. Pick up a free calendar of activities at a park visitor center or check the online calendar that is updated daily at **dayinthevalley.com**.

45　BLUE HEN FALLS

KEY AT-A-GLANCE INFORMATION

LENGTH: 1.2 miles

CONFIGURATION: Out-and-back

DIFFICULTY: Moderate

SCENERY: Two waterfalls, a meandering creek, deep ravine, deciduous forest, really big rocks!

EXPOSURE: Completely shaded

TRAFFIC: Moderate

TRAIL SURFACE: Dirt trail: rooty, rocky, and steeply banked in places

HIKING TIME: 45 minutes for hiking; allow extra dawdle time at the falls

DRIVING DISTANCE: 15 miles from I-77/I-480 exchange

ACCESS: Daily, 7 a.m.–10 p.m., but best done during daylight hours; tread carefully when wet or icy

WHEELCHAIR TRAVERSABLE: No

MAPS: USGS Peninsula; also available at park visitor centers and at nps.gov/cuva

FACILITIES: None

CONTACT INFORMATION: To inquire about possible road or trail closures or to find out more about Cuyahoga Valley National Park, stop at a visitor center (such as Boston Store, just east of Riverview Road at 1548 Boston Mills Road), call (330) 657-2752, or see nps.gov/cuva.

GPS Trailhead Coordinates

Latitude　41° 15.383577'

Longitude　81° 34.360199'

IN BRIEF

Sure-footed trekkers can follow the creek past quiet Blue Hen Falls down to the bottom of 20-foot-tall Buttermilk Falls.

DESCRIPTION

"Now I'm a *real* hiker!" my 5-year-old said soon after we started out. Her brother earned similar bragging rights a few years later. This short-but-steep trail offers kids an introduction to "real" hiking, while its beauty appeals to explorers of all ages.

Enter the trail at the north end of the parking lot. It was paved long ago, so gravel and dirt are more apparent than asphalt. You'll descend about 30 feet as you follow the path; then the ground levels out and the trail turns sharply right. (The long Buckeye Trail veers to the left here.) It continues gently sloping toward a sturdy wooden bench facing Blue Hen Falls. This picturesque point is an ideal conversation spot and about the only place to sit along the trail.

Blue Hen Falls tumbles 15 feet over the edge of a massive hunk of sandstone, landing in Spring Creek—which your feet will soon

----

Directions

From I-77 South take the Miller Road exit (147), turning left and then right onto Brecksville Road (OH 21). Turn left onto Snowville Road, right at Riverview Road, and then left onto Boston Mills Road. Entrance and parking areas are about 1 mile west of Riverview Road. Enter the small parking lot with the Blue Hen Falls sign, on the north side of Boston Mills Road. The parking lot on the north side of Boston Mills Road holds just a few vehicles; additional spots can be found in the overflow lot on the south side of the road.

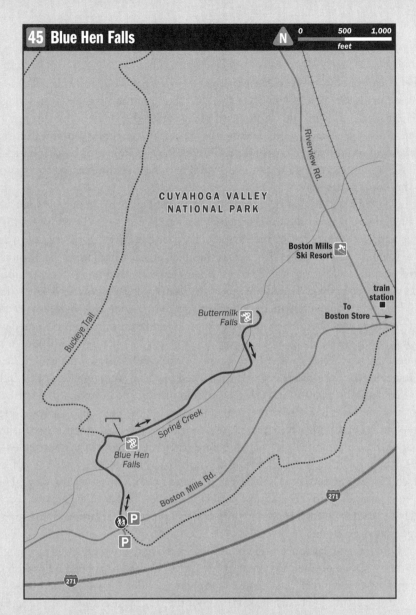

N

0   500   1,000
feet

CUYAHOGA VALLEY
NATIONAL PARK

Riverview Rd.

Boston Mills
Ski Resort

train
station

To
Boston Store

Buttermilk
Falls

Buckeye Trail

Spring Creek

Blue Hen
Falls

Boston Mills Rd.

271

P

P

271

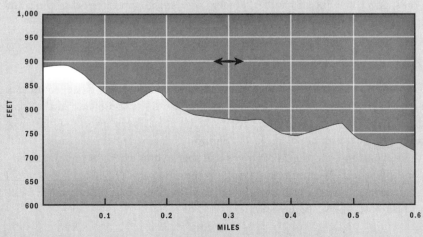

1,000
950
900
850
800
750
700
650
600

FEET

0.1   0.2   0.3   0.4   0.5   0.6
MILES

meet. Continue on the trail past the bench to a long wooden bridge. Follow it across Spring Creek and you'll see the blue blazes of the Buckeye Trail rising to the left. Instead, continue on the path as it veers right, descending through the deep, thickly forested ravine. During the spring, the pockmarked limestone and shale seem to glow with a green hue; in the fall, they appear to blush a bit under the reddening leaves. Many of the national park's moss and fern varieties thrive in this cool, moist hollow.

The path winds as it descends 50 feet or so. Fallen trees make it somewhat challenging to stay on the trail, which twists and bumps over the trunks of fallen trees and along the edge of the ravine. The trail is narrow in places, and you'll have to jump or splash your way across the creek at least three times, and you may cross trickles and runoff water several other times, depending on recent rainfall. The widest points you'll cross are 15–20 feet across, but don't worry—a slip here will land you in just a few inches of water. At the first wide crossing, look to your right (east) to see where layers of Bedford shale and Berea sandstone slammed into each other, forming the geological equivalent of a layer cake in the hillside. In the winter, when trickles of water freeze in place while falling down the wall, it's easy to imagine that cake has been recently frosted and is awaiting a giant's first bite.

Because the trail forms a crescent around the top and bottom of the falls, you can hear Buttermilk Falls before you can see it. Follow the trail as it bends right after the second wide creek crossing. The trail then heads down a final, sharp decline and a hairpin turn to the left before reaching the pool at the bottom of the falls. The pool at the point closest to the falls is several feet deep, so it is not safe for children to be unsupervised there. Whether or not you're willing to wade in, let your eyes adjust to the shadowy world under a few inches of water, and you are likely to see a small toad or tiny white crayfish playing hide-and-seek among the large, flat shale stones.

On your way back up, stop about 20 feet above the second creek crossing. If you didn't notice on the way down, pause on your climb to appreciate your avian companions—the creek has created a popular corridor for woodland birds.

After passing the bench near the top of the trail, pause again to take in Blue Hen Falls. After viewing her louder, longer sister at the opposite end of the trail, you'll appreciate Blue Hen's unique, quiet beauty from a different perspective.

NEARBY ACTIVITIES

If you want a snack, more hiking, or both, take Boston Mills Road about 0.3 miles east of Riverview Road to the Boston Store. On the south side of the road sits the old company store, dating back to 1836; it has been given new life as a visitor center in the national park. In addition to maps and information you'll find there, you can cross the street to a small snack shop where ice cream, beverages, and other trail essentials await, next to the Towpath Trailhead.

Also, just around the corner on Riverview Road you'll find Boston Mills Ski Resort ([330] 467-2242; **bmbw.com**).

CENTER VALLEY PARK TRAIL 46

IN BRIEF

Leapin' lizards! These trails offer salamanders, herons, forest, a creekside trek, a butterfly garden, and playground equipment. A flat, paved trail—perfect for bikes and blades—cuts through this wooded wetland corridor. Several rustic hiking paths shoot off the main trail, wind through the woods, and return to the center. In a word, this valley is versatile.

DESCRIPTION

The city of Twinsburg did something brilliant when it created this corridor of park that connects residential neighborhoods with city amenities—but you don't have to live in Twinsburg to appreciate the paved multiuse trail stretching more than a mile to connect Glenwood Avenue and nearby neighborhoods to Dodge Intermediate School. Twinsburg's thoughtful plan—featuring a playground, picnic shelter, benches, and several nature trails looping off the relatively straight north-south path—attracts area residents, city workers, and visitors.

The trail configuration allows you to tailor your hike to meet your needs. For a short,

KEY AT-A-GLANCE INFORMATION

LENGTH: 4 miles

CONFIGURATION: Out-and-back with loops

DIFFICULTY: Flat and easy; Green Heron Way is moderately strenuous

SCENERY: Thick deciduous forest, pines, wetlands, amphibians, birds

EXPOSURE: Paved path is exposed; dirt trails are shaded.

TRAFFIC: Paved path sees constant traffic; nature trails see far less.

SURFACE: Center trail is paved; foot trails are dirt with some wood chips.

HIKING TIME: 1–3 hours, depending on length

DRIVING DISTANCE: 18 miles from I-77/I-480 exchange

ACCESS: Daily, sunrise–sunset

WHEELCHAIR TRAVERSABLE: Yes, on paved path; nature trails not accessible

MAPS: USGS Twinsburg; also posted at trailhead

FACILITIES: Emergency phones at Dodge Intermediate School and Idlewood parking lots; restrooms in Idlewood parking lot

CONTACT INFORMATION: For information about various events in and around the park, see mytwinsburg .com or call (330) 963-8704.

Directions

Take I-480 East to Exit 36/OH 82/Aurora and turn left, toward Twinsburg. Turn left again onto Ravenna Road (at the center of town). Continue about 1 mile west to Dodge Intermediate School. Park in the school's lot (when school is out) and enter the trail by the school's ball fields.

(*Note:* During school hours, park at Idlewood Park, about 1 mile farther up Ravenna Road, or at the lot at the trail's northern tip, off Glenwood Drive—take Ravenna Road to Glenwood and turn right. Trailhead parking is 0.5 miles from Ravenna Road, on the right.)

GPS Trailhead Coordinates

Latitude 41° 19.447861'

Longitude 81° 27.090483'

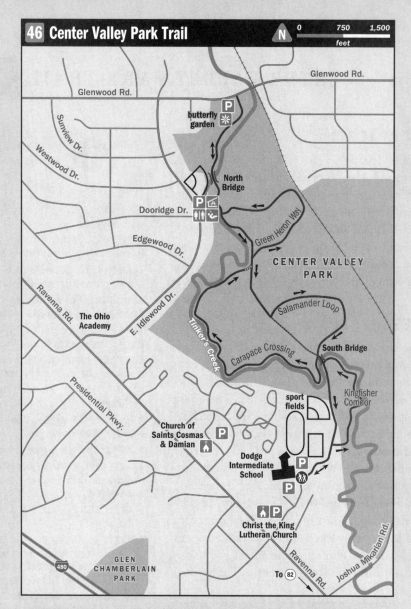

46 Center Valley Park Trail

N   0   750   1,500
            feet

Glenwood Rd.

Glenwood Rd.

Sunview Dr.

Westwood Dr.

butterfly garden

P

North Bridge

Dooridge Dr.

P

Green Heron Way

Edgewood Dr.

CENTER VALLEY PARK

Ravenna Rd.

The Ohio Academy

E. Idlewood Dr.

Salamander Loop

Tinker's Creek

Carapace Crossing

South Bridge

Presidential Pkwy.

Kingfisher Corridor

sport fields

Church of Saints Cosmas & Damian

P

Dodge Intermediate School

P

P

Christ the King Lutheran Church

P

GLEN CHAMBERLAIN PARK

480

To 82

Ravenna Rd.

Joshua Mikarian Rd.

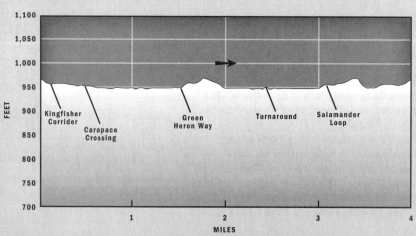

1,100
1,050
1,000
950
900
850
800
750
700

FEET

Kingfisher Corrider

Carapace Crossing

Green Heron Way

Turnaround

Salamander Loop

1   2   3   4
MILES

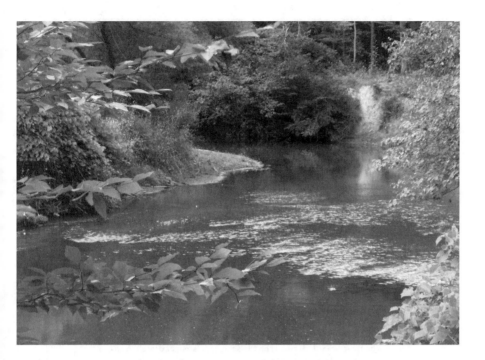

Near the southern end of Carapace Crossing

satisfying hike, leave the school parking lot on the paved path, follow Kingfisher Corridor, and loop back to the lot in less than a mile. (Just about right for the preschool set or those restarting an exercise program.) Or for a longer hike that strays farther from the pavement, follow Buttonbush Trace, which incorporates the Green Heron Way and the longer Carapace Crossing.

Begin from the southeast end of the Dodge parking lot, where a metal map of the entire park is posted. You'll see and soon smell that you're facing the Twinsburg wastewater treatment facility. But stop and think for a moment—isn't this a fabulous development for a strip of land that other cities might have discounted as mere right-of-way space? With that perspective (and knowing you'll soon leave the plant behind), hit the trail.

The wide, paved trail sees heavy traffic on warm days after school is dismissed, as students and teachers walk, jog, and blade away the day's cares. During the summer months, you're likely to encounter groups of parents and children on their way to or from the pool, the library, or a ballgame. The foot trails are generally less well traveled, and you'll find them quiet and shady.

Just beyond the trailhead sign, the path veers left. Soon, a sign on the right points to Kingfisher Corridor. Take this short loop as it twists alongside Tinker's Creek, about 4 feet above the water level, and you'll see that it's aptly named—kingfishers are often seen here. When the dirt path deposits you back

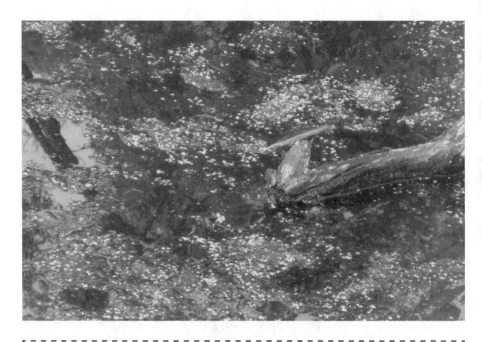

Who lives here? It depends on the season. (Listen, and you'll find out.)

on pavement, turn right and cross over South Bridge. Just north of the bridge, turn left onto Carapace Crossing.

With the woods to your right and Tinker's Creek now on your left, you will need to jump over the creek in a couple of spots as the trail winds. It's the perfect trail to whet the appetite of young hikers and to groom them for longer, more adventurous treks. As the path snakes back and forth, you find yourself nearly 50 feet from the water's edge. Then, at water's edge, carefully cross over a trickle of water on a makeshift log bridge or find a spot where you can step across. If you're willing to carry a small net along with you, this is a great place to dip in and see what you can find.

About a mile into your hike from the wooded path, you'll be able to see homes on the western side of the creek.

Amid the mud, Virginia creeper, and mayapples lives a dense population of birds, bugs, and small mammals. The carapace for which this trail is named refers to a hard covering, usually describing a turtle's shell. Even if you don't see a turtle on Carapace Crossing, you'll almost certainly see one along the Center Valley Park corridor somewhere (during the warmer months, at least). The calls of various birds, the rustle of chipmunks darting about, and frogs hopping through the valley accompany your every footfall. Many dragonflies and damselflies, a wide variety of beetles, and other insects (wear mosquito repellent in the evening!) call this park home. As you bend back to the center path, you'll cross over a wooden boardwalk to avoid a culvert and a ditch. Take the paved path to the left to find Green Heron Way.

In spite of its proximity to some of Twinsburg's residential areas, Green Heron Way could convince you that you were traveling in a vast forest. Interpretive signs point out the history of the area. When your feet hit pavement again, you're on the north side of the park. Of course, if you've had enough, you can turn left and head back to the school parking lot. But if you turn right and continue on the paved path, you'll soon reach the playground on the western side of the paved path, where a picnic shelter and restrooms are also available. As you continue your hike north/northeast from the playground, you'll soon reach a small butterfly garden, which must seem much larger to the winged population, as it attracts many different butterflies and other pollinators. From here you can continue to the northern terminus at Glenwood Avenue and turn back, retracing your steps or taking a slightly different path back to the Dodge parking lot.

As you head south on the center path, you can choose to follow Green Heron Way or Carapace again, or wait until you're near the trail's southern end to take a short turn around Salamander Loop on the left (east) side of the path.

Much of the year, Salamander Loop is a hard-packed dirt-and-grass trail, but during the amphibian's short mating and spawning season, it's a wet and perfect salamander habitat. Even then, smart trail design keeps the trail—for the most part—dry. The city's park staff offers seasonal programs that aim to strike a balance between the creature's need for protection and our natural curiosity about their habits. (Call in mid-March to inquire about program dates.) If you're not able to catch the salamanders in action, try to imagine them sizing you up from a distance. Emerging from the trees, your giant feet (well, that's how they look to salamanders!) find pavement again. With your tour of Twinsburg's valley complete, turn left and return to the school parking lot, or revisit any part of these trails at your leisure.

NEARBY ACTIVITIES

Twinsburg's city square is small but interesting. It has served as the center of town festivals since the early 1800s. A bandstand, historical church, and war memorial grace the square, located at the junction of OH 91, Ravenna Road, and Church Street.

The internationally famous Twins Days celebration is held each August. For information about the festivities, see **twinsdays.org**.

47 F. A. SEIBERLING NATURE REALM

KEY AT-A-GLANCE INFORMATION

LENGTH: 1.5 miles

CONFIGURATION: Three loops

DIFFICULTY: Easy

SCENERY: Fountain, small ponds, herb and flower garden, swingy suspension bridge

EXPOSURE: About half shaded

TRAFFIC: Moderate

TRAIL SURFACE: Paved or stone paths and mulched trails

HIKING TIME: 45 minutes

DRIVING DISTANCE: 21 miles from I-77/I-480 exchange

ACCESS: Grounds: Daily, 6 a.m.–11 p.m. Visitor center: Tuesday–Saturday, 10 a.m.–5 p.m. (open until 7 p.m. Thursday–Saturday, March–October); Sunday, noon–5 p.m.; closed holidays. Pets, bikes, and other recreational equipment not permitted.

WHEELCHAIR TRAVERSABLE: Yes, the visitor center and many trails

MAPS: USGS Peninsula; also available inside the visitor center

FACILITIES: Restrooms and water inside visitor center; restrooms also outside when building is closed

CONTACT INFORMATION: Call (330) 865-8065 or visit summitmetroparks.org.

IN BRIEF

Inside the visitor center, you can learn about as much about green building design as your brain can grasp—or handle a snake, or enjoy a puppet show. Outside, some of the gardens are as neatly buttoned-down as a Sunday school teacher—but when you reach the southern end of the nature trails, you'll find a bouncy suspension bridge sure to bring out your inner child.

DESCRIPTION

F. A. Seiberling founded The Goodyear Tire & Rubber Co., and if that was all he had done, you'd expect to find a park in Akron named after him. But Seiberling did much more. He served as an early member of the Board of Park Commissioners, and over the years he donated more than 400 acres to help establish the park system. In 1948 Seiberling donated the 100-acre plot on which the nature realm now sits; it was established as a MetroPark in 1964. Today the grounds of the nature realm offer the prettiest of plantings and well-groomed trails. Meticulous planning of the arboretum and surrounding trails provides constant changes of scenery—from the crabapples that bloom in the early spring to May and June's rhododendron blossoms to the rich explosion of fall perennials. You can always find color here.

GPS Trailhead Coordinates

Latitude   41° 8.360159'

Longitude   81° 34.546080'

Directions

Take I-77 South to Ghent Road, Exit 138. Head south (left) on Ghent Road and go to the light at Smith Road. Turn left on Smith Road. Travel approximately 2 miles to find the park entrance (1826 Smith Road) on your left.

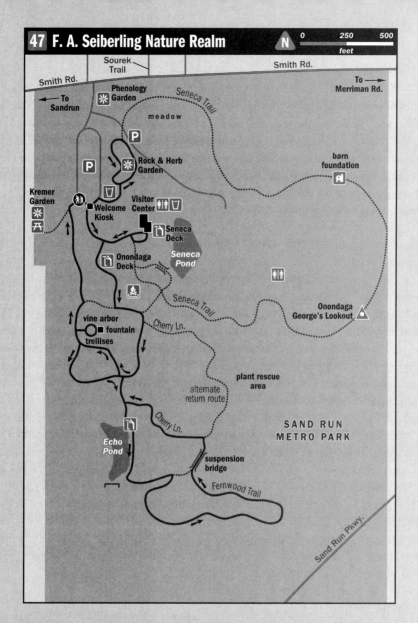

N

| 0 | 250 | 500 |

feet

Smith Rd.

Sourek
Trail

Smith Rd.

← To
Sandrun

To →
Merriman Rd.

Phenology
Garden

Seneca Trail

m e a d o w

P

Rock & Herb
Garden

barn
foundation

P

Kremer
Garden

Welcome
Kiosk

Visitor
Center

Seneca
Deck

Onondaga
Deck

*Seneca
Pond*

Seneca Trail

Onondaga
George's Lookout

vine arbor
fountain
trellises

Cherry Ln.

plant rescue
area

alternate
return route

S A N D   R U N
M E T R O   P A R K

Cherry Ln.

*Echo
Pond*

suspension
bridge

Fernwood Trail

Sand Run Pkwy.

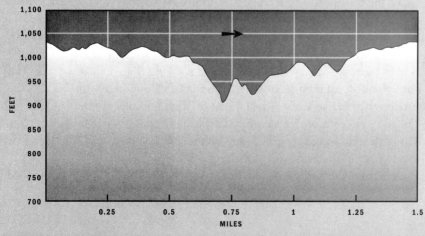

					1,100
					1,050
					1,000
					950
					900
					850
					800
					750
					700

FEET

0.25   0.5   0.75   1   1.25   1.5

MILES

When you enter the park from the southwest corner of the parking lot, wander into the herb and rock garden first. Like many of the 300-or-so tree and shrub varieties here, most of the herbs are labeled for easy identification.

Once you've looped around on the stone walkway encircling fragrant herbs and medicinal plants, you'll find yourself looking down on the visitor center. You're not looking down on it because the hill is steep—it's more of a gentle slope—but because it's partially underground. As you approach, you'll also notice some large solar panels near the building's entrance.

While the center was originally designed to be environmentally friendly, major renovations in 2009–2010 made the building a shining example of green building principles.

Go inside to learn more about those principles, and you'll also have an opportunity to meet a black rat snake and several other reptiles, amphibians, and other Ohio natives. Other educational opportunities await inside—for children and adults—but don't stay too long; there's much to see outside!

Leave the building by the same door in which you arrived. When you walk south by pines and crabapples, the decorative brick and stone–patterned path leads you through the arboretum to see first the flowering, then the weeping, then the vine trees. Less than 0.2 miles from where you start, towering white trellises lure you to a small fountain; three great blue herons (made of wrought iron) bathe in it. (This is a popular place for wedding pictures, and amateur photography is encouraged. Commercial photographers, however, must obtain a special permit.)

Continue on the paved trail, veering west (right) at the fork in the path just a few paces south of the fountain. You'll follow a planting of pines and deciduous trees before turning east, leaving the paved path. (*Note:* Wheelchairs and strollers can continue on the paved path, heading northeast through the middle of the park.) The wide, flat, mulched trail continues south to Echo Pond. A covered observation deck sits on the pond's north side; a park bench on the south side of the pond is tucked near a stand of cattails—an excellent place to watch for birds, butterflies, frogs, and fish.

Leave the south end of the pond and head east down a gentle incline. Turn right to follow Fernwood Trail (wooden trail markers display fern leaves). Fernwood winds its way south and then curves east through a thick deciduous forest, and, indeed, you'll find ferns here. This shady trail is farthest from the park entrance and where you're most likely to find solitude. The path straightens out at about 0.7 miles and then turns sharply to the left. From here, you wiggle your way northwest to arrive at the base of a bouncy suspension bridge.

The long wooden bridge supported by cables spans a 45-foot-deep ravine. You may find that you're torn between running across it to make it swing or stopping to take in the beauty of the ravine.

Once across the bridge, you'll find yourself on Cherry Lane (trail signs marked with carving of two cherries). Turn left and follow the path as it rises slightly to the west. Soon, the trail bends to the north where the mulch surface is replaced by pavement. The western portion of Cherry Lane is as straight as the tall pines it borders. Soon, you'll come to a fork in the trail. Here you must decide whether to go left, taking the path through the rhododendrons, or to go right, through the planting of fruit and nut trees on your way to the Anniversary Garden. Either way, you'll enjoy the view, and you'll have logged about 1.5 miles when you arrive at the underground visitor center.

NEARBY ACTIVITIES

On the northern side of the nature realm, the longer Seneca Trail leads guests over more than a mile of the woodlands and open field, starting from the Anniversary Garden on the south side of the visitor center. If you'd like to learn more about Mr. Seiberling, you may want to visit beautiful Stan Hywet Hall at 714 North Portage Path. The 65-room mansion with equally impressive grounds was the Seiberlings' home for many years. There is an admission fee to tour the house and grounds; call (330) 836-5533 for details.

If it's more hiking you want, Sand Run Metro Park (see page 263) has it, just about 2 miles south of the nature realm.

48 GORGE TRAIL

KEY AT-A-GLANCE INFORMATION

LENGTH: 2 miles

CONFIGURATION: Loop

DIFFICULTY: Moderate, with a few steep sections and lots of steps

SCENERY: Two small caves, a waterfall, large rock passes, river views, a 50-foot-high dam

EXPOSURE: Entirely shaded when trees have leaves

TRAFFIC: Moderate–heavy

TRAIL SURFACE: Dirt and rocks

HIKING TIME: Allow an hour, so you can investigate the cave and enjoy the rock passes

DRIVING DISTANCE: 34 miles from I-77/I-480 exchange

ACCESS: Daily, 6 a.m.–sunset; it's smart to avoid this trail when icy

MAPS: USGS Akron East; also available at trailhead

WHEELCHAIR TRAVERSABLE: No

FACILITIES: Restrooms at the trailhead; water at the picnic area

CONTACT INFORMATION: Contact Metro Parks Serving Summit County at (330) 865-8060 or summitmetroparks.org.

IN BRIEF

With pudding rocks, lucky stones, waterfalls, caves, and a Native American tale, this trail is irresistible to kids. Don't be fooled by its fun nature, though—Gorge Trail offers enough up-and-down rock rambling to qualify as a serious hike.

DESCRIPTION

The Cuyahoga River provides tremendous waterpower that has been put to good use here for well over a century. In 1882 High Bridge Glens Park opened on this spot, where patrons could enjoy a roller coaster and dance hall. Electric cable cars powered by the dam were added later. After the amusement park closed, the local electric company donated this 144-acre tract to the Metro Parks Serving Summit County. Several educational signs along the trail offer history and geology lessons.

From the northwest corner of the parking lot, head west on the wide dirt path. You'll follow the yellow circles on wooden signs that identify Gorge Trail. Pass three picnic shelters and the skating pond, all on your left, on your way to one of the area's great but unfortunately little-known historical sites.

About 0.4 miles into the trail, just beyond a small hill, you'll reach the Mary Campbell

GPS Trailhead Coordinates

Latitude   41° 7.244818'

Longitude   81° 29.609041'

Directions ⟶

Follow I-77 South to I-480 East, merging onto I-271 South. Follow the signs to continue south onto OH 8. Take Exit 5 at Broad Boulevard, turning right, and take the first left onto Front Street. The park entrance will be on your left.

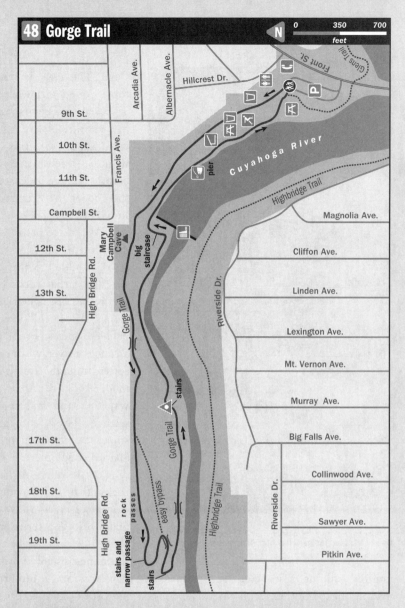

N

0   350   700
feet

Arcadia Ave.

Albernacle Ave.

Hillcrest Dr.

Front St.

Glens Trail

9th St.

10th St.

11th St.

Francis Ave.

Campbell St.

pier

Cuyahoga River

Highbridge Trail

Magnolia Ave.

12th St.

Mary Campbell Cave

big staircase

Cliffon Ave.

Linden Ave.

High Bridge Rd.

13th St.

Gorge Trail

Riverside Dr.

Lexington Ave.

Mt. Vernon Ave.

Murray Ave.

stairs

Gorge Trail

Big Falls Ave.

17th St.

Collinwood Ave.

Riverside Dr.

18th St.

High Bridge Rd.

rock passes

easy bypass

Highbridge Trail

Sawyer Ave.

19th St.

stairs and narrow passage

stairs

Pitkin Ave.

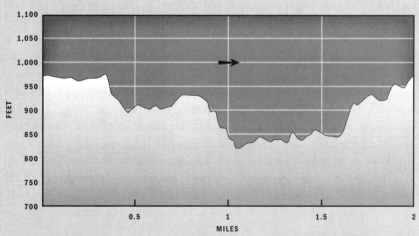

1,100

1,050

1,000

950

900

850

800

750

700

FEET

0.5   1   1.5   2

MILES

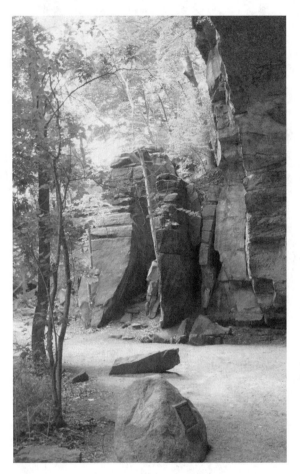

One of the few flat stretches of trail here in the gorge

Cave. The cave is named for a young girl who was captured in Pennsylvania by Delaware Native Americans. She lived in this cave with the tribe for five years before she was released at the end of the French and Indian War in 1764.

As the path goes downhill from the cave, it is studded with fist-size and larger rocks. The small ones are called lucky stones. These milky white pebbles were smoothed by an ancient river, while other softer minerals eroded into mud. As a result of the way the sand and pebbles settled, layers of lucky stones can be seen in the Sharon conglomerate. Pudding stone refers to larger rocks that contain lucky stones of various shapes and sizes. The term probably came into use because the stones resemble British-style chunky pudding. Mind your lucky stones, and then cross over a footbridge and head uphill to another small cave. The trail becomes rocky here, and water tumbles over a 20-foot drop from above, sometimes spilling across the trail.

Continuing west, you'll notice at least three unmarked trails to the left. They are shortcuts, to be sure, but if you were to follow them, you'd miss some great sites, including a gigantic oak tree on the south (left) side of trail. About 0.9 miles west of your starting point, you'll find yourself between two boulders, each nearly 20 feet tall. Climb up a short but steep hill between the rock walls and then turn left as the trail heads south through another rock pass.

This one is almost a cave—it's not a difficult climb, but it is a narrow passageway. (An alternate route is available to the left for those too wide or too claustrophobic to pass through it.) Twenty-two stone stairs have been laid inside the pass. At the top of the steps, turn around and watch as the hikers behind you emerge from what appears to be a tiny crack between the two rocks. As you continue west, you'll walk through a short "hallway" of dark gray and white-washed shale; lucky stones decorate the walls on both sides.

A Gorge Trail marker indicates a sharp left turn, and from there you'll slip-slide down a sandy hill. The trail curves right again, heading west for the last time before dropping down a log staircase, which is neatly stitched into the side of a sandy ravine. As the trail straightens out, you'll soon notice what looks like a root maze underfoot. From the large surface of exposed roots, you can over-look the shallow rapids of the Cuyahoga River. The trail earns its name here, providing beautiful views and sounds of the river gorge.

The trail bends left to cross over a long footbridge, and you may notice some fossil remains in the rock here. You'll cross another footbridge and hit a few more small hills as you continue east. Once over the hills, a short log stair-way takes you down to the dam overlook, where you can relax on a bench and enjoy the view.

Rested? Good. You'll climb up 105 wooden steps from the dam overlook before you veer right and east again. On your way back to the parking lot, you'll pass by a large wooden fishing pier. If you have time, hop onto it and enjoy a look at the water, so smooth here just above the dam. You'll pass by the south side of the picnic areas, and a water fountain, before returning to the trailhead.

NEARBY ACTIVITIES

If you're just getting warmed up after this hike, head south on Front Street and turn into the smaller Gorge Metro Park lot to venture onto Highbridge Trail. It's a 3.2-mile hike connecting to the Cascade Valley area of the Metro Parks Serving Summit County (see the Oxbow Trail on page 242). In cold weather, the skating pond is open, weather permitting. Watch the website **summitmetroparks.org** or call the seasonal information line at (330) 865-8060 for skating conditions.

49 GREEN LEAF PARK

KEY AT-A-GLANCE INFORMATION

LENGTH: 1 mile

CONFIGURATION: Loop

DIFFICULTY: Easy

SCENERY: Forest, fishing lakes, historical log cabin, and herb garden

EXPOSURE: About half shaded

TRAFFIC: Moderate

TRAIL SURFACE: Dirt, grass, and gravel

HIKING TIME: 30 minutes

DRIVING DISTANCE: 22 miles from I-77/I-480 exchange

ACCESS: Daily, 8 a.m.–sunset

WHEELCHAIR TRAVERSABLE: No, though most all-terrain strollers could manage when the trail is dry.

MAPS: USGS Wadsworth

FACILITIES: Portable toilets near fishing lake

CONTACT INFORMATION: Call (330) 722-9364 or visit medinacountyparks.com for more information or to reserve a shelter in the park.

IN BRIEF

Not so long ago, a gravel pit sat at the corner of Medina Line Road and OH 162. When a young park district converted the parcel into a 45-acre park, it became the first of many lovely Medina County Parks. Instead of gravel, visitors here now pick up bits of history. Green Leaf Park features an old log cabin, two picnic shelters, a fishing lake, and a nature trail that winds around a small herb garden.

DESCRIPTION

Start your walk at the north end of the main parking lot, in front of Willow Shelter. Your first few steps follow a low, pretty sandstone wall as it bends around the eastern side of the shelter. From there, follow the wide grass-and-gravel path north toward the fishing lake. As you walk, you'll pass a ball field and a grassy hill on your right. The tall, thick trees on your left offer afternoon shade.

Two park benches just west of the trail provide pleasant views of the little lake. From the north end of the lake, turn right onto a sandy path leading through the woods and to the old log cabin. The Hard family constructed this house in 1817, shortly after they arrived in Ohio. Abraham Hard and his wife, Rebecca, had left Vermont a year or so

GPS Trailhead Coordinates

Latitude   41° 5.456100'

Longitude   81° 41.387758'

Directions

Take I-77 South toward Akron, exiting at Exit 136 onto OH 21 south toward Massillon. Exit at OH 162/Copley Road and turn right, traveling about 0.2 miles before turning left onto Medina Line Road, where you'll see the northern entrance to Green Leaf Park.

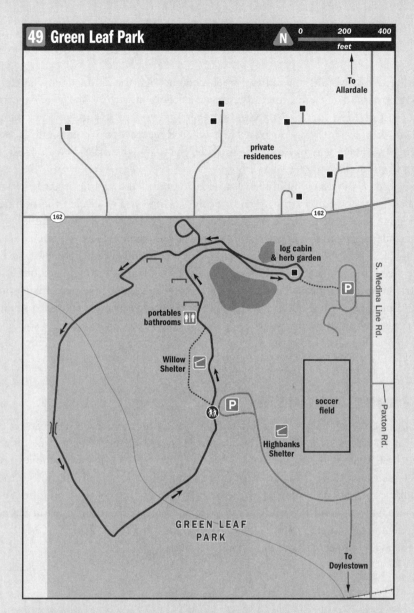

0   200   400
feet

N

To
Allardale

private
residences

162   162

log cabin
& herb garden

P

S. Medina Line Rd.

portables
bathrooms

Willow
Shelter

soccer
field

Paxton Rd.

P

Highbanks
Shelter

GREEN LEAF
PARK

To
Doylestown

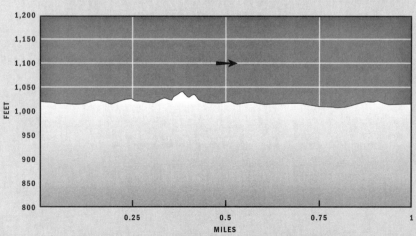

FEET				
1,200				
1,150				
1,100				
1,050				
1,000				
950				
900				
850				
800				

0.25   0.5   0.75   1

MILES

earlier, with five of their ten children. They headed for Tallmadge, where their son Cyrus had settled; eventually, they put roots down in what would become the eastern edge of Medina County. Here, they also expanded their family. Moses Knapp Hard was born in 1818, when Rebecca was 50 years old. It seems that Mrs. Hard was made of tough stuff, indeed—when she died in 1860, she had lived an amazing 91 years.

Today, the Hard family log house is surrounded by an herb garden, established by the Medina County Herb Society. Once you've circled the perimeter (or gone inside, if it is open), head back through the woods past the lake and continue west on the grassy path, eventually encountering a couple of short, unmarked paths that have been worn over several sandy knolls. Some of the hills are steep and slippery, but they are all short—so there's little chance of getting hurt, even if you slip. A park bench marks the spot where the path turns south, running under tall shade trees and over a footbridge to the park's two shelters. The path winds a bit before it takes you to Highbanks Shelter on the south side of the parking lot. From there, a path to the left leads you back to Willow Shelter, just 0.1 mile north of Highbanks.

NEARBY ACTIVITIES

Both of Green Leaf's picnic shelters have grills; shelters can be reserved by calling the Medina Park District. Fishing is permitted at the lake. While you're in the area, visit Allardale (see page 193) on Remsen Road, just a few miles north of Green Leaf Park. You can learn more about the Hard family and other tough cookies in Medina's past at the county's historical society. The John Smart House Museum and Research Center is located at 206 North Elmwood Street in Medina. The museum's hours vary with the seasons; call (330) 722-1341 or see **medinahistorical.com** to get the current schedule.

HAPPY DAYS, LEDGES, AND PINES **50**

IN BRIEF

This hilly combination of three trails visits some of my favorite spots in the Cuyahoga Valley National Park, including a pioneer cemetery, awe-inspiring caves and ledges, and (arguably) the best spot in the valley to watch a sunset. For beginning hikers, especially little ones, start with the Haskell Run Trail. You can also shorten this hike by taking the Ledges Trail to return to the Happy Days Lodge.

DESCRIPTION

From the parking lot, you'll cross under OH 303 through a 200-foot-long lighted tunnel; emerge to find yourself on the edge of the Mater Delorosa cemetery, which dates to 1869. Its inhabitants include a Civil War soldier who died in battle and his parents, a Mr. and Mrs. Coady, who lived to be 93 and 83 years old, respectively. (We'll never know the secret to their longevity, but we can guess that they walked a lot.) Many of the cemetery's other souls rest in mystery, as their names have long since faded from their sandstone markers.

The short-but-steep Haskell Run Trail abuts the southern edge of the cemetery. Step onto it. Soon the path turns to the right and drops about 30 feet, crossing a short wooden footbridge over the meandering creek for which the trail is named. From here, the trail bends sharply to the left, working its way up toward the base of the Ledges Trail. Arriving

KEY AT-A-GLANCE INFORMATION

LENGTH: 4.3 miles

CONFIGURATION: Bumpy loop

DIFFICULTY: Moderate, with difficult sections

SCENERY: Large rock outcrops, cave, valley overlook, forest, streams

EXPOSURE: Mostly shaded

TRAFFIC: Moderate–heavy near the cave on Ledges portion; lighter traffic on the Pine Grove portion

TRAIL SURFACE: Mixed—from large stones to dirt and gravel

HIKING TIME: 2 hours

DRIVING DISTANCE: 23 miles from I-77/I-480 exchange

ACCESS: Daily, 7 a.m.–11 p.m.

WHEELCHAIR TRAVERSABLE: No

MAPS: USGS Peninsula; also available at nps.gov/cuva and park visitor centers

FACILITIES: Portable restrooms located in Happy Days parking lot; restrooms and water available at Ledges Shelter and Octagon Shelter

CONTACT INFORMATION: Call the visitor information line at (330) 657-2752 or visit nps.gov/cuva.

Directions

From the I-77/I-480 exchange, take I-480 East to I-271 South. Take Exit 18 to take OH 8 south to OH 303. On OH 303, head west to find Happy Days Lodge parking lot, on the north side of OH 303, approximately 1 mile west of OH 8.

GPS Trailhead Coordinates

Latitude   41° 13.894258'

Longitude   81° 30.471060'

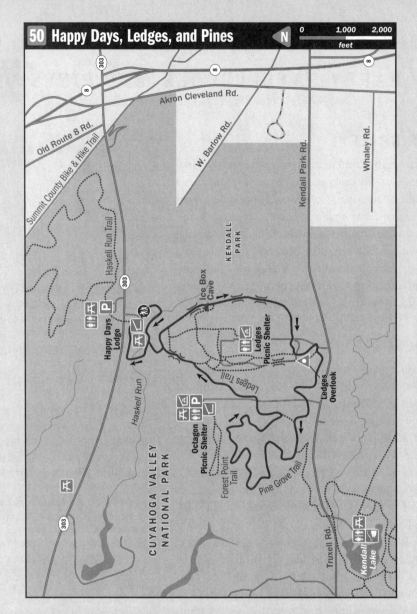

N

0   1,000   2,000
feet

303
8
8
Akron Cleveland Rd.
Old Route 8 Rd.
W. Barlow Rd.
Kendall Park Rd.
Whaley Rd.
Summit County Bike & Hike Trail
Haskell Run Trail
303
KENDALL PARK
Ice Box Cave
Happy Days Lodge
P
Ledges Picnic Shelter
Ledges Trail
Ledges Overlook
Octagon Picnic Shelter
P
Haskell Run
Forest Point Trail
Pine Grove Trail
CUYAHOGA VALLEY NATIONAL PARK
303
Truxell Rd.
Kendall Lake

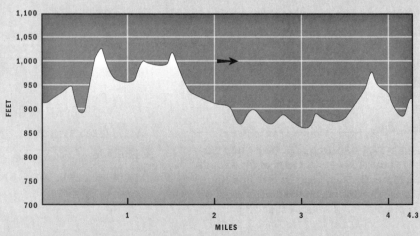

MILES
FEET
1,100
1,050
1,000
950
900
850
800
750
700
1   2   3   4   4.3

at the top of 20 or so steps, turn left onto Ledges Trail and follow the signs to Ice Box Cave. While the destination sounds refreshing (and it is!), getting there requires a bit of work. Footing can be challenging on Ledges Trail because you'll climb over too many rocks to count—some left by glaciers' work, others placed by human hands.

In the 1930s, the Civilian Conservation Corp (CCC) carefully created stairways out of the indigenous stones to provide hikers with a safer path. You will appreciate their work for both its form and its function. The CCC's mission, in part, was stated in a 1910 report of the U.S. Department of the Interior,

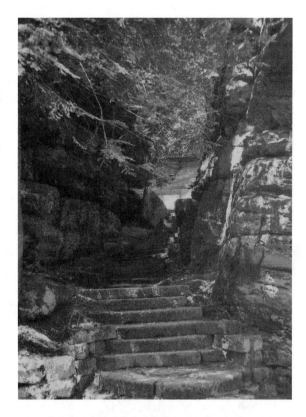

Another example of the Civilian Conservation Corps' hard work

declaring that "particular attention must be devoted always to harmonizing of these improvements with the landscape." Along this trail (and many other places in the park), you'll see evidence of the CCC's adherence to this goal.

Before you reach Ice Box Cave, you'll be called into one of the skinny, cool crevices along the right side of the path. Giant walls of Sharon conglomerate (300-million-year-old rock formed of cemented sand and small quartz pebbles) seem to have been dropped like a giant child's blocks, scattered across the Ledges area, creating a playground of sorts for average-size humans like us. Park signs prohibiting rock climbing and warning of the dangers of falling off the sometimes-slippery cliffs are posted here. Heed the signs but have fun.

While the entire Ledges Trail is naturally cooled thanks to the surrounding rocks, you'll notice a distinct drop in temperature as you approach Ice Box Cave. South of the cave you'll cross two tiny streams. Farther south, the trail veers right and leads you across the park's driveway to the Ledges Picnic Area. The trail rises a bit, revealing the south end of a large, open field where people on blankets often vie for space amid kite fliers and dogs chasing flying discs. Permanent restroom facilities are also here. Follow the path up another 30 yards to a sign directing you left (south) to the Ledges Trail or straight ahead to visit

Octagon Ledges overlook. The overlook is a sunset-watcher's paradise. Sitting on the flat expanse of rock, you're facing west, overlooking the valley. On most days, you can see well past the communities of Bath and Brecksville. Many nights, a crowd gathers here to catch the short sunset performance, and I've watched a few times when viewers actually applauded as the sun slipped out of sight. It is an almost magical spot in this beautiful valley. Move on for now (you won't want to finish the hike without the benefit of daylight) and plan to come back another time to enjoy the nightly show.

The Ledges Trail continues just south of the overlook point, veering west and dropping down 41 wood-reinforced steps into the forest. A sign at the bottom of the steps points right (north) to complete the Ledges Trail loop, but you should continue straight through the cool forest, toward Pine Grove Trail. You'll cross the park road to the Octagon Shelter and get a brief view of Truxell Road, about 200 yards to your left. Most days, the woodpeckers and the wind in the trees will distract you from any traffic noises that may come from the road.

Soon the trail turns right, heading north, where you'll notice a few pines amid the tall aspen, beech, and maple trees. About 2 miles into the trail, you'll see a sign noting the connector to Lake Trail, also part of the Virginia Kendall unit of the park.

Midway through the climbing, twisting Pine Grove Trail, you'll find yourself overlooking a deep ravine and a small footbridge. Two sharp left turns and a 30-foot drop later, you'll cross that bridge and climb up again, this time ascending 66 wooden stairs. (As you huff and puff, remember to thank the Cuyahoga Valley Trail Council volunteers who built them.) As soon as you catch your breath, you leave Pine Grove on the connector, heading east to cross over the Octagon Ledges access road again. Follow the signs to the Ledges Trail and Happy Days Lodge, veering left to complete your clockwise jaunt around this rocky place.

Your final quarter mile is the second half of Haskell Run. Your legs will get one more workout as you climb up a gravel trail and then a dozen stone steps to arrive on the western edge of the field adjacent to the lodge. Several grills and picnic tables here may seem rather inviting at this point, as you have likely worked up an appetite on the trail.

NEARBY ACTIVITIES

Happy Days Lodge (formerly a visitor center) is open for special events, including concerts and lyceum speakers, often discussing topics related to the national parks. To find out what's going on at Happy Days Lodge and elsewhere in the park, call (330) 650-4636 or visit **dayinthevalley.com.**

If you like, bring your bike—and helmet. Trailhead parking for the Towpath Trail is off OH 303 about 2 miles to the west (in Peninsula), and parking for the paved Summit County Bike & Hike Trail is located just east of here, at the intersection of OH 303 and Olde Eight Road.

HUDSON SPRINGS PARK 51

IN BRIEF

Bring the family: after circling the lake on the shady crushed-limestone trail, young hikers will be rewarded with a great view of a playground (including a hedge maze) on the northwest edge of this park. Those who've outgrown playgrounds can enjoy a picturesque sunset from one of many benches or decks on the lake's north side.

DESCRIPTION

Hudson Springs Park spans 260 acres, including a 50-acre lake. Fishing and small (non-motorized) boats are allowed here. Hudson residents can rent space on the lakeshore to keep their canoes and rowboats handy; non-residents may bring their own nonmotorized boats to enjoy the water for a small fee.

Although the lake is the park's largest feature, the trail seems to draw more visitors, and even though bicycles are allowed on the trail, you won't see many of them. That may be because the long, mostly paved Summit County Bike & Hike Trail runs nearby. The trail is well used, however, and you will certainly have company as you travel around the lake.

To follow the trail counterclockwise, head south from the parking lot, entering

KEY AT-A-GLANCE INFORMATION

LENGTH: 1.8 miles
CONFIGURATION: Loop
DIFFICULTY: Easy
SCENERY: Lake views, lush woods, a small island
EXPOSURE: Three-quarters of the trail is shaded
TRAFFIC: Moderate
TRAIL SURFACE: Crushed limestone
HIKING TIME: 50 minutes
DRIVING DISTANCE: 30 miles from I-77/I-480 exchange
ACCESS: Daily, sunrise—sunset
WHEELCHAIR TRAVERSABLE: No
MAPS: USGS Hudson
FACILITIES: Restrooms in the parking lot; three picnic shelters within the park
CONTACT INFORMATION: Contact the City of Hudson Parks & Recreation Department at hudson.oh.us or (330) 653-5201.

Directions

From Cleveland, take I-480 East to Frost Road (Exit 41). Turn right onto Aurora Hudson Road; then turn right on Stow Road. The park entrance is on the eastern side of Stow Road, just south of the Ohio Turnpike.

GPS Trailhead Coordinates
Latitude 41° 15.089278'
Longitude 81° 24.464700'

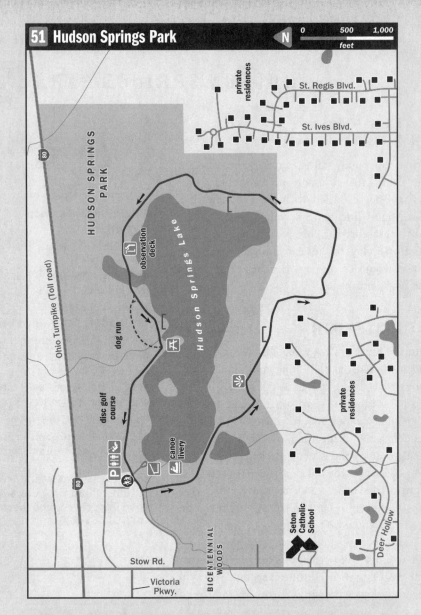

N

0   500   1,000
feet

private
residences

St. Regis Blvd.

St. Ives Blvd.

80

HUDSON SPRINGS PARK

observation
deck

Hudson Springs Lake

dog run

disc golf
course

canoe
livery

80

private
residences

Deer Hollow

Seton
Catholic
School

Stow Rd.

BICENTENNIAL WOODS

Victoria
Pkwy.

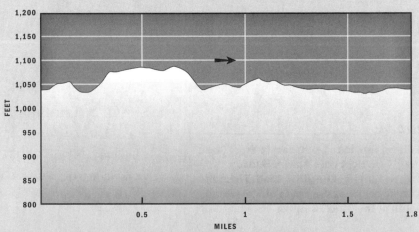

1,200
1,150
1,100
1,050
1,000
950
900
850
800

FEET

0.5   1   1.5   1.8
MILES

the trail just to the right of the shelter and boat launch area. The dirt-and-gravel path heads up a slight rise before it curves toward the east. From here, you'll have a good view of the entire lake and its little island.

The trail is wide and relatively flat. On the eastern side of the lake, the trail rolls up and down over a few hills, 10 feet or so at a time.

On the south side of the lake, you'll cross over a well-disguised culvert; soon after, you'll notice an unmarked path on your right, leading east to a nearby residential neighborhood. It's one of several such footpaths here, most of which are unmarked. Just past this one, however, on the left of the trail, a sign points visitors to an overlook. The 0.3-mile or so detour off the main trail is well worth it.

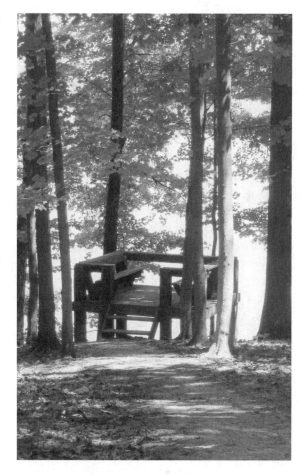

Have a seat, drop a line ... or just relax.

Follow the fairly steep descent and you'll find a wooden deck with built-in benches overlooking the lake's calm waters. Returning to the main trail and rounding the eastern edge of the lake, you'll come to another observation deck, this one raised and facing west, making it perfect for sunset viewing. For a less direct but equally beautiful view of the sunset, follow the loop a little farther northeast to a second lower, but slightly larger, deck.

As you continue (now west) on the trail, you'll come to a dog run area (it is posted as such) and then to a disc golf course. Both are used frequently. Just a few steps from here, on the west (south) side of the trail, two pieces of land jut into the lake. The park department wisely planted a couple of park benches and picnic tables here. They are situated so that you can enjoy a peaceful lake view, with your back to the action at the disc golf course and playground. Ah, but peaceful contemplation is only fun for so long. Heading west on the path again, you might find it hard to resist the playground's charm.

The northwestern corner of the park boasts play equipment for kids of all sizes. There's a small obstacle course, a tire swing, climbing equipment, and slides—and they're all fun. But perhaps most inspired is the little hedge maze, perfect for pint-size explorers. The maze was dedicated in 1988, "To all children . . . from the Hudson preschool parents." It was a very thoughtful gift, from people who clearly know kids. The playground is adjacent to the parking lot, so when you're done playing, you're free to leave. Bet you'll be back, though.

NEARBY ACTIVITIES

If the hedge maze, trails, bocce ball courts, disc golf course, and playgrounds don't tucker you out, cross Stow Road west to pick up the 0.5-mile Bike & Hike Trail through Bicentennial Woods. Or, if you prefer a bit of history with your hike, drive into the heart of Hudson and admire its many well-preserved century-old homes and other reminders of the city's Western Reserve heritage. Western Reserve College was established in Hudson in 1826. In 1882 the college moved to Cleveland, and Hudson took the loss hard. By 1906 Hudson had no water service, and the business district went bust. Then Hudson native James Ellsworth stepped in. He told local officials that he'd help out, provided that they rescind all liquor licenses in town. The officials complied and, by 1912, Hudson was once again a thriving town.

Thanks to Eric Hutchinson, City of Hudson Parks Superintendent, for reviewing this hike description.

INDIAN HOLLOW RESERVATION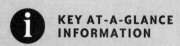

IN BRIEF

Hikers can observe the effects of glaciers as well as spy herons and myriad birds enjoying this shady stretch of the Black River. A gravel loop provides a different experience away from the river, along land that was once quarried for stones used to build bridges and mills.

DESCRIPTION

About 30 miles southwest of Cleveland, Indian Hollow Reservation lies under the flight path of Cleveland Hopkins' jets. Watching them fly over, you can't help but feel sorry for the people in the sky, for whom the Black River is just a tiny line wending north to Lake Erie. For you, here on the ground, the river is the beautiful, dominant feature of this hike.

Begin at the trailhead map posted by the picnic shelter and restrooms. From here, a connector trail to your left leads you down a short hill and across a bridge over the East Branch of Black River to the Beech-Maple Trail, a 1-mile loop. But before you follow that trail, take a few minutes to explore the banks of this beautiful river.

It's impossible to miss an unmarked but well-traveled dirt path to your left, drawing you toward the river's edge and into the woods. If you follow the narrow dirt-and-rock

KEY AT-A-GLANCE INFORMATION

LENGTH: 2.5 miles

CONFIGURATION: Loop and out-and-back spurs

DIFFICULTY: Easy

SCENERY: Black River, exposed sandstone walls, beech-maple forest, variety of wildflowers

EXPOSURE: Mostly shaded

TRAFFIC: Moderate

TRAIL SURFACE: Loop trail is crushed gravel; spurs are hard-packed dirt

HIKING TIME: 45 minutes–1 hour

DRIVING DISTANCE: 30 miles from I-77/I-480 exchange

ACCESS: Daily, 8 a.m.–sunset

WHEELCHAIR TRAVERSABLE: No

MAPS: USGS Grafton; also available online at loraincountymetroparks.com

FACILITIES: Two picnic shelters, grills, water, restrooms, and a small playground

CONTACT INFORMATION: Call (440) 458-5121 or visit loraincountymetroparks.com.

Directions

Take I-480 West to OH 10 West, exiting at OH 57 toward Medina. Turn left onto OH 57/John F. Kennedy Memorial Highway, continuing about 4 miles west before turning right onto Parsons Road. Indian Hollow Reservation's Sheldon Woods entrance is on Parsons Road, just east of Indian Hollow Road.

GPS Trailhead Coordinates

Latitude 41° 16.635597'

Longitude 82° 4.442160'

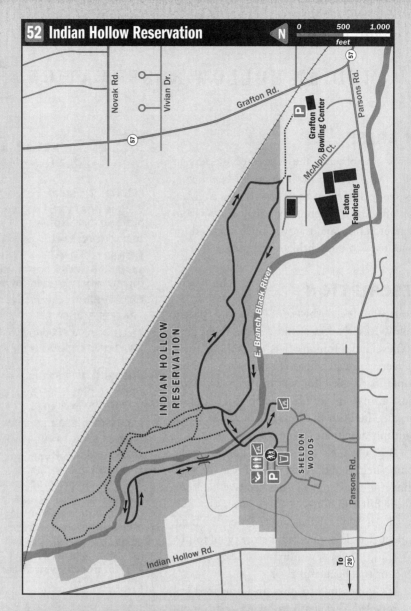

N

0   500   1,000
feet

Novak Rd.

Vivian Dr.

57

Grafton Rd.

P

Grafton Bowling Center

McAlpin Ct.

Parsons Rd.

57

Eaton Fabricating

E. Branch Black River

INDIAN HOLLOW RESERVATION

SHELDON WOODS

P

Parsons Rd.

Indian Hollow Rd.

To 20

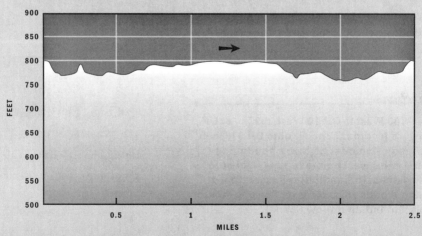

FEET

900
850
800
750
700
650
600
550
500

0.5   1   1.5   2   2.5

MILES

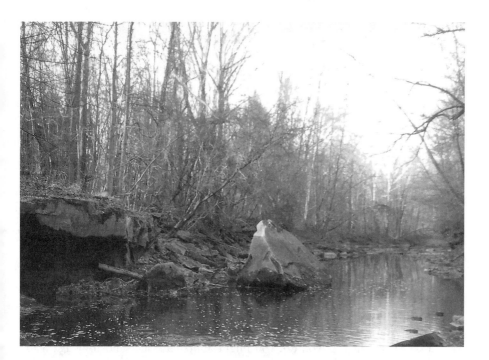

Before the large rock, known as jutting rock, broke in two, it sheltered a boy from a devastating tornado.

trail north-northeast, you'll be struck by how many shades of greens and grays the lichen and moss on the rocks along the river display. In at least two spots on this trail, the river appears easy to cross, and a path similar to this one calls enticingly from the other side of the river. Don't answer the call—the rocks are slippery, and the river runs several feet deep here. Continue on the dirt path on this side of the river, keeping an eye out for herons and other fishing birds.

You might also notice deep lines in the sandstone wall across the river. These lines were cut by a glacier called the Wisconsin Ice Sheet, creating a wall that looks much like a layer cake. It is especially striking as you approach an old railroad bridge. Before you reach the bridge, however, you'll find a no-trespassing sign. Heed it, retracing your steps to the base of the bridge. On your return, you'll notice a thick and fragrant stand of pines separating the trail from the private homes on your right.

Also as you head back to the loop trail, you'll have time to consider this river's long history. Local authors Chris Smith and Paul Justy dug into the area's industrial past and uncovered more than a few fascinating stories about the Indian Hollow and Willow Park areas in Grafton. (Smith graciously shared some of those stories with me as this book was in production, about the time his book was released. Look for many more stories in *The Lost Quarry Industry of Indian Hollow and Willow Park—Grafton, Ohio*.)

One of the large rocks placed just so in the river, for example, hasn't always been there. Apparently, it broke off around 1950. Prior to that, the jutting rock jutted out a bit farther into the river—and saved a young boy's life. According to Smith:

"About the time of the Revolutionary War, a young Native American boy saw an approaching tornado coming up the river from the south. He was north of the rock and ran south, toward the tornado, because he knew his only chance to survive was to get under the rock. Luckily a dry summer had reduced the river to a few inches of water, so he could easily run under the rock. Within seconds of reaching safety, the trees came crashing down. Not one tree on this bank of the river survived."

That's a pretty good legacy for a rock, but unfortunately, Smith found out that later, the rock also marked the spot of several tragic events. Quarries were dangerous places to work, and snapping derrick cables injured and killed many quarry workers near the same rock. Smith also learned that in 1899, a 14-year-old boy was hit by a quarry train and had to have an arm amputated.

While the rock has saved at least one life and been witness to many tragic events, it sits here quietly surrounded by great natural beauty, and here, on this unmarked trail, so are you.

When you get back to the connector to the Beech-Maple Trail, turn left and cross the bridge. As you do, you might appreciate the sandstone again for a different reason. Because the river bottom is sandstone, the water runs over it clear and bright. Crossing the bridge on a sunny day, the river fairly sparkles up at your shoes.

Across the bridge, the loop trail rises up a slight hill and splits. Veer left, following the gravel trail clockwise. The path is level and wide, with enough twists and turns to hold the interest of hikers and beginning mountain bikers. The trail lies under the shade of sugar maple and American beech trees. If you look closely, you may spot a tall cucumber tree. Indian Hollow is thought to be the only place in Lorain County where this particular member of the magnolia family grows.

Midway through the loop, a connector trail heads straight into the town of Grafton. In fact, you'll have to make a sharp right turn at a park bench to avoid going into town. After the turn, you're heading due west. This section is especially lovely in the late afternoon, when the sun bounces off the river and bleeds through the trees.

After completing the loop and returning across the bridge, head off the path again, this time to the left (south). Follow this unmarked, well-worn dirt trail to a large, flat rock. Perched just a few feet above the sparkling river, it seems custom-made for a picnic. Even if you're not packing a snack, stop, sit, and listen to the river rush by.

When you've heard enough, retrace your steps back to the paved connector trail; turn left and follow it back to the parking lot.

NEARBY ACTIVITIES

Mountain bike trails rolling into Grafton give visitors a chance to see remnants of many quarries on their way into the historical town. (A major upgrade to the trail was underway as this book went to press. During construction, some sections may be closed. Check the park website for trail updates.)

Also, while you're here, you're not far from another great chapter in American history. In 1858 nearby Oberlin earned the nickname "the town that started the Civil War," after townspeople foiled an attempt by bounty hunters to return a fugitive slave to his owner. In addition to the town's rich history, the Oberlin College campus boasts beautiful gardens and landscaping and a fine legacy of its own. To reach Oberlin, follow Parsons Road west about 8 miles.

I sincerely thank Chris Smith, author and dedicated historian, for sharing his tremendous research and enthusiasm for Lorain County and Grafton in particular. His work will be appreciated by countless visitors to Indian Hollow as they gain a greater understanding and appreciation for the impact generations have had on this land, and the role the river has played in the area's history. Thanks, Chris!

53 OXBOW TRAIL

KEY AT-A-GLANCE INFORMATION

LENGTH: 1.7 miles

CONFIGURATION: Loop

DIFFICULTY: Moderate, with all the climbing at once; not for weak knees

SCENERY: Marsh, river, woodlands, rumbling rapids of Cuyahoga River

EXPOSURE: Shady throughout, except for exposed steps

TRAFFIC: Moderate most days; bustling on evenings and weekends

TRAIL SURFACE: Dirt carpeted with leaves; first leg can be muddy; steps and bridge slippery when wet.

HIKING TIME: 45 minutes

DRIVING DISTANCE: 35 miles from I-77/I-480 exchange

ACCESS: Daily, 7 a.m.–11 p.m.; dogs allowed on leash

WHEELCHAIR TRAVERSABLE: No

MAPS: USGS Peninsula; also available at summitmetroparks.org

FACILITIES: Restrooms (closed in winter) and water; concessions during league ballgames; emergency phone at southernmost entrance

CONTACT INFORMATION: Report problems at park to Summit County Metro Parks Rangers at (330) 657-2131. For general info, contact the parks office at (330) 865-5511 or summitmetroparks.org.

- -

GPS Trailhead Coordinates

Latitude   41° 7.321o22'

Longitude 81° 31.228623'

IN BRIEF

Oxbow Trail winds through the Cuyahoga River Valley, north of Akron. From the burbling rapids of the Cuyahoga River to a cardiac climb to a fabulous vista, this hike offers variety over a short haul. Though a steep sledding hill and several ball fields are nearby, hikers can get away from the action in the center of the park to enjoy this remote wooded trail and the great views of the surrounding valley that it offers.

DESCRIPTION

If Oxbow Trail were a book—well, it would be a novella—you'd describe it to your friends by saying, "It started a bit slow, but before I was halfway through, I hoped it wouldn't end." In fact, Oxbow packs so much scenery in its little loop that you'll be glad you picked it up. It's also a great casual dining spot. Oxbow's many picnic tables are placed to provide comfortable space between diners. It's entirely possible to enjoy a picnic supper here, with the lifting of

- -

Directions ⟶

Cascade Valley Metro Parks South Chuckery/ Oxbow Area is located off Cuyahoga Street, between Uhler Avenue and Sackett Avenue, in North Akron. From Cleveland, follow I-480 East to I-271 South. From I-271 take Exit 18 onto OH 8 south and exit at Howe Avenue. Turn right to follow Howe, and then veer right to continue on Cuyahoga Falls Avenue. Follow Cuyahoga Falls Avenue about 2.5 miles to Cuyahoga Street; turn right. Follow Cuyahoga Street north about 1 mile; the park sign will be on your right. (*Note:* There are two entrances to the Oxbow/ Chuckery Area on Cuyahoga Street; take the northernmost entrance. An alternate entrance is available on Sackett Avenue.)

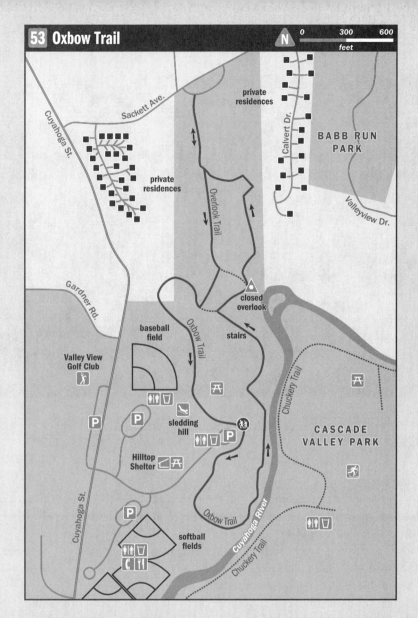

N

0   300   600
feet

Sackett Ave.

Cuyahoga St.

private
residences

private
residences

Calvert Dr.

BABB RUN
PARK

Valleyview Dr.

Overlook Trail

Gardner Rd.

closed
overlook

stairs

baseball
field

Oxbow Trail

Valley View
Golf Club

P

P

sledding
hill

P

Chuckery Trail

CASCADE
VALLEY
PARK

Hilltop
Shelter

P

Oxbow Trail

Cuyahoga River

softball
fields

Cuyahoga St.

Chuckery Trail

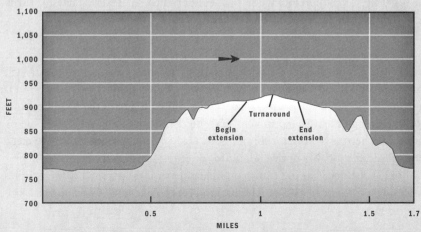

1,100

1,050

1,000

950

900

850

800

750

700

FEET

0.5   1   1.5   1.7

MILES

Turnaround

Begin
extension

End
extension

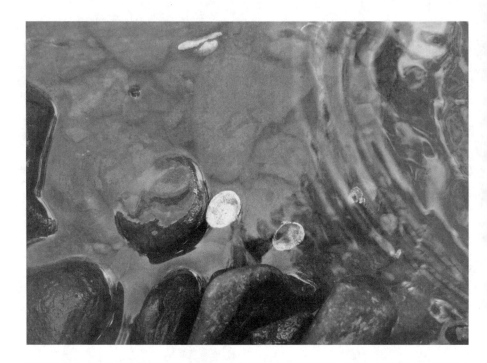

The Cuyahoga River is home to countless creatures.

the Cuyahoga to entertain you, and never catch wind of the dinner conversation at another table.

Because the trail is damp along the river and shady throughout, it's a great place for insects to hang out. It's advisable to apply some bug repellent when visiting Oxbow during mosquito or fly season. The insects attract birds, of course, and you're likely to hear, if not see, woodpeckers at work on some of the 60-foot-tall (and taller) trees along the way. Mostly deciduous varieties—tall oaks and black cherries—shade the trail.

The trailhead marker lets you decide to start out in either direction. Head south-southwest, counterclockwise, to meander through several marshy turns (in dry weather) or large puddles (in wetter times). In the spring and summer months, you'll be met by white trilliums (Ohio's official state wildflower) and a variety of violets that like the wet ground along the river.

About 0.2 miles into the trail, the path turns sharply left, heading north, and meets up with the Cuyahoga River. Traveling along the river's edge, you'll soon hear several rapids providing a musical accompaniment to the sound of your feet on the dirt and leaves. Approach very quietly and you may see great blue or green-backed herons fishing for dinner here. Crouch down to look into the clear water and you'll probably notice a handful of empty freshwater clamshells.

About 0.3 miles into the trail, you'll pass a small clearing with several picnic tables. (Here you can also see the parking lot to your left.) Continue past the tables and veer to your left to continue along the trail. It remains flat and almost entirely shaded until you come to a railroad-tie staircase. Take a deep breath—you're about to climb up 98 (or so) steps. At the top, pause, take another deep breath, and turn around. The view is worth it.

Once you've caught your breath, you're faced with a decision: to do the Oxbow Overlook extension or not. It's just 0.5 miles—do it! (If you skip the extension, you'll take several smaller stairways down the hill and encounter a small footbridge that may be slippery when snowy or wet. You'll also find a few more picnic tables along the way. The Overlook extension rejoins the main trail before too long.)

The Overlook Trail heads to the right a bit, and up a bit more, then to the right a bit, up a bit . . . and you soon realize how great the view is going to be from the overlook. (The overlook deck has been closed in the past. Erosion is the culprit here; the sandy soil just can't support the overlook's overhang.)

The trail itself ventures closely enough to the side of the cliff that you can see for miles, with feet planted safely on terra firma. Photographers, however, may have a harder time swallowing the news that the deck has been closed; trees obscure the view too much to get a great panoramic shot.

After a few minutes admiring the view, amble on along the path, which veers to the left and then proceeds to work its way down the trail, with a few stairs here and a handrail there.

As you descend, the sledding hill comes into view. During the winter and early spring, thanks to the lay of the land, you'll be able to keep an eye on the sledding hill—and your car in the parking lot—during most of the final third of the loop. In the summer, you'll have less of a view but will continue to enjoy the trees' air-conditioning effect.

When there's no snow and no ballgame, you won't have much company on the trail. Hilltop Shelter, above the sledding hill, is available for free on a first-come, first-serve basis. The shelter, which holds about 40 people, also can be reserved for a fee by calling (330) 687-5511.

NEARBY ACTIVITIES

Oxbow is popular in winter thanks to its sledding hill and in-ground toboggan runs. The hill is lighted for night use, and cross-country skiers frequent the trail. The park service maintains a 24-hour seasonal information phone line at (330) 865-8060.

During much of the year, the park's ball fields—three softball, one baseball, and two soccer—host league play. When the fields are not in use for league play, park visitors are free to use them.

Within a couple of miles, you'll find plenty of other hiking trails. Visitors can hike from the Oxbow Trailhead to Gorge Metro Park (see page 222) via the Highbridge Trail (3-plus miles) or head over to Babb Run Bird and Wildlife Sanctuary, about 2 miles to the north (see page 198).

54 PENINSULA HISTORY AND QUARRY TRAIL

KEY AT-A-GLANCE INFORMATION

LENGTH: 2.5 miles

CONFIGURATION: Loop and a cross

DIFFICULTY: Moderate (city portion, easy; Quarry, somewhat challenging)

SCENERY: Two canal locks, sandstone quarry, historical architecture, wildlife along the river

EXPOSURE: Trail, shady; sidewalks, exposed

TRAFFIC: Typically heavy in town and light on Quarry Trail

TRAIL SURFACE: Asphalt, sand, dirt, crushed limestone

HIKING TIME: 1.5 hours

DRIVING DISTANCE: 16 miles from I-77/I-480 exchange

ACCESS: Towpath and Quarry Trail: Daily, sunrise–10 p.m.

WHEELCHAIR TRAVERSABLE: Peninsula sidewalks, yes (most businesses, no); Quarry Trail, no

MAPS: USGS Peninsula; Peninsula architectural tour guide at Peninsula Library & Historical Society, 6105 Riverview Road

FACILITIES: Restrooms, water, and drink machine at Lock 29 parking

CONTACT INFORMATION: Learn more about the Towpath and national park at nps.gov/cuva or call (330) 657-2752.

IN BRIEF

Peninsula displays the well-preserved vestiges of a canal-era town and a railroad town, while serving as a portal into the Cuyahoga Valley National Park. Some folks say Peninsula has a lock on history. Actually, it has two—and visitors will see both on this hike.

DESCRIPTION

Change steamed through Peninsula in the form of a canal in the 1840s and rolled through again in the 1880s when the railroad came to town. The changes kept coming, with the dedication of the Cuyahoga Valley National Recreation Area (now National Park) in 1975. And when the federal government comes to town to claim more than 30,000 acres, *change* is putting it mildly.

While other towns might buckle under the strain of being a gateway to a national park, Peninsula thrives. The town is well suited to serve as a portal back in time; in some ways, Peninsula also serves as an extension of the park. Lock 29 along the Ohio and Erie Towpath Trail literally deposits thru-hikers and bikers into the heart of Peninsula. The local bike shop is an icon to regular Towpath riders and a welcome beacon to folks with flats. Peninsula's restaurants are so popular with

GPS Trailhead Coordinates

Latitude   41° 14.536257'

Longitude   81° 32.955780'

Directions

From Cleveland, take I-77 South to Exit 136/ OH 21. Continue south to OH 303 and turn left, heading east about 5 miles. To reach parking at Lock 29 Trailhead, turn left onto North Locust Street after crossing the river and then left again on Mill Street and into the lot. (A sign directs you to LOCK 29 TRAILHEAD PARKING.)

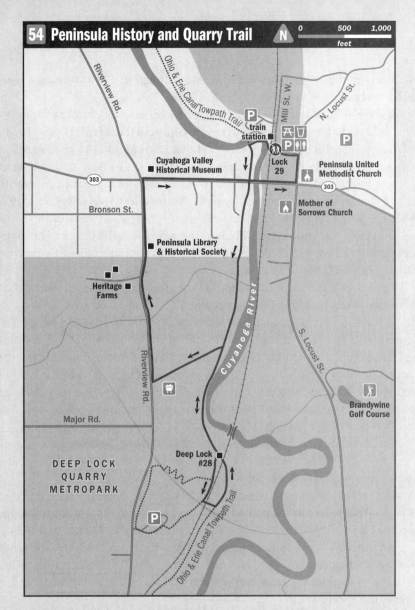

N

| 0 | 500 | 1,000 |

feet

Ohio & Erie Canal/Towpath Trail

Riverview Rd.

Mill St. W.

N. Locust St.

P

train station

Lock 29

Peninsula United Methodist Church

303

Cuyahoga Valley Historical Museum

Bronson St.

Mother of Sorrows Church

Peninsula Library & Historical Society

Cuyahoga River

Heritage Farms

Riverview Rd.

S. Locust St.

Brandywine Golf Course

Major Rd.

DEEP LOCK QUARRY METROPARK

Deep Lock #28

Ohio & Erie Canal Towpath Trail

P

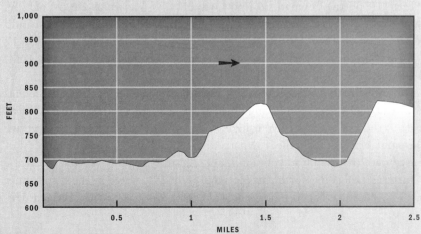

1,000
950
900
850
800
750
700
650
600

FEET

0.5   1   1.5   2   2.5

MILES

train riders that the Cuyahoga Valley Scenic Railroad (CVSRR) features a layover lunch stop here.

Start your tour at the trailhead sign and map at Lock 29. Take the steps up to the bridge that literally and figuratively connects the relatively new Towpath Trail and national park to the historical town of Peninsula. An interpretive sign on the bridge highlights the building of the Ohio and Erie Canal. When construction began in 1825, workers had to devise it so that boats could negotiate the 395-foot elevation difference between Akron and Cleveland. Locks 29 and 28 were key to leveling the ride, and the canal was key to Ohio's economy.

Go below the bridge and walk into the now earth-filled lock. The mason's marks on some of the blocks are still visible, indicating the quarry and the work group from which the stone came.

Once over the bridge, continue south on the Towpath and under OH 303, where the paved path gives way to crushed limestone. The river runs on your left; beyond it, the railroad tracks carry passengers on the Cuyahoga Valley Scenic Line north into the park and south into Akron. About 0.5 miles into the trail, a sign points to Deep Lock Quarry. Take the cue and venture off the Towpath heading west. Cross a narrow, wooden footbridge and then head up a steep hill. A bench at the top may be a welcome sight after the climb. Follow the dirt path under tall pines and right over the rocky but now level ground. You'll reach the quarry shortly.

Sandstone dug here helped build many local homes and businesses, as well as several locks along the canal. Today, trees cover the quarry's floor, but the sheer stone walls leave no doubt where you are.

The adventurous may want to climb into the quarry, and it's allowed, but all should take care near the edges, as gravel and sand make for slippery footing. The trail skirts the eastern side of the quarry and heads south. As you go downhill, you'll see Summit County Metro Parks trail markers (in yellow), pointing west to the Quarry Trail parking lot, off of Riverview Road. Unless you want to explore the park further, stay on the trail heading south and east to return to the Towpath.

Turn left on the Towpath to find Lock 28, also known as Deep Lock. As its name suggests, it is the deepest lock on the canal. While a typical lock would move a boat up or down 8 or 9 feet, Deep Lock could raise and lower boats 17 feet. For its hard work, Deep Lock was awarded a historical civil engineers landmark plaque, which is displayed inside the lock.

Continue north on the Towpath toward Peninsula. The calls of geese and other birds blend with the bubbling of the river, now on your right. Now you're heading to the city portion of your hike, where you'll get a different perspective on the same era. Veer off the Towpath toward your left on an unmarked but well-used path that will lead you uphill and deposit you on Riverview Road.

Turn right, heading north past Heritage Farms. Operated by the same family since 1848, Heritage Farms holds seasonal events and has a lovely herb garden.

Walk through the garden and enjoy the orchids and lilies—or pick out your Christmas tree, depending on the season.

On the north side of OH 303, you'll see the Boston Township Hall and its distinctive bell tower at 1775 Main. Built as a school in 1887, today it houses Boston Township offices, community meeting rooms, and the Cuyahoga Valley Historical Museum. Another stop along Riverview that's worth your time is the Peninsula Library & Historical Society. Stop in to get an architectural tour guide or to learn more about the area.

Turn right at OH 303 and head into the Peninsula Business District, listed on the National Register of Historic Places. As

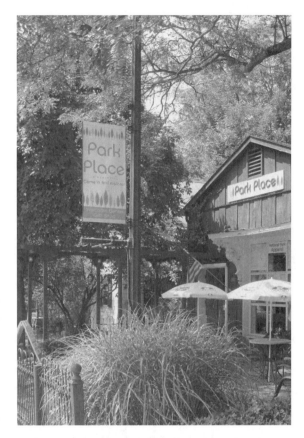

National park store in downtown Peninsula

you continue east, consider the girth of the maples that line the yards in this town. Most of them were planted at or about the time of construction—making these granddaddy trees several times over. And speaking of construction . . . notice the building located at 1663 Main, built in 1820. Like many homes here, it is a good example of the Western Reserve Greek Revival style.

Also stop to look at 1749 Main Street. Perhaps the biggest bargain on the block, this Vallonia model Sears and Roebuck kit home sold for $2,076 in 1926. Its steep roof and white columns have been maintained so carefully that you might say it looks brand-new, or fresh out of the box. It's estimated that about 100,000 kit homes were built in the U.S. between 1908 and 1940. Most models came entirely as precut and numbered pieces of lumber. The homes were inexpensive but not inferior, and were efficient to build too. The Sears catalog boasted that a kit home could be built in about 60% of the time required to build a traditional home.

As you cross the bridge and the railroad tracks, you'll pass a variety of antiques shops, cafés, and galleries. The sign for the Old Peninsula Night Club hanging at 1615 Main Street has been around for many years; the building was a nightclub and a dance hall in the 1930s and '40s. Today, the restaurant is the Winking Lizard, but the owners still display the cool antique sign (along with their own).

About a block east of the Lizard, turn right and walk one block south on Akron-Peninsula Road to Mother of Sorrows Catholic Church. Originally built in 1882, the church was enlarged in 1935 in a rather clever way. The building was literally cut in half, the west end was moved back, and the middle filled in to enlarge the sanctuary. Now turn around and go north on Akron-Peninsula Road. The street name changes to Locust, and you'll pass the Peninsula Village Hall, constructed with sandstone from the local quarry in 1851. Cost to the taxpayers? About $600. It's still used to house village services—talk about getting your money's worth!

Speaking of money, that concludes your nickel tour of Peninsula. You can continue north on Locust to Mill Street to return to the parking lot at Lock 29. Or continue to explore . . . you'll find plenty in Peninsula to pique your interest.

NEARBY ACTIVITIES

Peninsula's seasonal art walks are fun and friendly. See the schedule at **explore peninsula.com**. To explore the national park from here, you can leave town on foot or on bike, either north or south, on the Towpath. The National Park Service staffs Park Place, a visitor center and gift shop, on the corner of OH 303 and Locust Street. Prefer to take the train? Get schedules and ticket information at (800) 468-4070 or **cvsrr.org**. Heritage Farms, south of OH 303 on Riverview Road, is largely considered a tree farm, but it's also a farmer's market and is open on weekends all year long. Find out more about that valley business at **heritage farms.com** or call (330) 657-2330.

PLATEAU TRAIL 55

IN BRIEF

While Cuyahoga Valley National Park is full of great scenery, the Oak Hill area offers a special treat for the eyes. Here you'll encounter a series of S-curves that wiggle through the woods, following a ravine; a lovely change of scenery greets you at almost every turn on this loop trail. Don't be surprised if some of those breathtakingly beautiful scenes appear suddenly as you round a turn.

DESCRIPTION

Enter the trailhead at the eastern end of the Oak Hill parking lot. A trail map is posted there on a park bulletin board. Both the shorter Oak Hill Trail and the outer loop of Plateau Trail begin to the left, or north, of the sign. A few grassy steps and a short wooden bridge later, the trails diverge. Oak Hill Trail turns to the right and loops around the highest point of the plateau in just 1.5 miles. But to do the shorter loop is to miss most of the hills, and much of the fun, of the longer and varied trail.

So stay on Plateau Trail, heading north, as the trail bends left and climbs gradually

KEY AT-A-GLANCE INFORMATION

LENGTH: 4.7 miles

CONFIGURATION: Loop

DIFFICULTY: Moderate

SCENERY: Pine and deciduous forests, three ponds, lush hemlock ravine

EXPOSURE: Mostly shaded

TRAFFIC: Light

TRAIL SURFACE: Dirt, with short stretches of grass and gravel

HIKING TIME: 2 hours

DRIVING DISTANCE: 16 miles from I-77/I-480 exchange

ACCESS: Daily, 7 a.m.–10 p.m. Two restricted trails, one on either side of Meadowedge Pond, are clearly signed. They lead to the Cuyahoga Valley Environmental Education Center (CVEEC) and are authorized for CVEEC use only.

WHEELCHAIR TRAVERSABLE: No

MAPS: USGS Peninsula; also posted at trailhead kiosk and available at most of the national park visitor centers and at nps.gov/cuva

FACILITIES: Restrooms at trailhead

CONTACT INFORMATION: For the Cuyahoga Valley National Park, visit nps.gov/cuva or call (330) 657-2752. For information about CVEEC programs, see cvnpa.org.

Directions ⟶

From I-77, exit at Wheatley Road (OH 176/Exit 143 toward Richfield and I-271) and head east to Oak Hill Road. Turn left, going north about 2 miles. The entrance to Oak Hill Picnic Area is on your right. Turn right, following Major Road west 1.5 miles; then turn left onto Oak Hill Road. (Eastsiders may prefer to take OH 8 south to OH 303, heading west to Riverview Road, following it approximately 1 mile south to Major Road.) The entrance to Oak Hill Picnic Area (and the trails) is on the eastern side of Oak Hill Road. Turn left and follow the driveway 0.2 miles east to the parking lot.

GPS Trailhead
Coordinates
Latitude   41° 13.177199'
Longitude   81° 34.562523'

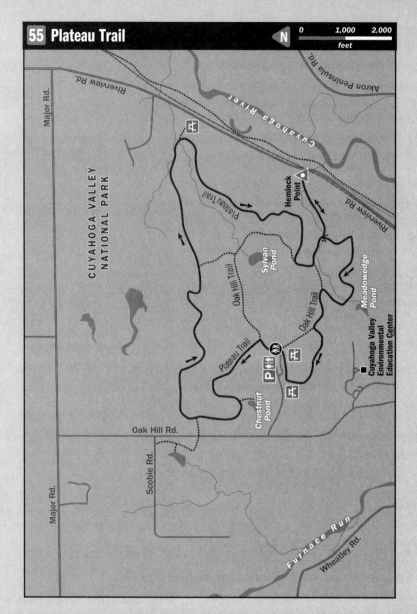

0   1,000   2,000
feet

N

CUYAHOGA VALLEY NATIONAL PARK

Major Rd.

Riverview Rd.

Akron Peninsula Rd.

Cuyahoga River

Plateau Trail

Hemlock Point

Oak Hill Trail

Sylvan Pond

Meadowedge Pond

Oak Hill Trail

Cuyahoga Valley Environmental Education Center

Plateau Trail

P

Chestnut Pond

Oak Hill Rd.

Scobie Rd.

Major Rd.

Furnace Run

Wheatley Rd.

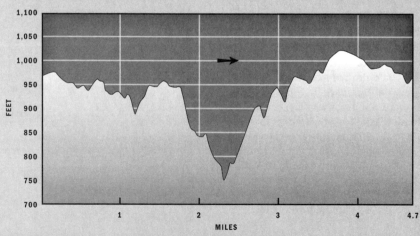

FEET

1,100
1,050
1,000
950
900
850
800
750
700

1   2   3   4   4.7

MILES

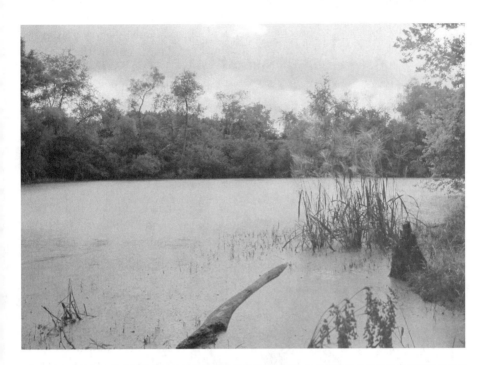

Chestnut Pond is a haven for green frogs.

beneath the cover of hemlock trees. For a few paces, the old trees give way to meadow bushes and growth. This is one of the few stretches of trail where you'll be able to see the sky, as much of the way is completely shaded by hemlocks and deciduous trees. Half a mile into the trail you'll cross another bridge and come to Chestnut Pond.

Small and easy to dismiss, the pond is a haven for amphibians who apparently take quite a bite out of the local insect population. (Translation: You can afford to stand on the pond's edge, looking and listening for frogs, without being bothered by mosquitoes!) As you turn and leave the pond, the trail turns sharply to the right. You're about to have one of those aha moments—or perhaps more accurately—an ooh-and-aah moment. Only a few steps from Chestnut Pond you'll find a long, long, long corridor of tall pines, as visually stunning as they are fragrant. As you stroll through the hallway of pines, try to keep your feet on the ground while you gaze up at their tops, 60 feet or so above you.

At the western end of the pine corridor, the path veers right again. Gravel and grass work together to keep this stretch of trail nice and dry. Heading north, you'll begin to see evidence of the hard work put into this trail, which was completed in 1997. More than a dozen small culverts have been created alongside and underneath the trail. Designed and laid with care, they are both unobtrusive and necessary. As you round the loop and head east, the ravine is only a few feet from the trail. It's worth a few careful sidesteps to peer over the edge (beware,

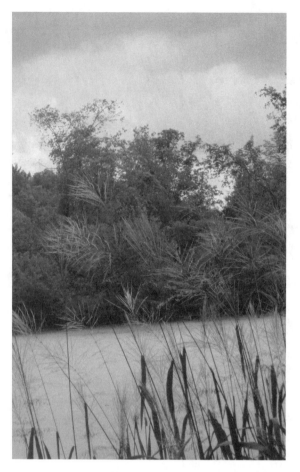

Plateau Trail is less used than many trails in this national park.

though—hearty poison ivy hides among the Virginia creeper and young oaks). The ravine is only about 10 feet deep here, but keep an eye on it; it grows wider and deeper as you continue on the trail.

At 1.5 miles, you'll pass a sign indicating a connector trail to Sylvan Pond. If you follow it, you'll also find the short (1.5-mile) inner loop, Oak Hill Trail. But for now, stay on the Plateau Trail . . . you have a lot to look forward to.

Less than 2 miles into the trail, tree buffs will find a special section of the path, loaded with multi-trunked trees. Is there a proper name for this occurrence? If there is, it's elusive, but children—who tend to name things more expediently than botanists—call them two-headed and three-headed trees. Call 'em what you will, but watching for them along this section may take your mind off the fact that you're heading uphill for most of the next 0.8 miles. As the trail bends to the right, you'll pass over a feeder stream to Sylvan Creek (unnoticeable during dry periods) and head south, easing downhill. Soon you'll cross another footbridge, this one high enough to warrant leaning over the railing for another look at the ravine.

Just past the 3-mile mark, you'll climb a bit more and veer left to Hemlock Ravine, where a sign directs you to a short side trip. The 0.2-mile, out-and-back trail to Hemlock Point is to your left. Unless you need to conserve your energy, you should take the opportunity to enjoy the overlook. Back on the main trail, you'll follow a series of S-shaped curves. In fact, the trail turns you this way and that, barely righting itself (and you) between the crooks as it slopes up slightly, and then takes you down a few feet, to the right. Here you'll see that the twisting served a purpose: directly in front of you is the beautiful Meadowedge Pond—and you didn't even see it coming.

To arrive at Meadowedge Pond in the late spring or summer is perhaps the hiker's equivalent of a carnival visitor leaving the midway's relatively constant panorama for a spectacular, if brief, sideshow. The pond vista is an oasis of color and song. Orioles, goldfinches, and yellow warblers spin colorful, dizzying circles around the pond. Frogs bound in with a splash as you walk by and then scold you for interrupting their day. Lily pads cover much of the pond's surface, and cattails stand like a stockade fence around much of the perimeter, as if protecting it from too-eager visitors.

Linger here and enjoy the show; the colors and sounds offer an amazing contrast to the quiet, forested trail behind you. When you're ready for yet another change of scenery, follow the wide grassy trail to the right, heading north into the shade of pines and hemlocks. The trail unfurls again in a series of S-shaped curves to reach a sign indicating the Oak Hill Trail straight ahead. You can follow it from here, back to the parking lot, or continue on Plateau Trail, by turning left. For the sake of finishing what you've started, stay on Plateau Trail.

The ravine is on your right at this point, and the trail is at its flattest. Still, it's not straight, snaking along the last three-quarters of a mile in the now-familiar S-shaped pattern. Near the end of the trail, you'll ease down a gentle slope, in the company of young hemlock trees, to emerge in an open grassy area, surrounded by picnic tables and—in the spring and summer, at least—a lovely show of wildflowers, including oxeye daisies, coltsfoot, and clovers. It's somehow fitting that Plateau Trail manages to get in this final change of scenery as the curtain goes down on your hike. The show is over and the parking lot is on your right; you can leave, but you probably can't forget what you've seen here.

NEARBY ACTIVITIES

Up for another hike with dazzling views? Nearby Salt Run (see page 259) offers exactly that. Hungry? You're also within a five- to ten-minute drive of several seasonal farmer's markets.

56 RISING VALLEY PARK

KEY AT-A-GLANCE INFORMATION

LENGTH: 1.5 miles

CONFIGURATION: Loop

DIFFICULTY: Easy

SCENERY: Broad expanse of valley, trickles of the East Branch of the Rocky River, thick young woodlands

EXPOSURE: About half exposed

TRAFFIC: Light

TRAIL SURFACE: Grass and dirt

HIKING TIME: 45 minutes

DRIVING DISTANCE: 15 miles from I-77/I-480 exchange

ACCESS: Daily, sunrise–sunset

WHEELCHAIR TRAVERSABLE: No

MAPS: USGS West Richfield

FACILITIES: Restrooms at each picnic area, well-water pump by southern picnic shelter, two picnic shelters with grills, small playground, ball diamond, soccer fields, sledding hill

CONTACT INFORMATION: To reach park managers, contact Hinckley Township at (330) 278-4181 or hinckleytwp.org.

GPS Trailhead Coordinates

Latitude   41° 15.666482'

Longitude   81° 41.000040'

IN BRIEF

This 227-acre park located on the southern end of the Cuyahoga Valley was nearly turned into a federal prison. Fortunately, contemporary visitors can enjoy this beautiful area beside the headwaters of the East Branch of the Rocky River. Here you might spy a variety of mosses, wildflowers, and "pieces of Canada."

DESCRIPTION

Parks come about in a variety of ways. Rising Valley was sort of a gift from the federal government. The land was originally part of the Cleveland Army Tank Plant proving grounds. The federal government had plans to turn the place into a prison when area residents started to protest. No one wants a prison built in their neighborhood, but this seemed especially poor planning—the adjoining property is a Girl Scout camp! In 1977 the U.S. government deeded the 227 acres to Hinckley and Richfield townships for the purpose of creating a public park and recreation area. Today, the two townships manage it through a joint park board.

Directions ⟶

Follow I-77 South to Exit 149B to OH 82 West/ East Royalton Road toward Broadview Heights. Follow OH 82 about 2 miles and then turn left onto OH 176/Broadview Road. Continue south about 4 miles; then turn right onto Newton Road, which veers left and becomes Oviatt Road. Alternatively, you can access the park from OH 303, less than a mile west of OH 176. Traveling West on OH 303, turn right onto Oviatt Road. Follow Oviatt north about 2 miles—the park is not marked or signed until you reach the end of the residential drive. Continue to the parking lot, located at the north end of the park.

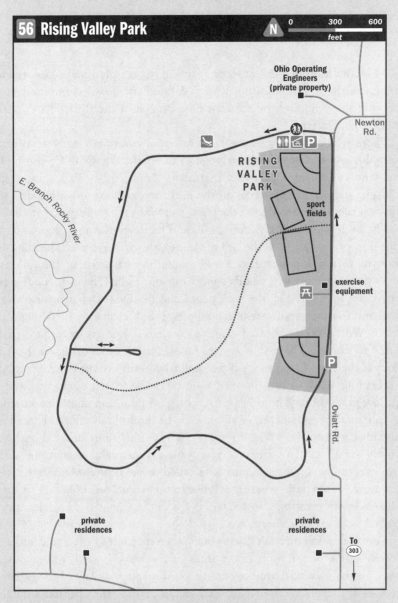

N

0   300   600
feet

Ohio Operating
Engineers
(private property)

Newton
Rd.

RISING
VALLEY
PARK

sport
fields

exercise
equipment

E. Branch Rocky River

Oviatt Rd.

private
residences

private
residences

To
303

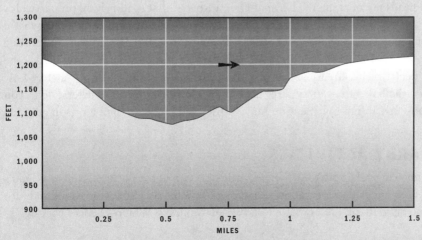

1,300
1,250
1,200
1,150
1,100
1,050
1,000
950
900

FEET

0.25   0.5   0.75   1   1.25   1.5

MILES

As a condition of the transfer of land, a master plan had to be developed and implemented. The resulting Rising Valley Park Board committed itself to preserving this land and the adjacent East Branch of the Rocky River corridor for future generations.

There are no trail signs here, but a rather obvious path leads west from the parking lot and shelter at the north end of the park. The Ohio Operating Engineers, who run a training facility that abuts Rising Valley Park, have donated much time, labor, and materials to the park over the years. With a nod to the facility on the northern edge of the park, step onto the wide grassy path.

The path is actually a sledding hill, and its steep downhill slope offers fantastic views of the valley. At the end of the hill, the path veers left, heading south. Before you turn to follow it, take a few minutes to really soak up the valley view.

As the path veers left, woods appear on your right. The wet woodlands and the river are monitored by the park board and the Ohio Department of Natural Resources. You may spot jack-in-the-pulpits, skunk cabbages, or trilliums along the way. Wild turkeys, pileated woodpeckers, great horned owls, and red foxes call this area home. The path is easy to follow for 0.3 miles or so, reaching a few trickles of the river. Once you're done exploring, return to the drier, grassy path.

Heading south again, the trail soon forks. Bear left, going east and up a long, low-grade hill. (The other path, going straight and south, soon lands in the residential development.) In the middle of the hill, an unmarked and little-used path cuts into the woods to your left. Take this short out-and-back to the relatively small stand of trees. If you want a shorter hike, continue walking north; eventually you'll emerge by a ball field or picnic area. Otherwise, return to the more beaten path, where you'll notice the woods on either side of the trail are littered with erratics, also known as "pieces of Canada," or rocks that were imported by glacier ice sheets.

Continue south through thick woods; then turn left as you come into a more exposed section of the trail. In the thick of the woods, you'll find a variety of mosses. In the spring, daffodils pop up amid maple, oak, and beech trees. (Be courteous and avoid the more exposed section, which runs behind a home and then heads north along the berm of Oviatt Road—that is all private property.) It's easy to appreciate the delicate wildflowers here but not hard to imagine what a great run it must have been for tanks, plowing through the thick mud and rolling over assorted large rocks. On your way back to the parking lot, you'll pass the ball fields, picnic areas, volleyball court, and playground. Still, no matter how rowdy the ball games, no matter how many picnickers fill the shelters, don't you suppose it's an improvement on tank traffic, and far nicer than a prison ground?

NEARBY ACTIVITIES

Lengthen this hike with the 4.7-mile Medina section of the Buckeye Trail to Whipp's Ledges at Hinckley Reservation (see page 270). Take OH 303 west 1 mile and turn left on State Road. Follow State Road about 4 miles to Whipp's Ledges parking.

SALT RUN TRAIL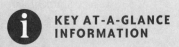

IN BRIEF

Hikers get a hilly workout while traveling through this former farm and estate of Hayward Kendall. Rolling meadows; shady creek crossings; and layers of moss, pine needles, and ferns provide a feast for the eyes. An optional 1.2-mile loop encircles beautiful Kendall Lake, built by the Civilian Conservation Corps (CCC) in the 1930s.

DESCRIPTION

Five rolling hills come together to greet you in the Pine Meadows parking lot. There are picnic tables aplenty here, and the view is always grand. On snowy days, the hills are alive with the sounds of little folks on sleds. Fog nestles in the lower areas in the morning; on a sunny afternoon, you can see acres and acres of . . . well, pines and meadows. Frankly, the parking lot vista is so pretty that you may have to pull yourself down to the lot's western end, where you'll find the trailhead. Come on. This is only the beginning.

Follow trail signs from the western end of the parking lot, over the rolling hills, and down about 10 feet to enter a dirt path. Turn left at the Salt Run sign to follow the trail clockwise. Meandering downhill, you'll soon

KEY AT-A-GLANCE INFORMATION

LENGTH: 3.3 miles

CONFIGURATION: Loop

DIFFICULTY: Moderate–difficult

SCENERY: Beech-oak forest with hemlocks and pines, rolling hills, meandering creek

EXPOSURE: Completely shaded

TRAFFIC: Moderate

TRAIL SURFACE: Dirt and clay, steeply banked in places

HIKING TIME: 90 minutes for Salt Run; allow 30 minutes more for Lake Trail

DRIVING DISTANCE: 20 miles from I-77/I-480 exchange

ACCESS: Daily, 7 a.m.–10 p.m.

WHEELCHAIR TRAVERSABLE: No

MAPS: USGS Peninsula; also available at the trailhead kiosk, park visitor centers, and nps.gov/cuva

FACILITIES: First-aid station, restrooms, and picnic tables at trailhead parking

CONTACT INFORMATION: Call (330) 657-2752 or visit nps.gov/cuva.

Directions

From Cleveland, take I-77 South, exiting at Wheatley Road (Exit 143/OH 176). Head east on Wheatley to Oak Hill, turning right; then follow it as it turns left and becomes Everett Road. Everett ends at Riverview Road; turn right. Turn left onto Bolanz Road, following it to Akron-Peninsula Road. Turn left (north). Turn right onto Quick Road. Pine Meadows parking lot is 0.4 miles east of Akron-Peninsula Road, off Quick Road.

GPS Trailhead Coordinates

Latitude   41° 12.890639'

Longitude   81° 31.916642'

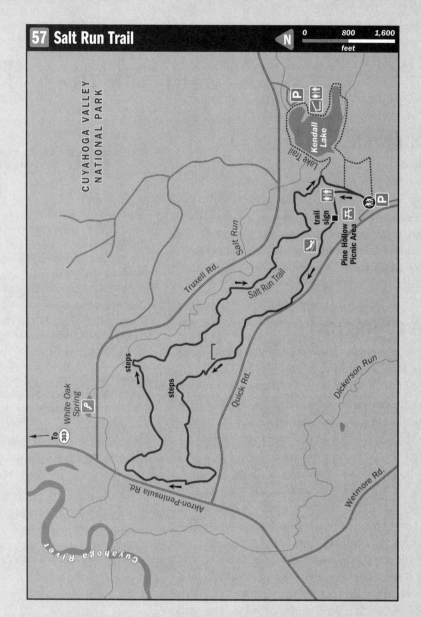

57 Salt Run Trail

N

0   800   1,600
feet

CUYAHOGA VALLEY
NATIONAL PARK

Kendall Lake

Lake Trail

Salt Run

Truxell Rd.

Salt Run Trail

trail sign

Pine Hollow Picnic Area

Dickerson Run

steps

Quick Rd.

steps

White Oak Spring

To 303

Akron-Peninsula Rd.

Wetmore Rd.

Cuyahoga River

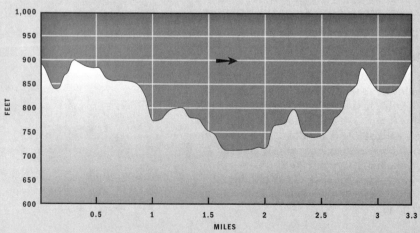

FEET

1,000
950
900
850
800
750
700
650
600

0.5   1   1.5   2   2.5   3   3.3

MILES

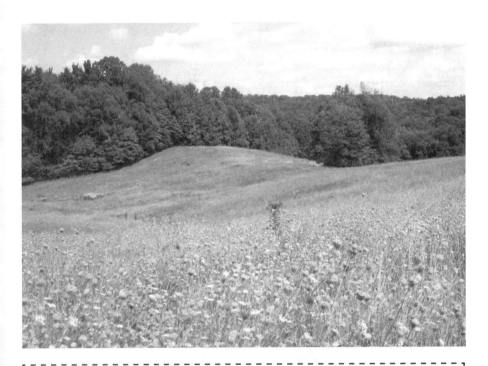

Prettier than your average parking lot view

cross a short footbridge. A shortcut to your right is best ignored—you'd miss much! Follow the trail as it bends left and heads uphill. For much of this hike, the trail rolls up and down, 10–30 feet at a time. The surface is rooty and uneven in places; this is a trail for sturdy boots, not sneakers.

Another curve to the left brings Quick Road into view, about 30 yards to the left of the trail. The road and the trail grow closer, then nearly together. The trail is covered with gravel for this short stretch. It's over soon—the white arrow on a trail marker beckons you off the road as the path darts back into the forest. And what a path it is—about 3 feet wide, it is the only level surface along the significant slope of the ravine. The ravine falls sharply to your right; you're beginning your descent into the densest part of the forest. A fork in the trail is signed—the right turn will lead you home sooner, via the shortcut trail (a loop of about 2.2 miles). Go straight instead, and you'll be rewarded with more gentle curves and steep drops, until you reach the bottom of an old field.

Enjoy the lower area of the Salt Run floodplain here, with its cool air and thick mosses; soon enough you'll be making up the difference with a series of short but steep climbs. Pine stands rise ahead of you, the flatland is below you, and you're in for another hill—this one, about a 30-foot climb.

Salt Run Trail is part of the former farm and estate of Hayward Kendall. He willed 420 acres to the state with the request that the land be used as a park and be named for his mother, Virginia. The CCC dammed and developed

Kendall Lake in the 1930s. The area was transferred to the National Park Service in 1978, becoming one of the first complete units in the Virginia Kendall National Recreation Area. Today the Pine Meadows and Salt Run area is a mix of successional forest and old meadow. You'll find a beech-oak forest with a hearty population of grapevines and the occasional spicebush (stop and smell it; it's like lemon, nutmeg, and cloves in a single leaf!). In the lower areas on the trail, you'll find a diverse population of ferns and mosses; in higher areas, where the sun can warm it a bit, you'll spot jewelweed. There's also plenty of poison ivy in these parts. The general rule to avoid contact is "leaves of three, let it be." Poison ivy, similar to Virginia creeper, likes to climb trees. If you are sensitive to poison ivy and know you'll be in a dense forest, it's a good idea to wear long sleeves and pants.

As you rise up with the trail, you'll cross several long, wide footbridges. They can be extremely slippery when wet (think ice-skating in your hiking boots). Hang onto the railing as you go. Once you've landed back on the dirt trail, you'll probably notice that you're surrounded by skunk cabbages.

As the path veers right to head west, you'll see a sign for the connector trail to Kendall Lake. If you follow it (left), you'll circle the lake and return to this trail in just over a mile. It's a narrow but fairly flat trail, pretty any time of year. To complete Salt Run from here, turn right. One more worthy climb awaits—punctuated by a half dozen railroad-tie steps notched into a steep hill of clay. Take special care here when the ground is wet.

Once you've reached the top, the remainder of Salt Run is relatively flat, and you'll finish your hike in the company of tall pines and hemlocks. Their needles lay a soft carpet on the trail, welcome after the harder trekking you've seen today. Take a deep whiff of pine and relax. You're done.

NEARBY ACTIVITIES

Of course, there's no lack of things to do here in the heart of the 33,000-acre national park. Nearby Kendall Lake is a beautiful place any time of year, so if you didn't take the extension trail to see it, consider driving over to have a look. Or, head up to Peninsula and check out Deep Lock (see page 246).

Or, if you'd prefer a different sort of walk, schedule a tee time at Brandywine Golf Course, just a couple miles north on Akron-Peninsula Road.

SAND RUN METRO PARK 58

IN BRIEF

Why not follow the crowd to Sand Run Metro Park? Akron-area residents and many area workers walk, jog, and talk along the 6-mile paved jogging path, and for good reason—it's pretty and mostly shaded, and the park staff even plows it after heavy snowfalls. There are many reasons to veer from the most obvious trail, however, and explore the rest of this park, the oldest in the Summit County system.

DESCRIPTION

Start from the trailhead at the Old Portage Area. Neither the map nor the long, grassy entrance to the trail gives you a good idea of what to expect. Consider it getting off to an easy start.

Here you'll follow signs for the Valley Link and Buckeye trails, just for a few hundred yards, to reach the hilly Dogwood Trail. The flat start will be good for your heart, providing you with a little warm-up time before the steeper trail gets your blood pumping considerably faster. Before the climbing really gets underway, though, you have a chance to admire the clear and gentle beauty of Sand Run, the stream. In fact, you'll have a chance to cross it a couple of times before you reach Dogwood Trail.

KEY AT-A-GLANCE INFORMATION

LENGTH: 4 miles

CONFIGURATION: Loop

DIFFICULTY: Moderate–difficult

SCENERY: Sparkling Sand Run and tributaries, salamanders and other amphibians during spring breeding season, tall pines and deciduous forest, beautiful ravine views

EXPOSURE: Mostly shaded

TRAFFIC: Moderate–busy

TRAIL SURFACE: Jogging path is paved; nature trails have dirt and rock surfaces.

HIKING TIME: Allow 2 hours or more

DRIVING DISTANCE: 27 miles from I-77/I-480 exchange

ACCESS: Daily, 6 a.m.–11 p.m.

WHEELCHAIR TRAVERSABLE: Jogging path, yes; nature trails, no

MAPS: USGS Akron West; also posted at trail kiosks throughout the park

FACILITIES: Restrooms and water fountains at picnic shelters and at trail kiosks found along the paved jogging trail extending throughout the park

CONTACT INFORMATION: For general information, contact the parks office at (330) 865-5511 or summitmetroparks.org.

Directions

Follow I-77 South toward Akron and take Exit 137A to merge onto OH 18 east (toward Fairlawn) and turn left onto Twin Oaks Road. Turn left again at North Portage Path. Follow North Portage Path north to the Sand Run Parkway, where you'll turn left to enter the park.

GPS Trailhead Coordinates

Latitude   41° 7.771440'

Longitude   81° 33.156717'

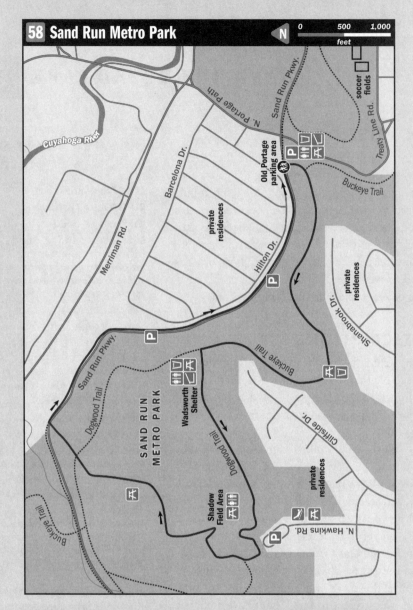

N

0   500   1,000
feet

Cuyahoga River

N. Portage Path

Sand Run Pkwy.

soccer fields

Treaty Line Rd.

Barcelona Dr.

private residences

Old Portage parking area

Buckeye Trail

Merriman Rd.

Hilton Dr.

P

Shanabrook Dr.

private residences

P

Buckeye Trail

Sand Run Pkwy.

P

Dogwood Trail

Wadsworth Shelter

Cliffside Dr.

SAND RUN METRO PARK

Dogwood Trail

private residences

Buckeye Trail

Shadow Field Area

N. Hawkins Rd.

P

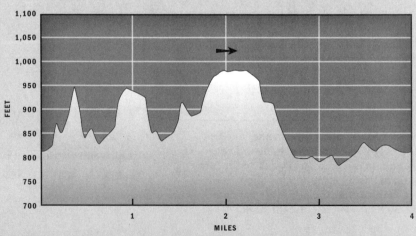

1,100

1,050

1,000

950

900

850

800

750

700

FEET

1   2   3   4

MILES

You'll know that you've reached Dogwood because it's clearly signed (leaf symbols mark the way), and the entrance is marked by a long set of wooden steps wedged into the sandy soil. At first, you'll admire the pretty hill; by the time you reach the top, however, you'll probably appreciate the bench as much as the view. If you don't need a break yet, you might soon. The trail narrows and turns to the right to reveal another set of stairs, just as steep. Once you reach the top of those, Dogwood flattens out a bit and you can keep your eyes open for signs posted here and there, identifying more than 20 trees you may not recognize otherwise, such as the cucumber tree. While the signs simply identify the trees by name, park naturalists (whom you can meet on many free, guided hikes offered year-round) can tell you much more about many trees. The tulip tree, for example, was often used to make dugout canoes, for the very practical reason that its trunks grow straighter than most other trees in the forest. (Many naturalists also call them dirty trees because their long-lasting blooms fall apart and can be seen littering the forest floor for several months out of the year.)

Dogwood Trail intersects with Mingo Trail, and your climbing is over for the time being. Follow Dogwood as it curves to the right (east) and brings you to the edge of Shadow Field, one of the few exposed pieces of trail in the park. In the summer, butterflies and other insects flit about, busy surveying the tall grasses and open spaces and avoiding birds that may be interested in a snack.

As you near the eastern edge of Dogwood, you'll start to head downhill at last on a wide, grassy path before heading back into the dark forest again. From here—and many spots along the nature trails in the park, including Mingo and Buckeye trails—you can see both Sand Run stream and the paved jogging path that runs along Sand Run Parkway. Many park visitors take the opportunity to veer off trail and into the stream to cool their feet, let their dogs have a drink, or allow their children to skip rocks and look for small fish in the shallow water.

However you choose to enjoy Sand Run, you won't be alone. The park system states that, on average, about 1,000 people step out on the jogging path every day, and it's probably not just for the exercise—this busy park is a calming spot seeped in natural beauty. While it's not always smart to follow the crowd, in this case, it's a very good idea.

NEARBY ACTIVITIES

Don't leave yet! There are more trails to enjoy here. If you must leave, why not take the 2.8-mile Valley Link Trail that connects to Schumacher Valley area in Cascade Metro Park? From there, if you dare, you can continue on to pretty Oxbow Trail (see page 242) to get a look at more of these beautiful sandstone cliffs, from on high.

Also nearby (off Smith Road on Sand Run's north side) you'll find F. A. Seiberling Nature Realm (see page 218), featuring a very educational nature center and more formal gardens and landscape design.

59 | SPENCER LAKE

KEY AT-A-GLANCE INFORMATION

LENGTH: 2 miles

CONFIGURATION: Loop

DIFFICULTY: Easy

SCENERY: Lake, river, marsh, woods, foxes, muskrats, pheasants, waterfowl, possibly eagles or wild turkeys

EXPOSURE: Mostly exposed

TRAFFIC: Light

TRAIL SURFACE: Dirt and grass

HIKING TIME: 45 minutes

DRIVING DISTANCE: 41 miles from I-77/I-480 exchange

ACCESS: Spencer Lake is a popular public hunting area—hunting, fishing, and trapping are allowed by permit. This area is closed to all other activity 8 p.m.–6 a.m., September 1–May 1; and 10 p.m.–6 a.m., May 2–August 31. Wear bright colors and avoid early-morning hours during hunting season.

WHEELCHAIR TRAVERSABLE: No

MAPS: USGS Lodi; also available from Buckeye Trail Association and at dnr.state.oh.us

FACILITIES: Two boat ramps, two fishing/observation decks

CONTACT INFORMATION: For more information, see dnr.state.oh.us or call the district office at (330) 644-2293.

IN BRIEF

Want to get away from it all? Spencer Lake is probably as far away from it all as you can get 40 miles from Cleveland. Once here, chances are fairly good that you won't meet another hiker on the trail. (But if the catfish are biting, you won't be alone.)

DESCRIPTION

From the parking area on the western side of the lake, head west on the park access road (Spencer Lake Road). About 0.1 mile west of the lot, turn left into the woods, where the only marker is a blue blaze on a fence post. The wide, flat trail under the shade of tall oaks soon bends to the left because it has to—otherwise, it would lead you into the river.

The east branch of the Black River snakes by, about 20 feet below you and to your right. The edge of the trail is unforgiving here, but if you stay a foot or two back, you'll have lovely views of the shady river for the next half mile. The view is best enjoyed while from a standstill, of course. While you're moving, you'll want to keep your eyes on the trail—you're likely to find a large log, or a whole tree, lying in your path. If you're quiet (and lucky), you may also catch a glimpse of some of the many songbirds that inhabit this area. The variety

GPS Trailhead Coordinates

Latitude   41° 6.751320'

Longitude 82° 5.277543'

Directions

Follow I-77 South to I-271 South to I-71 South, taking OH 18 (Exit 281) toward Akron/Medina. Follow OH 18 to Medina; follow OH 3/OH 162 southwest approximately 5 miles, through the small town of Chatham, and continue west on OH 162 to Root Road, where you'll turn right. A sign for Spencer Lake Wildlife Area is about 0.5 miles north, directing you to turn right onto Spencer Lake Road and into the parking area.

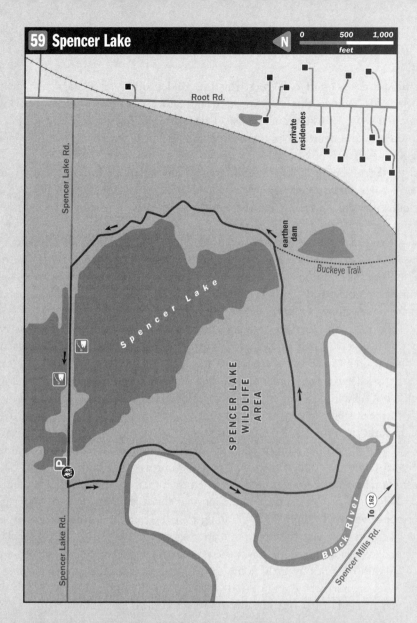

N

| 0 | 500 | 1,000 |

feet

Root Rd.

private
residences

Spencer Lake Rd.

earthen
dam

Buckeye Trail

S p e n c e r   L a k e

SPENCER LAKE
WILDLIFE
AREA

P

B l a c k   R i v e r

To (162)

Spencer Lake Rd.

Spencer Mills Rd.

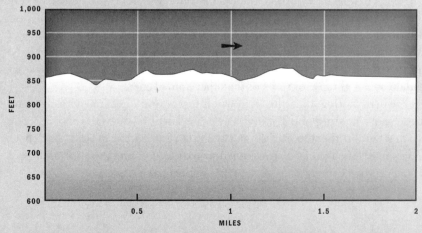

1,000				
950				
900				
850				

FEET

800
750
700
650
600

| | 0.5 | 1 | 1.5 | 2 |

MILES

of food sources—tall oak trees, thistles, goldenrods, marshlands, and nearby open fields—makes this spot very attractive to a rich assortment of birds and mammals. Wild turkeys and a host of waterfowl frequent the area too. (So do mosquitoes and deerflies, in their respective seasons—wearing insect repellent is a good idea!)

The trail bends left again and leads you by a field and some young-growth trees—their rustle entertains you as you continue east to the dam. This area can be quite wet during spring, but the wildflower display is worth getting a little bit of mud on your shoes.

If you really don't like squishy along a trail, though, plan to come during a dry spell or, even better, in the winter, when you're likely to see people ice fishing on the lake. In the summer, when you emerge from the woods, you'll pass ironweeds, goldenrods, milkweeds, and other popular bird food before you land on the wide, grassy walkway to the dam.

You reach the earthen dam about 0.9 miles into the hike. The grassy path continues east 100 feet or so and then turns right, crossing railroad tracks and ending at OH 162. Don't go there—instead, turn left, into the woods. Here the narrow path hugs the lakeshore and then darts into the woods, heading north. You'll roll up and down a few hills, rising slowly through bramble (and wildflowers, in the spring), until you reach a spot in the woods where it seems as if you might walk right into the lake. You don't, of course, but the view here is lovely.

The path wiggles a bit through the woods, and in a couple of spots you may need to climb over fallen trees to continue your hike. In one such spot, hikers beat out a secondary path around the fallen tree; then another tree landed on that path. Philosophers on the trail might consider this a good example of man versus nature; others will simply enjoy climbing over the tree. At various points around the lake, you may have to step around another visitor who is fishing. Channel catfish and largemouth bass are two varieties that anglers enjoy finding here.

About 0.5 miles from the southern dam, you'll reach the eastern parking lot and a newer, northern dam (a flood washed away the original in 1969; this dam was constructed in 1970). You'll also find the trailhead for the Buckeye Trail. Turn right if you're itching to go farther—but know before you follow the Buckeye Trail that it travels the entire state. (To learn more about Buckeye Trail and to purchase maps, visit the website at **buckeyetrail.org**.) Otherwise, turn left to continue your walk here at Spencer Lake. Cross the road and walk along the well-beaten path on the north side of the dam. It's a great spot to observe ducks and other migratory birds and catch a glimpse of some of the other animals here.

It's worth noting that this is a wildlife restoration area, actively managed for sport hunting and fishing. The state acquired the land in 1956 and built dams here in the 1960s. Fish and wildlife reclamation projects have been ongoing since. (Such projects are funded in part by hunting and fishing license sales, so everyone can enjoy more sporting opportunities.)

Over the years, grass carp have been stocked to control aquatic vegetation to improve the quality of fishing, and bass length limits and other measures are often in place. Heed any posted limits and work within program guidelines; they're created with all of Ohio's residents in mind. (*All* meaning the plants and animals, including *you*.) Hang out, quietly, and you may catch a glimpse of the mink and muskrat populations that attract sportsmen. Hang out until well after dark (hunting and fishing can go on here all night), and you'll also appreciate how dark the sky can be here, far enough away from major population centers so that the stars can *really* shine.

To complete your hike, cross the causeway and return to the western parking lot for a round-trip of nearly 2 miles. Before you go, you may also stop at one of the two fishing/observation decks for another perspective on the lake.

NEARBY ACTIVITIES

Looking for a long day trip? You can follow the Buckeye Trail west from Spencer Lake all the way to Findley State Park, about 9 miles from here. For maps and more information about the Buckeye Trail, call (800) 881-3062 or visit **buckeyetrail.org**. Just east of Spencer Wildlife Area, off of OH 162, you'll find two Medina County parks: Schleman Nature Preserve and Buckeye Woods, which offer hiking trails, picnic facilities, and play equipment. To learn more about those facilities, visit **medinacountyparks.com**.

With thanks to Ohio Department of Natural Resources Wildlife Officer Brennan Earick, who graciously agreed to review this hike description and provided many helpful details about Spencer Lake.

60 WHIPP'S LEDGES

KEY AT-A-GLANCE INFORMATION

LENGTH: 1 mile

CONFIGURATION: Loop

DIFFICULTY: Short but difficult

SCENERY: Giant rock boulders and mini-caves of Sharon conglomerate, a spectacular view from the top

EXPOSURE: Mostly shaded

TRAFFIC: Moderate–heavy

TRAIL SURFACE: Dirt and rocks

HIKING TIME: 30 minutes, plus gawking time

DRIVING DISTANCE: 18 miles from I-77/I-480 exchange

ACCESS: Daily, 6 a.m.–11 p.m. except where otherwise posted

WHEELCHAIR TRAVERSABLE: No

MAPS: USGS West Richfield; also available at ranger station on Bellus Road and posted at the boathouse

FACILITIES: Restrooms, water fountain, picnic shelter, grills

CONTACT INFORMATION: To learn more before you go, call (440) 526-1012 or visit clevelandmetroparks.com.

IN BRIEF

If you like to climb and gawk at great distances, Whipp's Ledges is for you. If buzzards are your bag, you'll want to visit this Medina County outpost of the Cleveland Metroparks in March. You need to be cautious while climbing. To be blunt, a drop off the edge of one of these ledges could prove fatal—but with reasonable care, you'll enjoy the hike and the views tremendously.

DESCRIPTION

Hinckley Reservation has attained considerable fame as "the home of the buzzards," although the buzzards are actually turkey vultures. Regardless, the raptors return to roost—quite predictably—in mid-March, and an annual party is held to celebrate the occasion. But all the fuss about the birds shouldn't suggest that they are the only ones who might be attracted to the park year after year. Hinckley Reservation is full of reasons to return. Challenging hiking at Whipp's Ledges is one good reason. Start your steep climb on Whipp's Ledges Loop Trail from the eastern end of the parking lot. You'll huff and puff from the get-go, and the fact that you'll have some roots and a few stone stairs to aid your climb is a mixed blessing. These steps—from root to root and

GPS Trailhead Coordinates

Latitude   41° 13.137360'

Longitude   81° 42.182937'

Directions

Hinckley Reservation is located in Hinckley Township, just south of OH 303. From Cleveland, take I-77 to Exit 147/Miller Road. Turn left onto Miller, then right onto Brecksville Road, and right again onto OH 303. Follow OH 303 west about 3 miles to State Road. Turn left. Whipp's Ledges parking lot is about 1 mile south of OH 303 on the left (east) side of State Road.

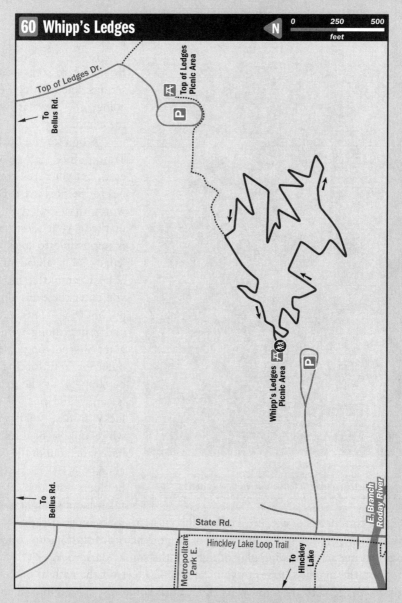

N

0   250   500
feet

Top of Ledges Dr.

To
Bellus Rd.

Top of Ledges
Picnic Area

P

To
Bellus Rd.

Whipp's Ledges
Picnic Area

P

State Rd.

E. Branch
Rocky River

Hinckley Lake Loop Trail

Metropolitan
Park E.

To
Hinckley
Lake

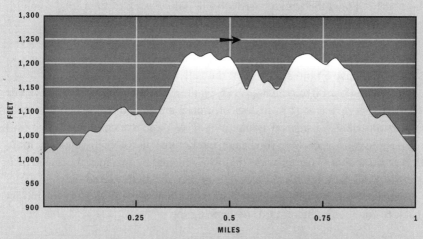

FEET

1,300
1,250
1,200
1,150
1,100
1,050
1,000
950
900

0.25   0.5   0.75   1

MILES

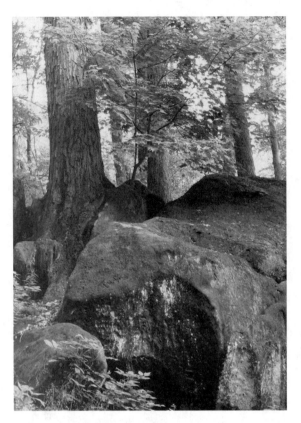

The trail is hard to follow but worth the effort.

from step to step—require serious knee lifting. Keep going; the view is worth the climb.

A sign for the Buckeye Trail points right (southeast), but your trek continues to the northeast. Don't worry that your path isn't marked; your destination is impossible to miss. The ledges loom ahead of you almost from the moment you enter the trail. Up you go, huffing and puffing and rising along with the giant Sharon conglomerate outcrops. Your footing may be slippery, as the ground is sandy and pocked with lucky stones, small milky white quartz pebbles that have fallen out of the larger conglomerate rock. Giant boulders—some 100 feet tall—loom straight ahead.

The trail bends to the left. Look at the massive stones on your right. Notice how the lichen grows in the indentations or pockmarks of the Sharon conglomerate, making an interesting play of light on the smoky dark rock.

Soon the massive stones to your left, 10–20 feet off the path at one point, begin to merge with those on your right, until you are squeezed into making a decision: either crawl through a narrow tunnel or sidestep to the right, climbing up and on top of the boulders.

Whether you tunnel through or crawl up, just don't miss the view from the top of the ledges—you'll stand about 350 feet above Hinckley Lake, and, looking west, you'll have a fantastic view of the valley.

As you ease down from the big rocks, you'll probably need to use your hands as well as your feet to steady your descent. Loose gravel and leaf debris on top of the sandy soil makes for slippery going, in both wet and dry conditions. The trail bottoms out just north of where you began, but before you complete this short loop, you'll walk through a 4–6-foot-wide "hallway" created by two massive rocks, each about 20 feet tall. Though it's not a cave, you may feel quite boxed in.

From here, the path winds west a bit and then veers to the left to find its way back to the picnic shelter and the parking lot.

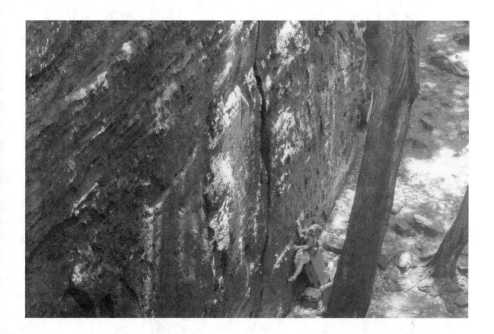

Climb with care.

NEARBY ACTIVITIES

Although you've reached the end of this short trail, plenty of Hinckley Reservation remains to be investigated. The reservation covers 2,700 acres. Consider visiting Worden's Ledges to see the stone carvings there or head off for the lake. You'll find boaters there in summer, skaters in the winter, and ducks and other wildlife year-round.

While in Hinckley, you're likely to see some rock climbers. The reservation requires those who use top ropes to obtain a climbing permit before they start scaling the walls here. While visitors are not required to obtain permits for bouldering, caution is advised—climbing is considered an adventure sport for good reason.

Want to log some hilly miles without the climbing element? Hit the paved, accessible All Purpose Trail here for a 3.3-mile trek around Hinckley Lake. Also inside the reservation, you can rent various watercraft at the boathouse, located on the south end of the lake off West Drive. Swimming is another option. Take your pick of Ledges Pool (off Ledges Road at the southern end of the reservation), open seasonally (a day-use fee applies), or the lake swimming area (off Bellus Road at the northern end), where admission is free. Both are on the north side of the lake and can be reached off Bellus Road.

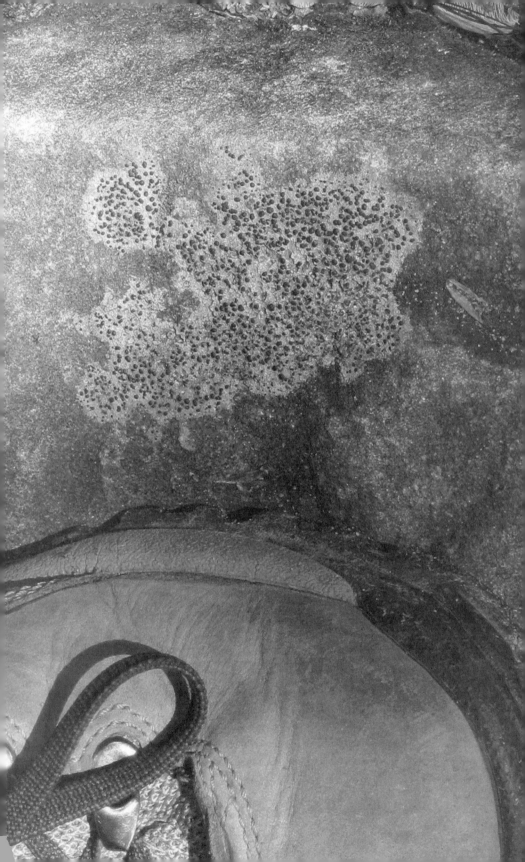

60 HIKES
WITHIN 60 MILES

CLEVELAND
INCLUDING
AKRON AND CANTON

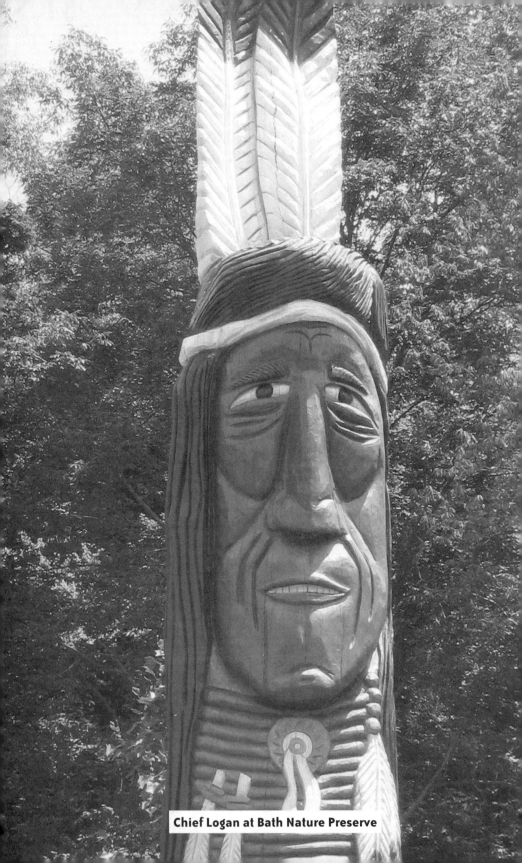

Chief Logan at Bath Nature Preserve

APPENDIXES
AND INDEX

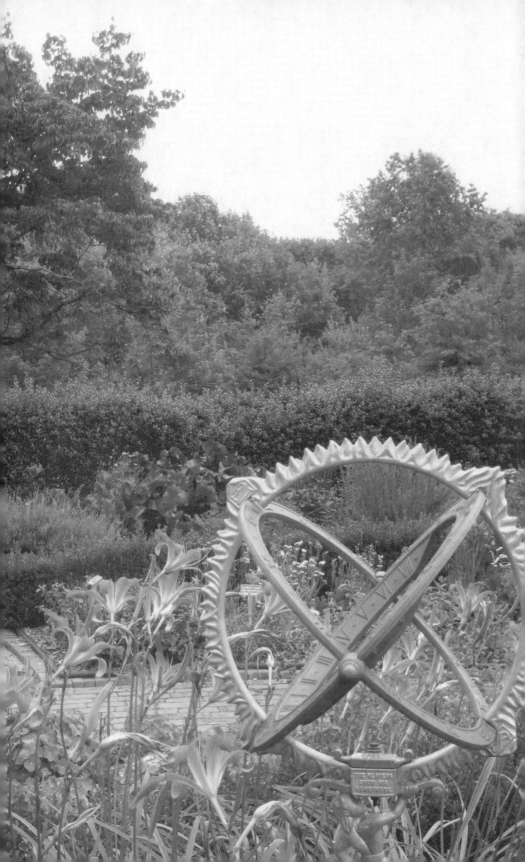

APPENDIX A:
OUTDOOR SHOPS

APPALACHIAN OUTFITTERS
60 Kendall Park Road
Peninsula, OH 44264
(330) 655-5444
appalachianoutfitters.com

THE BACKPACKERS SHOP
5128 Colorado Avenue (OH 611)
Sheffield Village, OH 44054
(440) 934-5345
(888) 303-3307
backpackersshop.com

GANDER MOUNTAIN
gandermountain.com
2695 Creekside Drive, Suite 100
Twinsburg, OH 44087
(330) 405-2999

5244 Cobblestone Road
Elyria, OH 44035
(440) 934-8222

9620 Diamond Centre Drive
Mentor, OH 44060
(440) 639-8545

Left: **Quail Hollow State Park**

APPENDIX B:
PLACES TO BUY MAPS

APPALACHIAN OUTFITTERS
60 Kendall Park Road
Peninsula, OH 44264
(330) 655-5444
appalachianoutfitters.com

GANDER MOUNTAIN
gandermountain.com
2695 Creekside Drive, Suite 100
Twinsburg, OH 44087
(330) 405-2999

5244 Cobblestone Road
Elyria, OH 44035
(440) 934-8222

9620 Diamond Centre Drive
Mentor, OH 44060
(440) 639-8545

CUYAHOGA VALLEY NATIONAL PARK
nps.gov/cuva
Boston Store Visitor Center
1548 Boston Mills Road
Peninsula, OH 44264
(330) 657-2752

CANAL VISITOR CENTER
7104 Canal Road
Valley View, OH 44125
(216) 524-1497 or
(800) 445-9667

EARTHWORDS NATURE SHOPS OF CLEVELAND METROPARKS
NORTH CHAGRIN RESERVATION
3037 SOM Center Road
Willoughby Hills, OH 44094
(440) 449-0511

ROCKY RIVER RESERVATION
24000 Valley Parkway
North Olmsted, OH 44070
(440) 734-7576

F. A. SEIBERLING NATURE REALM
Metroparks Serving Summit County
1828 Smith Road
Akron, OH 44313
(330) 867-5511
summitmetroparks.org

APPENDIX C:
HIKING CLUBS AND EVENTS

AKRON BICYCLE CLUB
(hikes off-season)
akronbike.org

CLEVELAND HIKING CLUB
clevelandhikingclub.com
(440) 449-2588

PORTAGE TRAIL WALKERS
(330) 673-6896

APPALACHIAN OUTFITTERS
60 Kendall Park Road
Peninsula, OH 44264
(330) 655-5444
appalachianoutfitters.com

APPENDIX D:
BIBLIOGRAPHY

Abercrombie, Jay. *Walks and Rambles in Ohio's Western Reserve*. Woodstock, VT: Backcountry Publications, 1996.

Bartush, William W. *Lake View Cemetery Historical Trail*. Eagle Scout project, Troop 656, Cleveland Heights, OH (undated).

Bobel, Pat. *The Nature of the Towpath*. Akron, Ohio: Cuyahoga Valley Trails Council, Inc., 1998.

Cuyahoga Valley Trails Council. *Cuyahoga Valley National Recreation Area Trail Guide Handbook*. Akron, OH: Cuyahoga Valley Trails Council, 1996.

Directory of Ohio's State Nature Preserves. Columbus, OH: Ohio Department of Natural Resources, 1998–2000.

Gross, W.H. (Chip). *Ohio Wildlife Viewing Guide*. Helena, MT: Falcon Publishing, 1996.

Hallowell, Anna C. and Barbara G. *Fern Finder*. Rochester, NY: Study Nature Guild, 1981.

Hannibal, Joseph T. and Schmidt, Mark T. "Rocks of Ages." *Earth Science*, Spring 1998.

Latimer, Jonathan P., and Nolting, Karen Stray. *Backyard Birds* (Peterson Field Guides for Young Naturalists). Boston, MA: Houghton Mifflin Company, 1999.

Leedy, Jr., Walter C. "Cleveland's Terminal Tower—The Van Sweringens," *Afterthought*. (Cleveland State University) 28 July 1997.

Manner, Barbara M. and Corbett, Robert G. *Environmental Atlas of the Cuyahoga Valley National Recreation Area*. Monroeville, PA: Surprise Valley Publications, 1990.

Ohio & Erie Canal Corridor Coalition, *Towpath Companion*. Akron, OH: Ohio &Erie Canal Corridor Coalition, 2001.

Path Finder—A Guide to Cleveland Metroparks. Cleveland, OH: Cleveland Metroparks (undated).

"Peninsula Village Architectural Tour." Peninsula Area Chamber of Commerce: Peninsula, OH (undated).

Sacha, Linda Hoy. "Area Cemeteries Rich in Historic Milestones of City," *Sun Newspapers*. 4 June 1998.

Watts, May Theilgaard. *Tree Finder*. Rochester, NY: Nature Study Guild, 1998.

Wright, Caryl. "Eccentric Russell 'caveman' was no hermit," *Russell Historical Society Newsletter*, Vol. I Issue 9. March 19, 1990.

Zim, Herbert S. (PhD) and Cottam, Clarence (PhD). *Insects*. New York, NY: Golden Books, 1997.

OTHER RESOURCES
CLEVELAND METROPARKS
clemetparks.com

CUYAHOGA VALLEY NATIONAL PARK
dayinthevalley.com

GEAUGA COUNTY PARKS
geaugaparkdistrict.org

LAKE COUNTY PARKS
lakemetroparks.com

LORAIN COUNTY METROPARKS
loraincountymetroparks.com

MEDINA COUNTY HISTORICAL SOCIETY
medinahistorical.com

MEDINA COUNTY METROPARKS
medinacountyparks.com

METROPARKS SERVING SUMMIT COUNTY
summitmetroparks.org

OHIO OUTDOOR SCULPTURE
INVENTORY (OOSI)
tinyurl.com/2vz9oyk

OHIO DEPARTMENT OF NATURAL RESOURCES, OHIO STATE PARKS
ohiodnr.com

PORTAGE COUNTY
HISTORICAL SOCIETY
history.portage.oh.us

STARK COUNTY PARKS DISTRICT
starkparks.com

SUMMIT COUNTY HISTORICAL SOCIETY
summithistory.org

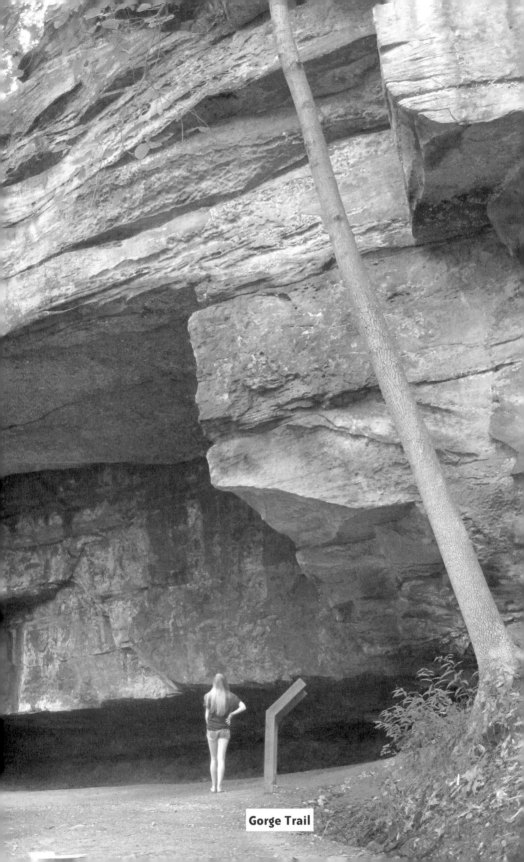

Gorge Trail

INDEX

Check out this other great title from
Menasha Ridge Press!

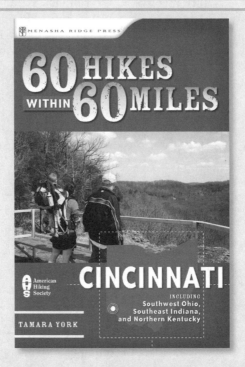

60 Hikes Within 60 Miles: Cincinnati

by Tammy York
ISBN: 978-0-89732-705-3
$17.95, 1st Edition
320 pages, 6x9, Trade paper
maps, photographs, index

60 Hikes Within 60 Miles: Cincinnati uncovers paths where
no guidebook has gone before and hits classic trails as well.
This is the essential guide to southwest Ohio, southeast Indiana, and Northern Kentucky. Treks range from easy strolls
not far from home such as Eden Park with sculptures and
specialty gardens near downtown Cincinnati to the challenging trails at Clifty Falls State Park in Indiana.

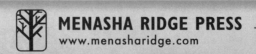

MENASHA RIDGE PRESS
www.menasharidge.com

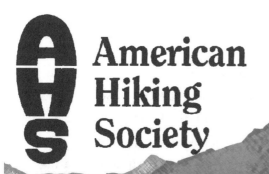

American Hiking Society

THE VOICE OF THE AMERICAN HIKER... THE HEART OF THE HIKING COMMUNITY.

Join the national voice for America's Hikers.

Visit **www.AmericanHiking.org**

or send a $25 check to:

American Hiking Society

Attn: Membership

1422 Fenwick Lane

Silver Spring, MD 20910

establishing, protecting and maintaining foot paths since 1976

Looking For More Info?

Menasha Ridge Press has partnered with Trails.com to provide additional information for all the trails in this book, including:

- Topo map downloads
- Real-time weather
- Trail reports, and more

To access this information, visit:

http://menasharidge.trails.com

In Partnership With

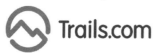 Trails.com

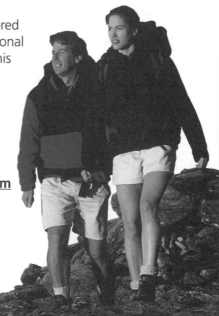

DEAR CUSTOMERS AND FRIENDS,

SUPPORTING YOUR INTEREST IN OUTDOOR ADVENTURE, travel, and an active lifestyle is central to our operations, from the authors we choose to the locations we detail to the way we design our books. Menasha Ridge Press was incorporated in 1982 by a group of veteran outdoorsmen and professional outfitters. For many years now, we've specialized in creating books that benefit the outdoors enthusiast.

Almost immediately, Menasha Ridge Press earned a reputation for revolutionizing outdoors- and travel-guidebook publishing. For such activities as canoeing, kayaking, hiking, backpacking, and mountain biking, we established new standards of quality that transformed the whole genre, resulting in outdoor-recreation guides of great sophistication and solid content. Menasha Ridge continues to be outdoor publishing's greatest innovator.

The folks at Menasha Ridge Press are as at home on a white-water river or mountain trail as they are editing a manuscript. The books we build for you are the best they can be, because we're responding to your needs. Plus, we use and depend on them ourselves.

We look forward to seeing you on the river or the trail. If you'd like to contact us directly, join in at www.trekalong.com or visit us at www.menasharidge.com. We thank you for your interest in our books and the natural world around us all.

SAFE TRAVELS,

Bob Sehlinger

BOB SEHLINGER
PUBLISHER